HEALTH
FOR
SENIORS

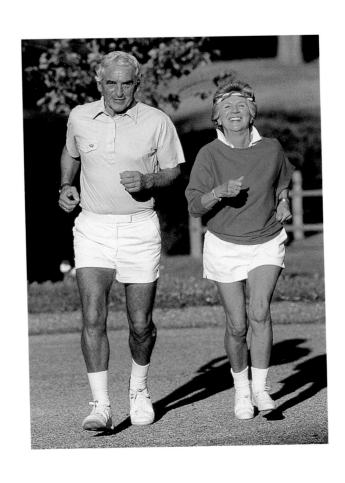

HEALTH
FOR
SENIORS

PROFESSOR PETER ABRAHAMS

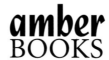

This edition first published in 2010

Published by
Amber Books Ltd
Bradley's Close
74–77 White Lion Street
London N1 9PF
United Kingdom
www.amberbooks.co.uk

Copyright © 2010 Bright Star Publishing Plc

Material previously published in the part-work *Inside the Human Body*

ISBN: 978-1-906626-77-8

Project Editor: Sarah Uttridge
Additional Design: Hawes Design
Jacket Design: Keren Harragan

Printed in Thailand

Contents

Introduction   6

How the Body Ages   8

Bone Disorders   26

Heart Disorders   46

Mental Health and the Nervous System   84

Cancer   108

Sight and Hearing   120

Common Conditions for Older People   130

Staying Fit   156

Index   174

Introduction

Medical advances and an improved diet have meant that we are all living longer and living a better quality of life. It is no longer rare in the twenty-first century to live to be 90 or even 100 years old.

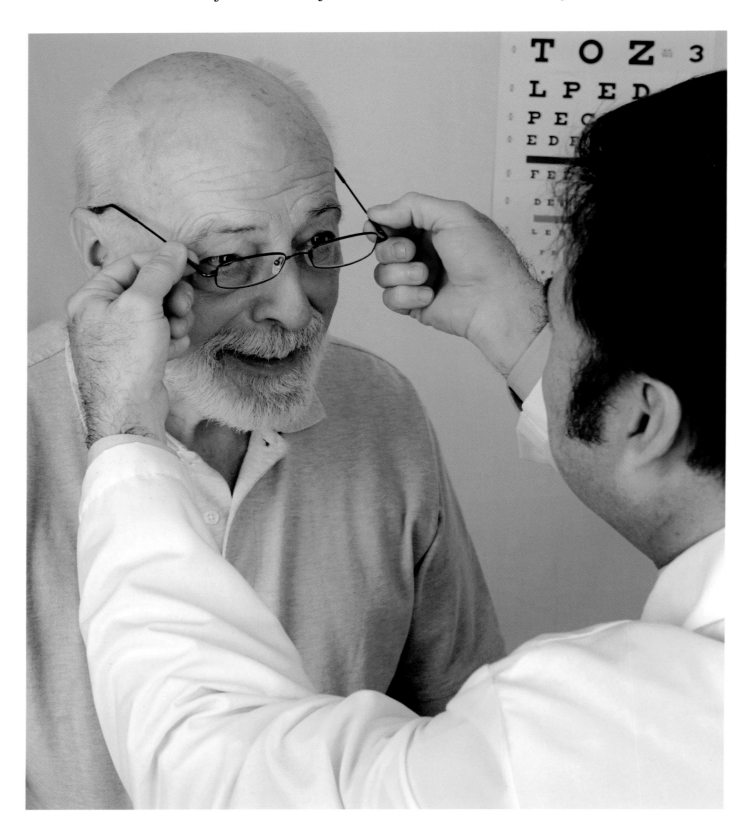

How we live our lives is significant: living well means having regular health checks, eating healthily, exercising two or three times a week. We can no longer regard our material needs - a home and a pension, say - and our working lives as the largest proportion of our life. If we are to live some 30, even 40, years beyond retirement, we need to focus as much on our physical health and our emotional and mental needs.

QUALITY OF LIFE

As we age, our bodies inevitably become less agile, less supple, and our senses, especially our vision and hearing, become less sharp.

Stiff, aching joints and fatigue are perhaps the hallmarks of increasing age. However, there is huge scope for improving our general health and fitness - through healthy eating and exercise - and for health monitoring to pick up early signs of disease and disorder. Early detection and diagnosis of illness pays off handsomely: the earlier a disorder is treated, the better the outcome is likely to be. This applies to conditions such as cancer and heart disease just as much as to illnesses such as depression and anxiety.

We all have an important role to play in the lives of our friends and family members, offering support and friendship and, when necessary, a sympathetic ear as the senses diminish, the aches and pains become more than an irritation, or the necessity for an operation looms.

Left: Regular eye tests are important as diseases such as diabetes are often first detected in the eyes.

PAIN-FREE LIFE

Pain is a symptom and not a disorder in itself. Pain should never be ignored and should always be investigated without delay. There is always a reason for pain. Medical advances both in surgery and medicine mean that a good resolution to pain is often available. There is now no need to continue suffering pain, even though pain typically increases with age.

Two-thirds of people aged 65-plus are in chronic pain and many people in long-term care homes suffer pain all the time. Pain management is a speciality in medicine that has existed for over 20 years and yet many people remain unaware that they can be referred to pain management clinics through their family doctor. Relief from chronic pain represents a major medical advance in improved quality of life for the middle aged and elderly.

HOW TO USE THIS BOOK

You will see the book is divided into easy to use sections as shown below:
- How the body ages
- Bone disorders
- Heart disorders
- Mental health and the nervous system
- Cancers
- Sight and hearing
- Common conditions in older people
- Staying fit

The book is fully comprehensive and includes, to take examples from each section, detailed and clearly illustrated features on the menopause, osteoarthritis, angina, heart attack, heart disease, dementias including Alzheimer's dementia,

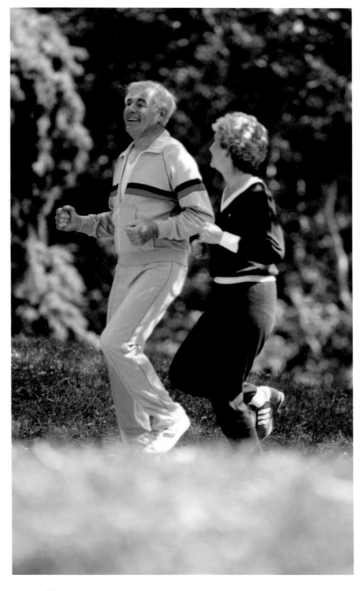

stroke (the single largest cause of disability in middle aged and elderly people), prostate cancer, cataracts and glaucoma, and some of the conditions of increasing age such as impaired mobility, diabetes, incontinence and chronic bronchitis. Finally, the book includes a section devoted to maintaining a healthy lifestyle entitled Staying Fit. (If you do not immediately spot the information you want, consult the index where you will find the relevant page numbers for the condition you seek.)

LIVING YOUR LIFE WELL

With this book and with regular health checks, below, you should be able to enjoy a good quality of life for many, many years.
- Eye test (diseases are often observed first in the eyes)

Early detection and diagnosis of illness is more likely to provide a better outcome. Always consult a doctor with any health worries.

Regular exercise can be of huge benefit to the elderly, minimizing the risk of cardiovascular disease and strokes.

- Blood pressure monitoring (vital to detect the possibility of heart disease and stroke)
- Cholesterol levels measurement
- Prostate check
- Mammogram
- Cervical smear
- Dental check up
- Hearing test

A strong focus on positive thinking - "I can walk, so I will", "I can run, so I will", "I enjoy eating well, so I will"- is essential. With preventative health in the form of regular health checks as listed above, positive thought is vital not only to securing a long life but, even more importantly, an excellent quality of life.

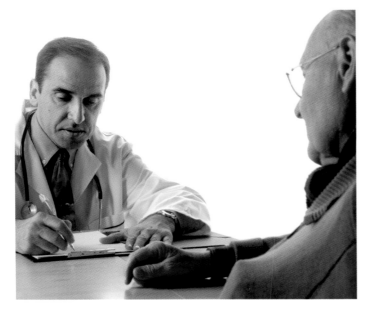

Entering middle age

In middle age, people tend to become aware for the first time of the ageing process. There are compensations, however, in the form of financial stability, increased self-confidence and widening horizons.

The period in life known as 'middle age' is considered to run from the ages of 40 to 65. As people enter middle age, they may become aware for the first time of the subtle changes that time has wrought on their appearance, memory and their relationships with others.

MORTALITY

For people who have always considered themselves to be invulnerable, middle age may be a time when they become aware of their own mortality for the first time. They may experience the onset of aches and pains and the early death of friends.

However, middle age also has many positive aspects. Middle-aged people often find that they can express themselves more freely and have acquired a liberating lack of concern for other people's opinion of them.

Older people have other advantages over the young. They are much more aware of the need to take advice, and more able to judge the priorities of the different tasks competing for their attention.

WIDENING HORIZONS

For mothers, middle age can be a time of widening horizons. Once their children have become more independent, non-working mothers may wish to return to their careers or to explore new possibilities. This can sometimes

In mid-life, many adults find themselves responsible for the welfare of their parents. This can be a good opportunity to develop the relationship further.

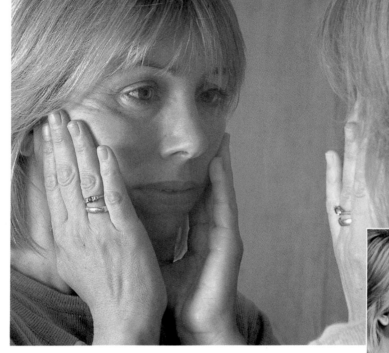

Middle age is a time when the ageing process begins to become apparent. Visible changes include the appearance of facial lines and grey hairs.

promote tension in a partnership, as some men find it hard to adjust to their partner's new-found independence.

This is also a time when children grow up and leave home. While this can cause a momentary sadness, it tends to be a problem for only a small number of parents, usually those for whom their children fulfilled a sense of being needed.

Instead of regretting that their children have left, most parents feel a sense of having accomplished one of life's major tasks and they can now afford to concentrate their energies on themselves once again.

FRICTION

It can happen that, particularly today, the high costs of housing force some children in their twenties to return home to live for a period of time. This can sometimes cause friction; the combined responsibilities of caring for a home, family and ageing parents can make the middle-aged feel that they are caught between the needs and desires of two generations.

ROLE-REVERSAL

Adults looking after elderly, infirm parents can feel confusion over the reversal of roles. Once their parents were all-powerful beings, but now they need help and protection. The practical problems of taking care of an ailing relative mean that this can be a demanding time – physically, emotionally and financially.

Children commonly leave home as parents reach middle-age. This can be a time for parents to pursue new ventures or dedicate more time to their careers.

RELATIONSHIPS

Couples who have devoted their lives to their children may find that, once the parental imperative is over, their relationship falters. They may be left to face each other and to work out difficulties that have been lying dormant for years. On the other hand, for many, this may be a time of new-found freedom and an opportunity to take up new interests, either independently or as a couple.

Today, men and women can look forward to 30 to 50 years of productive life after their

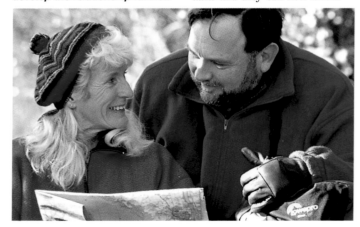

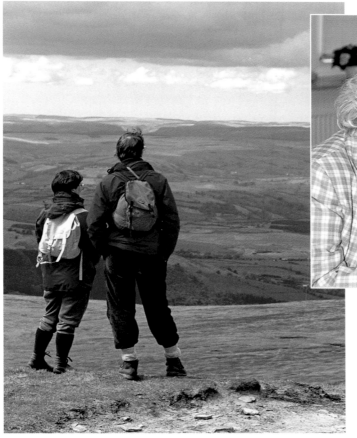

children have reached adulthood, in which they can return to putting themselves first.

As they are freed from the imperatives of earning a living and raising children, middle-aged people can focus their energies on personal development and on obtaining what they really want from life.

At this time, middle-aged men and women may go through post-parental psychological shifts that mark an increased androgyny. Men may become more openly sensual, dependent and emotional. Women can

While early adulthood can be a stressful time, middle-age tends to be a time of financial stability. Couples have more freedom to pursue shared interests.

become more assertive, less needful of love and more ready to risk losing love.

AMBITIONS
It is probably true to say that middle-aged people are searching for an accommodation between their long-held dreams and aspirations and the reality of their present situation.

'Nobel Prize' syndrome describes the realization that many people have in middle age that they are unlikely to achieve their longed-for hopes and dreams. Their chances of writing a bestseller, launching their own company or finding the perfect partner can begin to look increasingly remote.

Even for the extremely successful, it is rare for a person to succeed to a point that fulfils their early fantasies. In addition, those women not in a steady relationship may also have to come to terms with the fact that their chance of motherhood is gradually slipping away.

INDEPENDENCE
Many women, however, choose not to become mothers and these women often experience a sense of freedom and independence. They are free to concentrate on their careers or leisure interests, without the constraints of caring for a family.

Older employees may begin to find it difficult to relate to younger colleagues. This is usually caused by differing outlooks and views on life.

FINANCIAL STABILITY
As people become older, they tend to become more established in their careers. This is a time when they are generally more financially stable than in their youth and so are able to reap the benefits of their hard work.

It is also a time, however, when individuals may find that their employment horizons begin to narrow. And, if they lose their jobs, older people tend to remain unemployed for longer than younger people.

In the workplace, people may gradually become aware of the widening gap between themselves and their younger colleagues or employes. They may feel as though some boundary has been crossed and may feel a slight sense of alienation from their more youthful colleagues, particularly if they are outnumbered.

INTELLIGENCE
It is not that older people are any less able, however. Psychologists used to believe that a person's intelligence peaked at the age of 16 and gradually declined after this point. Now, it is thought that intelligence peaks at around 35 and that there is no great decline until the early sixties, when one's intelligence is comparable to the level it reached in the twenties.

As middle-age approaches, couples may find that they have more time to spend together. This can be a good opportunity to revive their relationship.

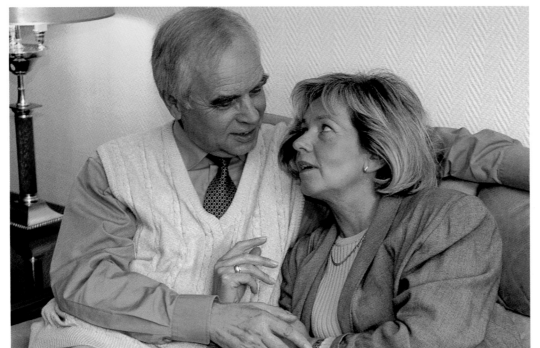

9

Coping with the menopause

The menopause is the time when a woman's menstrual cycle ceases. Women have different experiences of the menopause; some notice no changes, while others suffer unpleasant symptoms.

The term *menopause* is a combination of two Greek words – *menses* (periods) and *pausis* (stop) – and indicates the time in a woman's life when her menstrual periods have come to an end. This development is due to the inability of the ovaries (the female reproductive organs) to manufacture the sex hormones oestrogen and progesterone when they run out of their supply of eggs at around the age of 50. However, about one per cent of women experience a premature menopause before the age of 35.

LOSS OF FERTILITY
Menopause is as natural as puberty, pregnancy and childbirth and will happen to all women if they live long enough.

For some women, the end of fertility represents a major blow to their image of femininity and womanhood. There is a big difference between not wanting to become pregnant and no longer being physically able to do so. In coming to terms with menopause, women have to learn that femininity does not equal fertility.

PHYSICAL SYMPTOMS
The experience of menopause is different for each woman. About 20 per cent of women notice nothing at all, other than the end of their menstruating life,

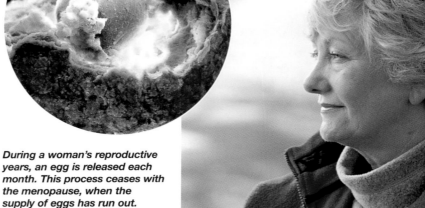

During a woman's reproductive years, an egg is released each month. This process ceases with the menopause, when the supply of eggs has run out.

and sail through the experience. Around 60 per cent are aware of changes and around 20 per cent experience severe, disabling symptoms resulting from hormonal imbalances.

For many women, the most uncomfortable symptom is the hot flush. These feelings of extreme warmth result from chemical shifts in the brain that cause blood vessels to dilate and constrict irregularly. Other common symptoms include night sweats, loss of libido and irritability.

Long-term symptoms include the thinning and drying out of the vaginal and genital skin and urinary problems.

HRT
Hormone replacement therapy (HRT) masks the passage through menopause and has been found to relieve hot flushes and night sweats and can be effective in restoring vaginal tissue. However, HRT has risks associated with long-term use, and may result in side effects such as breast tenderness, leg cramps, bloating, weight gain, depression and headaches.

PSYCHOLOGICAL CHANGES
Psychological changes are common around menopause. The most frequent complaints are depression and anxiety. Personality changes may occur,

Hormone replacement therapy is the use of female hormones to relieve menopausal symptoms. This is often prescribed in the form of skin patches.

The menopause marks a new stage in a woman's life. This usually occurs in a woman's 50s and brings about certain physical and emotional changes.

bringing rapidly changing moods, irritability, loss of confidence, and even panic attacks in women who have never experienced such symptoms before.

It is debatable whether these psychological symptoms are due to cessation of the production of oestrogen or the result of sleep disturbances, hot flushes and the negative attitude of a society obsessed by youth and beauty.

The physical changes that occur at the menopause can increase awareness and anxiety about the ageing process. In addition, at this time in their lives women can have numerous other stresses, such as having adolescent children, caring for elderly parents, or experiencing the 'empty nest syndrome', which is associated with children leaving the family home.

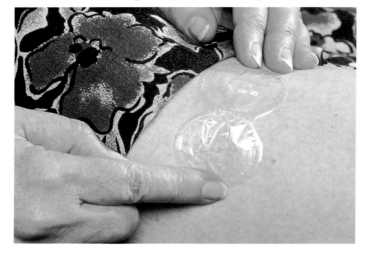

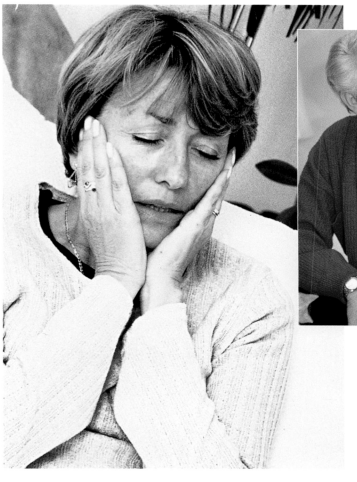

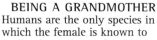

The menopause can be a difficult time for marital relationships. Women may feel they are not receiving enough support from their partners.

Some women find it hard to come to terms with the menopause. Many experience depression accompanied by a loss of confidence.

RELATIONSHIPS

Relations with partners can be strained around the period of the menopause. This is particularly true if men are experiencing the male mid-life transition, when they may feel that they have not achieved as much as they would have liked to from life.

At a time when women would particularly appreciate the support of a partner, men may be finding it hard to cope with their own problems. Conflicts at this time can be a recipe for disaster in the relationship.

Feelings of upheaval are by no means universal. Some women find the cessation of hormonal highs and lows associated with monthly menstrual cycles makes their menopause a time of tranquillity and composure.

VULNERABLE GROUPS

It has been shown that women of lower socio-economic groups have more psychological menopausal problems. The reasons for this are unclear, but it may be associated with financial security.

The post-menopausal period is when many women become grandmothers. This new role in the family can be a source of great enjoyment.

Particularly vulnerable to the symptoms of menopause are women who have defined their role in life in terms of pregnancy and motherhood. For these women, the menopause can take away part of their identity and make them feel without purpose.

VALUES IN SOCIETY

Studies of different cultures around the world have shown that the psychological impact of menopause is influenced by how much a society values the older woman.

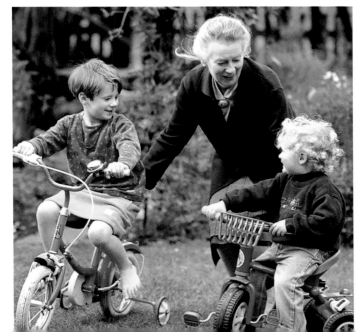

In societies like Papua New Guinea, where women enjoy increased status as they age and where their communities have positive attitudes to ageing and the menopause, women report few uncomfortable symptoms. In Rajasthan in India, women are able to take their veils off at menopause and are free to chat with men in their village.

Western society, on the other hand, tends to acknowledge the desirability of the younger female – at the expense of older women.

BEING A GRANDMOTHER

Humans are the only species in which the female is known to outlive her capacity for reproduction. One theory is that the menopause has evolved to provide grandmothering support to the next generation.

Once past child-bearing age, some women have their second chance at mothering – becoming a grandmother. Grandparents can experience enormous rewards from their relationships with grandchildren. Unlike mothers who are involved in day-to-day parenting, they can spend time on activities that are fun, rather than routine.

BENEFITS

Many women discover a sense of liberation after the menopause. They are no longer troubled by premenstrual syndrome, menstrual problems, child-rearing responsibilities, worries about pregnancy, or the gender stereotypes associated with youth.

In addition, they are the least likely of all women to suffer depression and often have a greater sense of their own well being than at any other time in their lives.

ACHIEVING GOALS

It is important for a woman to come to terms with her menopause since, with the average woman today living to over 80, she will spend at least 40 per cent of her life in a post-menopausal state.

Post-menopausal life should be viewed in a positive light, as a new stage in which women can look forward to new family roles and challenges.

Male mid-life transitions

In mid-life, men undergo changes related to the ageing process. In some men, these transitions may trigger emotional problems, such as depression, or relationship difficulties.

Men do not undergo an equivalent of the vivid physiological transition of the female menopause – the emphatic physiological change that is likely to cause a transformation in self-image. However, issues related to ageing do begin to affect men at this time, and the fact that there may not be an underlying physiological basis can make them all the more disturbing.

TRANSITIONS
Men undergo a range of transitions between the ages of about 35 and 55. Many experience a 'mid-life crisis', typically between the ages of 35 and 45. Some believe that such crises are largely emotional or psychological in origin, but if severe or extended, they may have physical consequences.

More physiological in basis is the so-called andropause, which becomes symptomatic between age 45 and 55. The andropause is probably due to a gradual decline in the levels of the hormone testosterone and is analogous to the menopause.

Although there is much debate in the medical community about the nature of the mid-life crisis, its connection to the andropause, and even whether the andropause exists at all, the testimony of the many men who have experienced severe mid-life transitions and the experience of the few medical professionals who are prepared to treat the andropause are sufficient for

male mid-life transitions to be taken seriously.

ANDROPAUSE
The term andropause refers to a group of symptoms caused by declining testosterone levels in ageing men. Some scientific studies of the andropause (also called the 'male menopause') have linked a variety of

Some middle-aged men have been shown to benefit from treatment with testosterone. A hormone implant can be inserted under the skin.

Men may experience a serious emotional crisis in their middle years. They may need counselling and support to help them at this time.

symptoms experienced by men in mid-life with a decline in the levels of testosterone available in the body. These include reduced libido, erectile dysfunction, emotional and psychological changes including irritability and depression, and muscular pain and weakness. However, the existence of the andropause is still hotly debated.

TESTOSTERONE
Decreases in hormone levels vary dramatically in the population, with some men affected at age 40 and others remaining unaffected by age 80. The onset of the andropause is unpredictable and its symptoms can be vague and variable.

In addition to reduced testosterone levels, there may be a range of underlying causes for the various symptoms. For example, erectile dysfunction

Excess alcohol consumption may cause erectile dysfunction. This problem may also be caused by a gradual decrease in testosterone levels.

may be caused by anxiety or excess alcohol consumption. Nevertheless, some medical professionals advocate the use of testosterone replacement therapy to restore hormonal levels, and many men have found it to be an effective treatment for their symptoms.

REPLACEMENT THERAPY
The suggested treatment for the andropause is testosterone replacement therapy. Treatment is administered in the form of injections, tablets, skin patches or implants that are inserted under the skin. In the latter two methods, small amounts of the hormone are continuously released over a period of months. Some men report a great improvement in both mood and libido.

Low testosterone levels are a risk factor for the development of osteoporosis in men and can increase the risk of cardiovascular disease; testosterone replacement therapy may therefore have a protective effect.

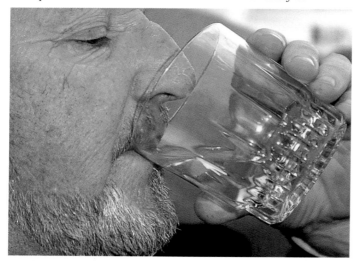

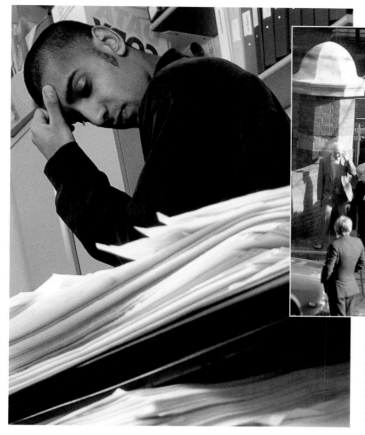

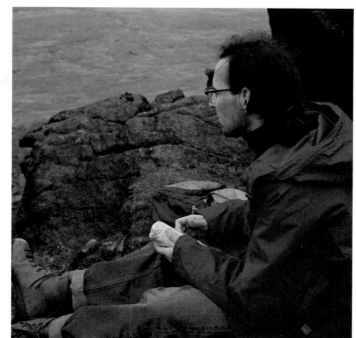

Mid-life crises may also have their origins in the 'crisis of masculinity' that some social observers note – a crisis precipitated in part at least by the decline in the importance of men's role as breadwinners for the family.

Some men try to deny the fact that they are ageing. However, significant life events, such as the death of a parent, may force them to accept their mortality.

physiological problems such as erectile dysfunction.

THE 'MID-LIFE CRISIS'
Problems in mid-life may be unrelated to hormonal changes but a form of 'mid-life crisis' affects many men. To some, the 'crisis' is simply a concomitant of the ageing process, the extent and severity of the crisis depending on how gracefully a man can accept that he is getting older.

For a woman, the transition from child-bearing years is very profound, because of the changes in her fertility and menstruation – essential parts of her identity. Such dramatic physical changes force her to come to terms psychologically with ageing.

By contrast, a man lacks this marked physiological change, meaning that he can choose to deny that he is getting older. Then, at some critical point, he is brought face to face with the passage of time and his own mortality. Triggers for such a crisis might include the death of a parent or close friend, the loss of a job, separation or divorce, children leaving home and becoming a grandparent.

EFFECTS OF MODERN LIFE
Some have suggested that the male mid-life crisis is essentially a side effect of a contemporary lifestyle of increased wealth and leisure with self-fulfilment as a major goal. Liberated from the constant toil of previous

Men who are strongly immersed in their careers may feel the pressures of work. Overwork can lead to feelings of stress and exhaustion.

generations, men now have time to engage in introspection. One negative outcome is a feeling of dissatisfaction with the shape of their lives compared with long-standing ideals.

Strongly career-driven men may feel a different set of pressures, and the constant pressure of performance in the workplace can easily lead to stress and emotional exhaustion.

EMOTIONAL PROBLEMS
Whatever the triggers and causes of mid-life crises, those experiencing them may suffer irritability, nervousness, anxiety, low self-esteem and other psychological and emotional disturbances. Depression can be triggered by and exacerbated by a tendency to reassess the past and berate oneself for unfulfilled goals. Emotional problems may put strain on existing relationships, and may even precipitate extramarital affairs. If the emotional and psychological problems become serious enough, they can precipitate

SEEKING HELP
Men who are going through a fundamentally emotional crisis may find it difficult to seek help, or even to admit to themselves that there is a problem. If a man is in the habit of keeping his feelings private and not sharing them with friends, particularly other men, then he may quickly become emotionally isolated at critical times.

MID-LIFE OPPORTUNITIES
Just as the pace and expectations of modern living may be factors in precipitating a 'mid-life crisis', so the general opportunities available may provide a route out of the crisis. Increased affluence and new working practices may allow a man to cut back his working week in mid-life. Opportunities also arise to explore lifelong interests or to travel.

The beginnings to a solution for a mid-life crisis may lie in simply recognizing which changes must simply be accepted, and which can be ameliorated by adapting personal expectations and goals and by recognizing that, as one mode of life is perhaps passing by, so another awaits.

New working practices and more disposable income mean that some men are able to reduce their working hours. They are free to enjoy life and to travel.

Entering old age

Many people fear old age, seeing it as a time of
mental and physical decline. With good health however, a
stimulating and fulfilling lifestyle can still be enjoyed.

Many people feel that they are
entering the period of their lives
described as 'old age' once they
pass their 70th birthday.

However, chronological age
should not be regarded as an
infallible guide to the division
between young old age (the
period just after retirement) and
old age. People who have led an
active life continue to think of
themselves as vigorous
individuals, rather than old
people well into their seventies.
Others can behave as though
they are old from a relatively
young age.

A CHANGING PERSPECTIVE
Society's attitudes towards
ageing varies enormously.
Young children seem indifferent
to age changes, while young
adults at the height of their
physical strength and beauty
often fear the decline that they
see as part of old age. Attitudes
formed in youth often influence
how people view the ageing
process as they go through life.

AGEISM
Ageism occurs when people
apply the stereotypes of ageing
to elderly people, and view them
as unattractive, incompetent,
and weak. Even well-meaning
people can hold such negative
attitudes, unknowingly acting
with condescension.

One of the principal problems
facing the old is that their role

*Attitudes towards ageing are
influenced by upbringing.
Children who have contact with
grandparents tend to be more
understanding of older people.*

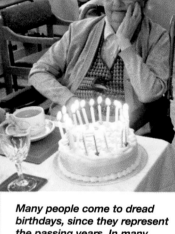

*Many people come to dread
birthdays, since they represent
the passing years. In many
cultures, however, increasing
age is seen in a positive light.*

has been eroded in Western
society. The respect once given
to older people for their
knowledge and experience was
largely tied in with oral
tradition. Civilizations that once
relied on older people to pass on
their learning and experience
can now access information
through books instead, leaving
older people without a clearly
defined role.

PHYSICAL DECLINE
People start to experience
physical decline with old age
and are more susceptible to a
number of chronic conditions. In
addition, the immune system
deteriorates with age, which
means that older people are
more vulnerable to infection.

The senses often decline,
becoming less sharp. People no
longer hear, see, smell or taste so
clearly. Eye conditions, such as
cataracts and macular
degeneration, may arise. A
cataract is a clouding of the eye
lens so that vision becomes hazy
and bright lights are dazzling;
macular degeneration is caused
by deterioration of the cells at
the back of the retina.

*Certain conditions and diseases
are more likely to affect the
elderly than other sections of
the population. Deterioration of
sight and hearing is common.*

In old age, a person's ability
to detect high-frequency sounds
is reduced as the 'hair cells' of
the inner ear become damaged.
This results in difficulty in
hearing consonants like 't' and
's', and therefore speech begins
to sound indistinct.

There is a gradual loss of lean
muscle tissue and bone mass. If
there is too much bone loss, the
bones become osteoporotic (a
condition in which the bones
become brittle) and are more
likely to break. Joints may
become stiffer, losing flexibility
and causing pain, especially low
back pain.

MEDICATION
Many older people find that
they are more sensitive to the
effects of medication than when
they were younger. This is
because detoxification by the
liver is slower, as is the
clearance of waste from the
body by the kidneys. Certain
drugs are therefore more likely
to cause side effects in older
people than in the remainder of
the population.

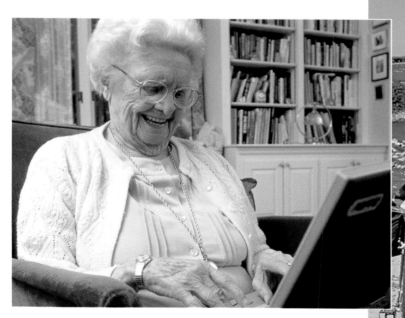

THE BALTIMORE STUDY

In 1958, the Baltimore Longitudinal Study was commenced. This set out to uncover the nature of the normal ageing process, by following the lives of thousands of people living in Baltimore, USA.

The study found that many of the accepted changes of ageing are apparently the result of disease. It also found that some of the expected declines, both physiological and intellectual, did not appear in very old individuals who retained their general good health.

Experts agree that if older people abandon unhealthy habits (such as smoking or over-eating) and acquire healthy ones, they can substantially improve their health prospects into old age.

POSITIVE ASPECTS

For many people, old age is an enriching experience. It offers an opportunity to step back and take an overview of their existence, seeing the shape and meaning of their life as a whole.

Moreover, some people are able to view old age not as a process of inevitable decline, but as a phase in their lives when they can continue to develop. Many take up new hobbies and learning opportunities.

In addition, the characteristics of the sexes seem to blend with old age, with beneficial results. Men can be surprised to discover sensitive feelings in themselves and women may acquire a new-found sense of assertiveness.

There comes a time, however, when many elderly people have to face the fact that they can no longer cope on their own. The daily chores of shopping,

Rather than being a time of mental decline, old age can allow people to learn new skills. New technologies can be mastered with a little practice.

cooking, cleaning and bathing can become too difficult.

At such times, the parent/child relationship undergoes a role reversal and the adult children become the carers. Many children feel a sense of loyalty and affection for their parents and want to repay the kindness that was shown to them.

However, several factors can make it difficult for the children of elderly parents to take on the caring role. The migration

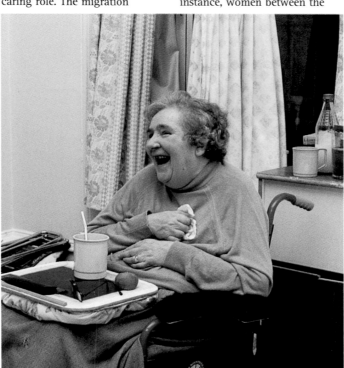

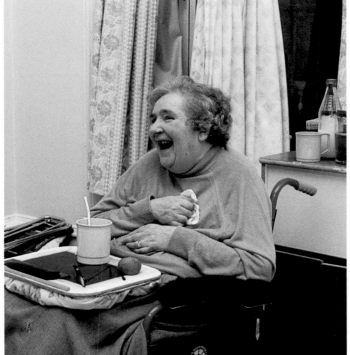

patterns of young people to the cities for work means that many children live great distances from their parents, making it hard for them to provide ongoing care.

In addition, the trend for smaller families means that there are fewer children to look after parents. Social changes have also meant that people who traditionally acted as carers are no longer able to do so. For instance, women between the

Many older people relish the increased leisure time of post-retirement. They view this time as a wonderful opportunity for personal development.

ages of 45 and 55, who have long played this role, have returned to the workplace in large numbers.

CHOOSING WHERE TO LIVE

For those elderly people who are able to move in with their children, this option has both advantages and disadvantages. It provides security and a support system, but offers little privacy and the older person can lose existing local friends and networks.

Other options include sheltered housing and residential/nursing homes. Sheltered housing can represent a half-way option, where independence is coupled with the reassurance of support when necessary.

Older people requiring more constant attention may choose to live in residential or nursing homes. Both options are expensive, and run the risk of institutionalizing the older person. In all cases, the mental and physical well-being of the older person must be paramount in the decision-making.

Nursing homes offer the reassuring protection of full-time care. This may become a desirable option if daily tasks become too difficult to manage.

How the body ages

Ageing is the gradual degeneration of the body with time.
Biological processes, such as cardiovascular system functions,
become less efficient until they can no longer fulfil their role.

Ageing is the term used to describe the physiological changes that take place in the body as it slowly degenerates with time. This process occurs gradually over a number of years, beginning in the third decade of life (age 20–30).

LIFE EXPECTANCY
The longest lifespan recorded by the *Guinness Book of Records* is currently 122 years. With advances in lifestyle, medicine and sanitation, however, this record is likely to be broken. On average in the UK, life expectancy is 74 years for men and 79 years for women.

'STOPPING THE CLOCK'
Extensive research has been carried out into the biological mechanisms behind ageing, in an attempt to delay its effects, and even reverse the process.

Though much progress has been made in our understanding of the ageing process, what holds true is that ageing is an inevitable biological state and is as much a part of life as infancy, childhood and adolescence.

Ageing occurs gradually, over a period of many years. Medical advances have helped to ensure that people are living longer today than ever before.

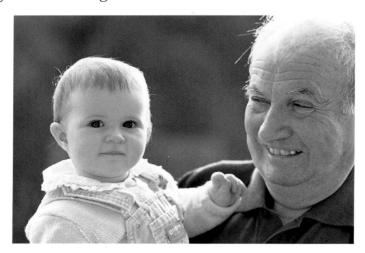

Cell ageing

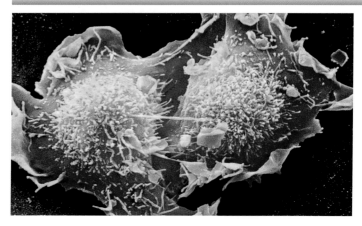

In order to understand the ageing process, it is necessary to investigate the biological mechanisms that occur at the cellular level. Cells are the individual building blocks, functioning together, that form the tissues which make up the body. These cells are replenished through the process of replication (cell division).

Cells divide a finite number of times before dying. It is likely therefore that cellular genes are programmed to stop functioning at a predetermined time.

CELL DEATH
Research has shown that cells divide a finite number of times before undergoing apoptosis (programmed cell death). In addition, the remaining cells may not function as efficiently as those in the young.

Certain cellular enzymes may be less active, so more time may be required for chemical reactions to occur that are essential to the basic functioning of the cell. As the cells fail to reproduce, the organ becomes less efficient, until it can no longer fulfil its biological role.

External changes

Ageing is most commonly characterized by the external changes that take place in the body.

HAIR CHANGES
Perhaps the most obvious change that takes place during the ageing process is the alteration in hair colour. Around the age of 30, grey or white hairs often begin to appear as the hair follicles lose their source of pigmentation. This greying becomes increasingly obvious as pigmented hairs are shed and replaced by grey hairs.

In both sexes, the hair thins considerably, and many men may experience balding.

SKIN CHANGES
The skin loses its elasticity with age, and wrinkles develop. This is due to changes in collagen (a structural protein) and elastin (the protein that gives the skin its elastic quality).

CHANGES IN STATURE
Middle age is often associated with an increase in weight as the metabolism slows, followed by a significant decrease in weight as old age progresses.

Muscle tissue may be replaced by fat, particularly around the trunk, while the arms and legs generally become thinner.

Older people tend to shrink in height, owing to compression of the spinal vertebrae.

As the body ages, the hair loses its colour and turns grey. The skin becomes less elastic and wrinkles develop due to changes in collagen and elastin.

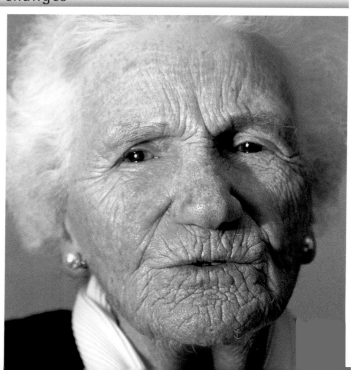

Internal changes

Physiological studies reveal that the performance of many of the body's vital organs – such as the heart, kidneys and lungs – declines with age.

Changes associated with ageing also take place internally. Many internal organs, such as the liver, kidneys, spleen, pancreas, lungs and liver, shrink in size and function less efficiently, as the cells that comprise them gradually degenerate.

The circulation of blood by the heart is also affected by ageing. The heart's pumping action is greatly reduced and the body's response to exercise or stress by increasing the heart rate is much more extreme. The blood vessels (veins, arteries and capillaries) throughout the body lose some elasticity and tend to become convoluted.

The bones become more brittle, as the calcium content decreases, making older people more liable to fractures, even after relatively minor falls.

There is a general decline in the body's regulating mechanisms, resulting in the body being less adaptable to external changes. Older people are more sensitive to extremes of temperature, and may take longer to recover from illness.

The gradual decline of the immune system also means that older people are more vulnerable to infection and disease.

Calcium and protein are progressively lost from the bones with age. This can lead to the condition osteoporosis, in which the bones become brittle.

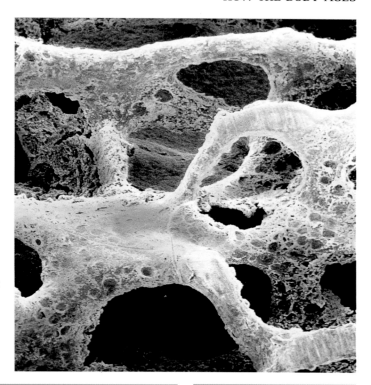

Changes in the nervous system

The ageing brain undergoes a gradual loss of neurones (brain cells), which are not replaced.

MENTAL ABILITY
However, although the number of brain cells decreases throughout life, this represents only a small percentage of the total number of cells in the brain. There is no conclusive evidence that intelligence deteriorates with age; rather it seems to be closely associated with education and lifestyle.

AGE-RELATED DISEASE
Brain cells are extremely sensitive to oxygen deficiency. It is likely that, when deterioration of the brain does occur, this is caused not by ageing itself, but by age-related diseases, such as arteriosclerosis.

Such diseases affect the cardiovascular system and

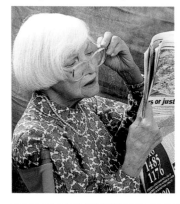

Mental stimulation plays a part in countering the effects of ageing on the brain. Activities such as doing crosswords help to keep the brain active.

reduce oxygen supply to the brain. The efficiency of the brain is therefore reduced, and there may be a decline in intellectual performance. Logic, mental agility and the ability to grasp new ideas can all be affected.

BRAIN FUNCTION
Functions related to the brain also lose their efficiency. Reflexes and physical movements become slower and the memory may deteriorate, especially for recent events.

SENILE DEMENTIA
In severe cases, this can lead to senile dementia. This condition is characterized by a loss of memory, childlike behaviour, incoherent speech and a lack of awareness.

Senses

There is a gradual deterioration of the senses with age:
■ Vision – beyond the age of around 20, there is a decline in visual acuity, which deteriorates at an even greater rate after age 50. The size of the pupil also reduces with age, with the result that night vision is affected. The eyes are also increasingly susceptible to disease
■ Hearing – there is a gradual reduction in the ability to hear tones at higher frequencies. This can interfere with the identification of individuals by their voices, and the ability to follow group conversations
■ Taste – the number of taste buds is gradually reduced, and the sense of taste is dulled
■ Smell – this may deteriorate with age, also affecting the sense of taste.

Genetics of ageing

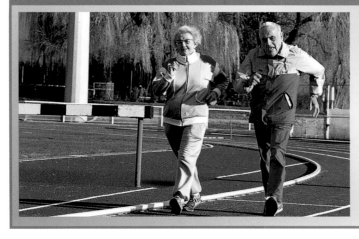

Medical advances have served to increase the average life expectancy, although these have not yet extended the maximum lifespan.

Laboratory research has shown that cells replicate themselves a certain number of times before dying, and that the quality of each cell gradually deteriorates. This suggests that human beings may

The rate at which a person ages is determined by both genetic and environmental factors. Taking regular exercise can help to delay the effects of time.

be programmed to age and die at some pre-determined point and that genes may carry instructions to cease functioning at a certain time.

Environmental factors
In reality, how a person ages is determined not solely by genes, but by environmental factors such as lifestyle and diet.

A person who smokes, has a generally poor diet and does not take any exercise is more likely to age more quickly, become ill and die before their genetically determined time.

Internal body changes in old age

As people age, numerous bodily changes take place.
Some are inevitable, but others depend on factors such as lifestyle
and the state of health during youth and middle age.

As the body ages, the cells of which it is made up degenerate. As a result, vital cellular processes slow down, and the internal organs become less efficient, affecting the way in which the body functions. The exact cause of these internal changes is unknown, although there appear to be a number of factors at play.

THEORIES OF AGEING
One important factor is genetics. It appears that the cells which make up the body are genetically programmed to stop replicating after a limited number of divisions, so that the number of cells gradually declines. Another theory is that free radicals (toxins that occur as a by-product of chemical reactions in the cells) build up and damage the cells, causing them to die.

SECONDARY AGEING
Although these body changes are a normal part of ageing, ill-health, loss of mobility and a decline in mental agility are not an inevitable consequence of growing old. These tend to be a result of various lifelong processes involving disease and lifestyle, which exacerbate the natural degeneration of the body that takes place during old age.

Keeping active is essential to help maintain good health in old age. If people look after themselves, many are capable of staying fit into their eighties.

Mental stimulation is important in elderly people to keep the mind active. Activities such as reading and doing crosswords can act as mental 'jogging'.

BRAIN
With age, the brain appears to shrink, and brain cells are lost in some areas, especially those that coordinate voluntary muscle activity. However, research has indicated that shrinkage may not be an inevitable consequence of ageing. In healthy elderly people, researchers have found no neuronal loss with age, only a shrinkage of neurone size.

The autonomic nervous system, which regulates body systems, can become slow or weakened with age. The result is that the body takes longer to react to changing conditions – for example, the increase in heart rate during exercise – and may not respond as effectively to stress.

VISION
In middle age, everyone experiences a loss of elasticity of the lens of the eye, resulting in long-sightededness.

Cataracts are more common with increasing age. A cataract is the result of change in protein of the lens of the eye, which gradually becomes cloudy and eventually opaque. Vision is at first blurred and colours seem muted, but large, central changes in the lens can severely impair sight. Treatment is by removal of the lens and the insertion of an artificial one.

HEARING
Presbyacusis is hearing loss that many people experience in old age. It is caused by atrophy and degeneration in the cochlea of the hair cells (structure in the inner ear) that convert vibrations in the inner ear into electrical impulses that travel to the brain to be perceived as sounds. As people develop presbyacusis, they tend to miss certain high-frequency sounds, such as birds singing, the ticking of a clock and the ring of a telephone.

Statistics from the Medical Research Council National Study of Hearing show that 55 per cent of people over 60 are deaf or hard of hearing. This rises to over 90 per cent for people over 80 years old.

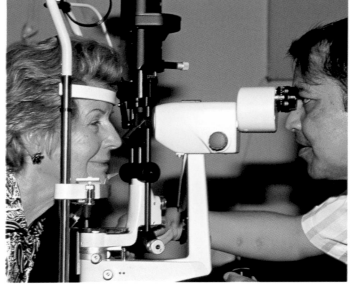

Vision often deteriorates as part of the ageing process. The lens of the eye becomes less elastic, with the result that long-sightedness is increasingly likely.

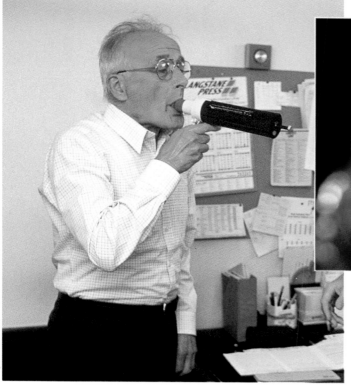

Lung function tests measure the volume of air in litres when a person takes a full breath. With increasing age, maximum breathing capacity is reduced.

In atherosclerosis, fatty plaques build up in arterial walls (shown). The condition is found in most elderly people, particularly if they have eaten a high-fat diet.

CARDIOVASCULAR SYSTEM

Age has an important effect on the appearance of the heart. Fat deposits collect on its surface and the collagen that surrounds the heart's fibres loses its elasticity. This means that under conditions of stress, even healthy hearts are less effective than they once were.

During exertion, heart rates increase in order to deliver oxygen to the body. When young men exercise vigorously, their hearts may beat as rapidly as 200 times per minute, but in men aged between 70 and 90, the heart can beat no faster than 125 times per minute under the same workload.

In addition, the cardiovascular system may become impaired by a condition known as atherosclerosis, in which hard, yellow, fatty plaques are deposited in the arterial walls. This is a common cause of heart attack, but is not an inevitable consequence of ageing.

LUNGS

Similarly, with increasing age, the lungs and chest wall become less elastic, and maximum breathing capacity is reduced.

In addition, the mechanisms protecting the lungs from infection – such as ciliary action (tiny hairlike cells preventing foreign particles from entering the lungs) and normal mucus production – become less effective. This results in an increased susceptibility to developing chest infections.

Older people find that, for a given level of physical effort, they have to breathe harder to maintain satisfactory blood oxygen levels. The result is that older people become breathless more rapidly when they are exercising.

BLADDER AND KIDNEY FUNCTION

The capacity of the bladder diminishes with age. This seems to be the result of muscle weakness and changes in the connective tissue. The result is that the average bladder of an older person holds less than half as much as a young person.

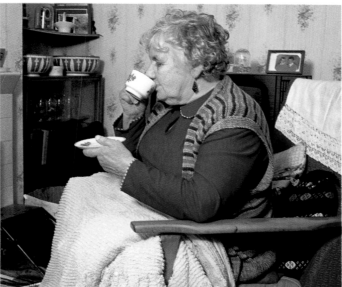

Signals from the ageing bladder also change. When young, the sensation of bladder fullness, which produces the urge to urinate, is felt when the bladder is about half full. However, among older adults, the urge is not felt until the bladder is nearly full.

Moreover, each kidney contains millions of tiny filtering units called nephrons, which cleanse the blood of impurities. The function of the kidneys declines as nephrons die off and the blood supply to the kidneys is reduced.

IMMUNE SYSTEM

The thymus, an endocrine gland that is a major component of the immune system, is important in the ageing process. As the thymus shrinks, there is an increase in the bloodstream of immature T-cells (white blood cells responsible for fighting infection), and the functioning of mature T-cells become less efficient while B-cells produce fewer antibodies.

Consequently, the body is less capable of mounting an immune response against invading organisms, making the body more vulnerable to infection. Whether such changes are an inevitable consequence of ageing is, however, still a matter for debate.

FERTILITY IN MEN AND WOMEN

Women lose their fertility with the onset of menopause, which usually occurs in the late forties or early fifties. Among men in their fifties, 68.5 per cent have active sperm in their semen, but among men in their seventies the proportion has decreased to 48 per cent.

In most men, normal ageing of the prostate gland is difficult to follow because abnormal but harmless cell growth enlarges the gland. Among men who reach their seventies, it is not uncommon for the prostate gland to have doubled in size. Often, the gland becomes so enlarged that it interferes with the function of the bladder and has to be removed.

In old age, the heart and lungs do not function as well as they should. As a result, mobility is restricted and many elderly people become house-bound.

External body changes in old age

Outward signs of ageing take place gradually over several decades. Although no-one can escape these changes, factors such as lifestyle and genetics can influence the rate at which they occur.

The first visible signs of ageing can be detected in the body while people are still young. A few grey hairs start to appear, wrinkles form at the corners of the eyes, and the flesh becomes less firm.

The changes progress so slowly that, at first, people are not really aware of them. However, by the time people have reached their late 50s and 60s, the cumulative effects of external body changes have become impossible to ignore.

RATE OF AGEING
Changes occur in hair colour, hair thickness and consistency, skin quality, body fat distribution, height and, sometimes, the shape of the spine. A person's precise rate of ageing depends on their genetic inheritance, which is modified by circumstances such as their early upbringing, lifestyle and environment. For example, a person who drinks, smokes and sunbathes is likely to look older than their identical twin who abstains from these practices.

EFFECTS ON THE HAIR
Hair begins to grey when the production of pigment in the hair follicles starts to slow down. It is a very variable process that can start as early as the 20s for some people and as late as the 60s for others. Genes play an important role in determining the age at which grey hair replaces the natural colour.

Each sex undergoes characteristic localized changes in the quality and quantity of their hair. In men, hair in the nostrils, eyebrows and ears that was once fine, short and colourless becomes coarser, longer and darker. In women over the age of 65, hair on the chin and above the lips may undergo a similar transformation.

BALDNESS
In male pattern baldness, hair on the scalp changes in the opposite way. Here, dark, coarse hair is replaced by fine, short, colourless hair. The familiar male-balding with receding hairline may also affect women, but this tends to happen only if women live into their 80s and 90s.

HOW THE SKIN CHANGES
The skin in older people has a slower cell turnover than in younger people. The cells are smaller in size and number, the result being thinner and drier skin. It is the increased laxity of the skin that leads to the formation of wrinkles.

The dramatic changes in the appearance of the skin are largely due to a progressive destruction of the delicate architecture of the connective tissue components – collagen and elastin (a tissue rich in elastic fibres) – that are found in the deeper layer of the skin (dermis). Elastic fibres maintain normal skin tension, but as people age, these fibres decrease in number, which means that the skin loses its elasticity.

Inhaled free radicals – highly reactive molecules in the atmosphere – have the unfortunate effect of attacking the skin's collagen. Their effects on the collagen contribute to an aged, leathery appearance.

Ageing skin can be exacerbated by sunbathing and smoking because both activities produce greater quantities of free radicals.

Wrinkles in the skin are usually the first sign of ageing. These occur because of a reduction of collagen in the skin; this results in loss of elasticity.

One of the most noticeable signs of ageing is greying of the hair. This occurs due to a decline in the production of pigment in the hair follicles.

Ageing has a dramatic effect on hair colour and consistency. In men, there may be increased hair growth in the ears and nostrils, and eyebrows.

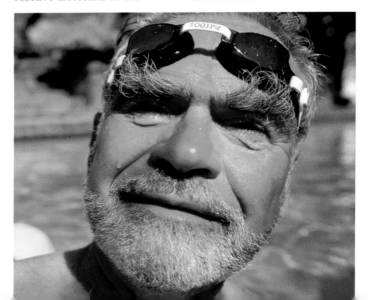

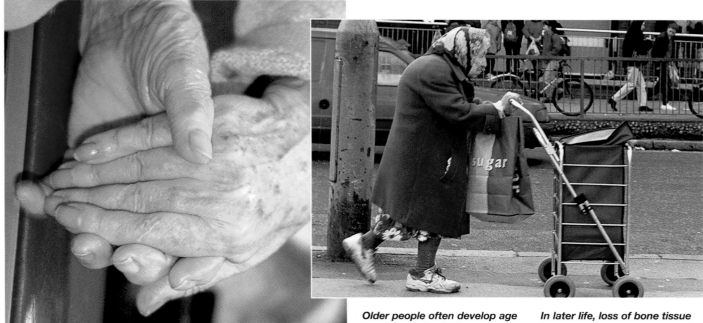

Older people often develop age spots (lentigines). These flat brown spots contain increased numbers of melanocytes (melanin-producing cells).

In later life, loss of bone tissue can lead to a change in posture and height. The spine can gradually become curved as the vertebrae are damaged.

FACIAL APPEARANCE

The facial appearance of older people changes because the amount of subcutaneous fat – the fat just beneath the skin – steadily decreases. When combined with the reduced thickness of the dermis and the diminished elasticity of the skin, this causes the skin to sag and make wrinkles more pronounced.

In addition, the contraction of facial bone allows skin to fold away from underlying muscles. The effect of gravity pulling this skin down can then lead to sagging jowls.

WRINKLES

Wrinkles develop gradually over many years. First to appear are horizontal furrows, or frown lines, across the forehead in the 20s, followed by crow's feet around the eyes at 40, wrinkles at the corner of the mouth from 50, and creases around the lips from 60.

AGE SPOTS

Although pigment-containing cells in the skin decrease with age, those that remain increase in size and sometimes cluster to form age spots, also known as liver spots.

The ageing of skin in women begins about 10 years earlier than in men. This is because the oil-producing glands in women's skin begin to atrophy (waste away) after the menopause when the levels of the hormone oestrogen decline. Because men's oil-producing glands continue to function, their skin is thicker and oilier, postponing the appearance of wrinkles.

ALTERED PHYSIQUE

Unlike skin cells, muscle cells cannot replace themselves. Muscle density increases until about the age of 39; muscle mass then begins to shrink as the muscle fibres decrease in number and diameter.

Fat replaces some of the muscles as it starts to infiltrate between them. This means that even if a person's weight is the same at age 60 as it was at 25, their body will generally contain more fat than it once did. The loss of muscle mass is accompanied by the loss of muscle strength, tone, flexibility and speed of movement.

After the menopause, when levels of oestrogen and progesterone are low, women start to notice that fat becomes more concentrated around the waist, abdomen and breasts. This shape begins to assume a more masculine outline than before.

BONE DENSITY AND LOSS OF HEIGHT

Osteoporotic changes in bone density can lead to the development of a 'dowager's

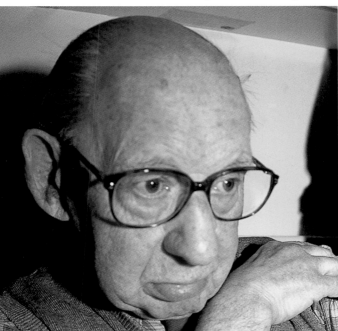

hump' as the back becomes curved. As the bones of the spine lose their density, the collapse of the vertebrae causes the ribcage to tilt downwards towards the hips.

A curvature in the upper spine creates a second curve in the lower spinal column, pushing the internal organs outwards. Due to the compressed spinal column, up to seven or eight inches in height can be lost. Internal functions are impaired as the organs shift position and obstruct other organs and systems.

Even for older people who do not have osteoporosis, there is a loss in height of just over an inch in men and two inches in women. Loss of height is due to altered posture, thinning of the cartilage discs that provide cushioning between the spinal vertebrae and a loss of water in the discs.

COMING TO TERMS WITH AGEING

For people, particularly women, who have set great store by good looks in their youth, the changes in body appearance that occur with age can be devastating. It is little wonder that face creams and cosmetic surgery have become billion dollar businesses as people try their hardest to forestall the march of time.

Ageing brings facial changes other than wrinkles. The bones in the face contract, leading to sagging jowels as skin pulls away from underlying muscles.

Sensory changes in old age

Many of the sensory changes experienced in old age may be due to a reduction in general circulation and the deterioration of the bodily structures governing sight, smell, hearing, touch and taste.

During the ageing process, the senses, which give us information about the world, tend to become less acute. Some of these changes can have a tremendous impact on the lives of elderly people.

DETERIORATING SENSES

Hearing, smell, taste, touch and sight are an important part of life. We use these senses to discover what is happening around us and to interact with other people. Deterioration of these senses affects the way in which people behave and is also likely to make communication more difficult.

These problems can be made worse by the elderly person's reluctance to seek help, which may have developed from a fear of being thought senile, or complaining too much. In many cases, there is a simple fear of the possible diagnosis.

HEARING PROBLEMS

Many people lose the ability to hear clearly as they get older. In fact, some hearing loss is almost inevitable and it is estimated that 30 per cent of people over the age of 65 have significant hearing impairment.

Total or even severe partial deafness can have a major effect on a person's life, as they are losing an important means of communication. Deafness can be a very isolating disability.

Hearing is reduced as people get older because the structures

The range of frequencies heard by the ear reduces after the age of 65. This makes it difficult to hear voices against background noise.

Many elderly people incur a deterioration in sight as the lens of the eye loses elasticity, resulting in difficulty in focusing. Bifocals may become necessary.

that make up the ear deteriorate with ageing. The eardrum itself often becomes thicker and there are changes in the bones of the middle ear (which are responsible for transmitting sound to the inner ear). The semicircular canals that control balance may also be affected.

AUDITORY NERVES

Sensorineural hearing loss involves changes in the inner ear, auditory nerve or brain. High-frequency sounds often become more difficult to hear as the part of the cochlea that responds to these frequencies ceases to work properly. This condition is called presbyacusis.

Hearing sound against a background noise, as at a party, also becomes more difficult. This is because the ear is not able to detect such a wide range of frequencies, making it more difficult to distinguish sounds from different sources. The overall effect can be one of jumbled sounds.

Changes in the auditory nerve may cause loss of auditory

acuity (sharpness), while changes in the brain may lessen its ability to process information from the ears and 'translate' it into meaningful information.

Tinnitus (ringing in the ears) occurs when the inner ear transmits signals to the brain without being first stimulated by sound from outside; often, there is no obvious cause for this.

There is, unfortunately, no cure or treatment for any of these conditions, although sometimes a modern hearing aid can ease some of the problems associated with presbyacusis.

CONDUCTIVE HEARING LOSS

Conductive hearing loss occurs when the structures of the outer and middle ear no longer transmit sound efficiently to the inner ear. A hearing aid or, sometimes, surgery can help with this type of hearing loss, depending on the specific cause.

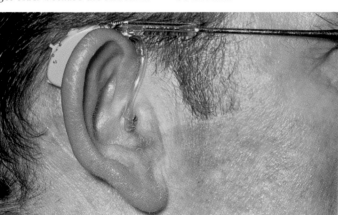

Many hearing problems can be discreetly and easily corrected. This air conductor hearing aid is small enough to fit on top of the arm of a pair of spectacles.

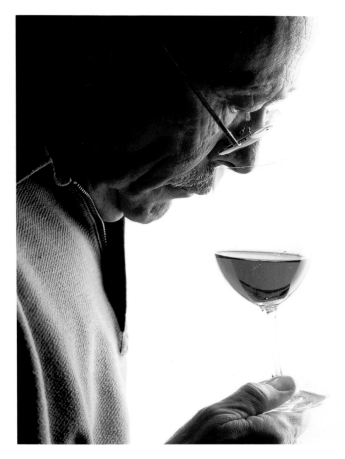

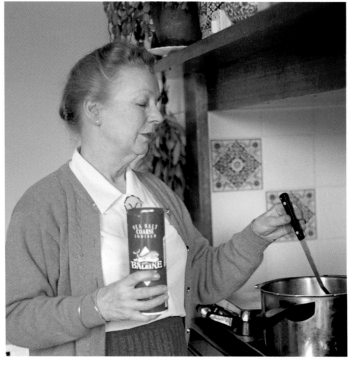

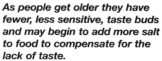

Smell receptors in the nose begin to thin out after the age of 30. This may explain why older people find it harder to distinguish smells.

As people get older they have fewer, less sensitive, taste buds and may begin to add more salt to food to compensate for the lack of taste.

LOSS OF SMELL AND TASTE

According to some research, people start to lose their sense of smell at the age of 30. However, the deterioration takes place so slowly that people are rarely aware that it is happening.

The causes are not fully understood, but it is known that the patch of nerve endings which act as smell receptors in the nose begin to thin. At the same time, the olfactory bulb (the part of the brain responsible for interpreting the signals from the smell receptors) becomes smaller. Consequently, older people can find it harder to distinguish smells.

At the same time, food may start to appear more bland. This is probably partly because the sense of taste is to some extent dependent on the ability to smell and partly because the taste buds also change.

A young person has around 9000 taste buds in the tongue. At the age of about 40-50 years in women and 50-60 years in men, the number of taste buds starts to decrease. At the same time, the remaining taste buds start to lose mass (atrophy).

Even so, the sensitivity to the four different taste sensations (sweet, salty, sour and bitter) does not seem to decrease until after the age of 60, if at all. There is also some doubt as to whether loss of taste and smell is actually related to ageing itself. The loss, if it occurs, may be more concerned with other factors, such as disease, smoking and a lifetime's exposure to chemicals in the environment.

TOUCH AND PAIN

The skin of the body is covered in receptors that are sensitive to touch, pressure, vibration, cold, heat and pain. There are also receptors inside the body that inform the brain about the condition and position of internal organs. As people age, their sensitivity to these sensations tends to be reduced. The cause is uncertain. It may be that the reduced circulation of old age leads to a corresponding reduced blood flow to the receptors, making them less efficient. Changes in the brain or spinal cord may also play a part.

Equally, though, the loss of sensitivity may be a result of the disorders that occur more often in the elderly. Minor dietary deficiencies, such as a decreased thiamine level, may play a part.

The sense of fine touch decreases up until the age of about 70, when it seems actually to increase again, due to the skin becoming thinner.

A reduced ability to detect touch, pain and heat means that there is a greater risk of injury. Loss of pressure sensitivity can lead to pressure sores that can become ulcerated, while loss of sensitivity to cold increases the risk of suffering from hypothermia and frostbite.

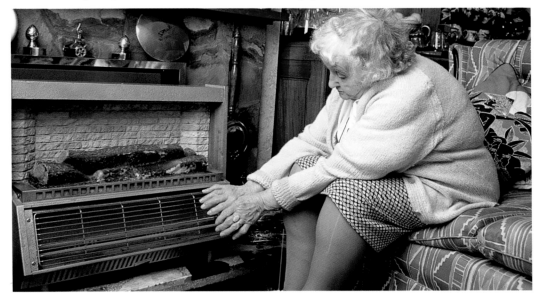

The skin is covered in receptors that are sensitive to touch, heat and pain. These lose efficiency with age, and require greater stimulus to register an effect.

Life expectancy

Human beings are never likely to become immortal. However, scientists are looking for ways of slowing the ageing process, and future generations may have life expectancies of over 100 years.

Life expectancy depends greatly upon a person's general health and the care that they receive when they are sick. In most parts of the world, living conditions and medical care have improved dramatically in the last 50 years and most people now live longer than did their ancestors.

MEDICAL ADVANCES
In 1900, the average life expectancy worldwide was just 48 years. Today, it has risen to 67 years, having increased by 10 years just since 1970. This increased life expectancy is due to improved access to nutritious food, and improvements in primary healthcare, particularly the provision of safe water, good sanitation, immunization, and antibiotics and other medicines.

However, as yet, relatively few people live to see their hundredth birthday. Even in Japan where, statistically, people live longer than anywhere else, the average lifespan for men is only 71.9 years and 77.2 years for women. In the UK, these figures are 69.7 and 73.7 years respectively, while in the US they are 67.5 and 72.6 years.

REDUCED EXPECTANCY
In some parts of the world, life expectancy has actually fallen during the last 20 years. Infectious diseases such as tuberculosis and AIDS, as well

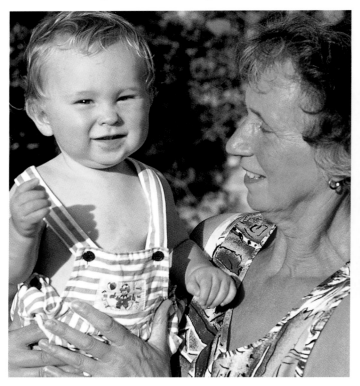

Life expectancy has increased dramatically in recent years. A child born today is expected to live to at least age 67, compared to 48 back in 1900.

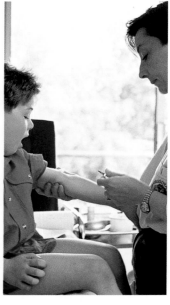

Immunization has been an important contributory factor to increased life expectancy. At an early age, children are vaccinated against a range of diseases.

as smoking, excessive alcohol consumption, high-fat diets and stress-related illnesses are all factors that reduce life expectancy. In the nations that formed part of the former Soviet Union, economic depression has caused a decline in living conditions. Moreover, in many sub-Saharan countries, where infant mortality is high and one

in three adults is infected with HIV, average life expectancy has declined by 15 years since 1987; today, in Sierra Leone, Niger and Malawi, average life expectancy is less than 30 years.

FEMALE LONGEVITY
In parts of the world where life expectancy is highest, women tend to outlive men by five to eight years. The reason for this is not clear, but it may be linked to the female menopause. This involves reduced hormone levels due to the cessation of egg production, compared to hormone levels in men, which remain high and are associated with increased chances of heart disease and prostate cancer.

Life expectancy actually increases with age. Children who

reach the age of five have a better chance of surviving into adulthood because their bodies are better able to fight off disease. And, the longer a person lives, the greater their chances of reaching older ages. For example, those who live beyond the age of 70 have a greater chance of surviving into their eighties or nineties. Furthermore, anyone who reaches the age of 100 is more likely to reach the age of 101 than someone in their nineties, even though they have a greater and increasing chance of dying in subsequent years.

DNA
Even if an individual survives to a healthy old age, they die because their bodies simply wear out. Human beings are not, however, actually programmed to die. Ageing and death are, it seems, simply the accidental consequence of errors in cellular DNA. These errors are the result of damage caused by chemical processes and subsequent errors in replication and protein production.

Although the body has repair mechanisms that deal with much

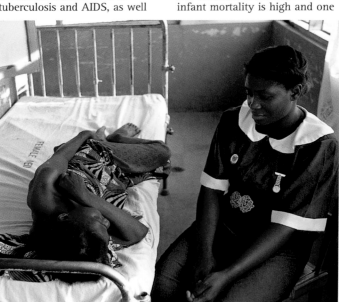

Diseases such as AIDS have adversely affected life expectancy in some parts of the world. In certain sub-Saharan countries, it is now less than 30 years.

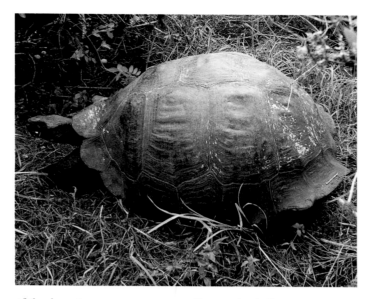

of the damage, some errors persist, with the result that permanent errors gradually accumulate. During the reproductive years, errors normally have no marked effect and thus are not selected against by the evolutionary process. However, as a person ages, the accumulation of DNA errors in genes that would otherwise prolong life expectancy causes these genes to fail, and human beings therefore become more prone to disease and disability.

Humans already live to ages well beyond the point at which they are capable of producing and rearing children. In fact, the maximum lifespan for a human being appears to be about 120 years. The oldest recorded person was Jeanne Calment of France, who was born in 1875 and lived for 120 years and five months. However, this is exceptional; according to at least one researcher, the average human lifespan is unlikely to reach 100 for several centuries to come.

FREE RADICALS
Nevertheless, it is now known that the ageing process can be controlled. Scientists have established that free oxygen radicals (potentially damaging molecules that are introduced into the body through exposure to UV radiation and inhaling pollutants and cigarette smoke) are one of the main causes of ageing. It has been shown that using antioxidant drugs to remove these free radicals can slow down the ageing process. The lifespans of mice have been greatly increased in this way, and the antioxidant drug SCS (synthetic catalytic scavenger) can cause earthworms to live for twice their normal lifespan.

Free oxygen radicals are impossible to avoid. We need

Some animals live to a great age; this Giant Galapagos tortoise can live for over 100 years. The oldest recorded human survived until age 120.

oxygen to survive, and free radicals are created during many of the body's metabolic processes. However, it is possible to reduce their production by the simple expedient of eating less food and thereby, it is presumed, reducing the amount of oxygen consumed. A restricted diet has been shown to dramatically increase the lifespan of monkeys. In addition, certain foods, such as fruit, fresh vegetables, tea, red wine and even chocolate, contain antioxidants that block the action of free oxygen radicals.

MELATONIN
Other research has looked at the effects of melatonin, a hormone that is secreted by the pineal gland in the brain and which has a rejuvenating effect on the body. Some researchers believe

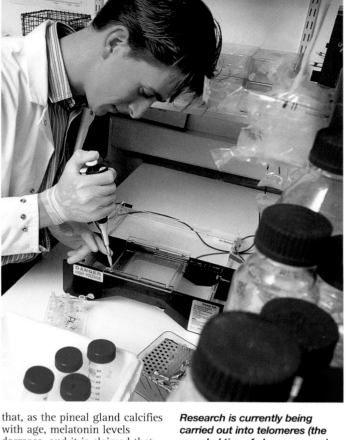

that, as the pineal gland calcifies with age, melatonin levels decrease, and it is claimed that injections of melatonin can provide protection against almost every disease of old age.

TELOMERES
Another line of research is the study of telomeres, the rounded tips of chromosomes. It has been shown that, as cells grow older, telomeres become shorter, until a point is reached at which the chromosomes cannot replicate. Cancer and reproductive cells, on the other hand, have intact telomeres, due to the presence

Research is currently being carried out into telomeres (the rounded tips of chromosomes). Activating telomeres in body cells could prevent cells from ageing.

of the enzyme telomerase. Researchers are looking at ways of activating the telomerase gene in body cells. If this can be achieved, it could prevent cellular ageing, and consequently increase the lifespan of the body.

In time, therefore, the human lifespan may increase. However, even if the ageing process is eventually overcome, true immortality is virtually impossible. Accidents would still happen, after all, and it is estimated that few people would survive longer than about 600 years.

And, even extending average life expectancy by a shorter period – say 50 years – would create new challenges, putting pressure on population levels, housing, and the worlds of work and leisure. Furthermore, in a world in which an increasing proportion of the population would be over 70, social attitudes to old age would have to change dramatically.

Human lifespan is increasing all the time due to improved lifestyle and healthcare. Jeanne Calment (pictured here) survived until she was 120 years old.

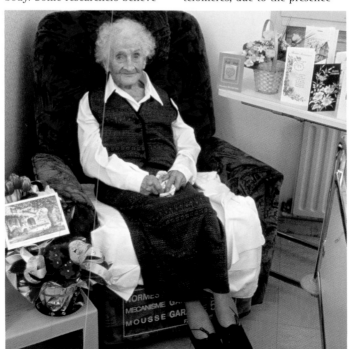

Acute arthritis

Up to a third of all people who attend casualty have acutely painful or swollen joints. This is often symptomatic of arthritis, but other conditions must be excluded before a firm diagnosis can be made.

Arthritis is a common condition that affects one or more joints in the body (monoarthritis or polyarthritis respectively). It is characterized by inflammation, swelling, pain and decreased mobility. There are over 200 causative diseases, including infection, rheumatoid and osteo-arthritis, gout and tuberculosis. A doctor must therefore carry out extensive tests to ascertain the correct diagnosis.

EMERGENCY ASSESSMENT
The most important emergency assessment is to detect or exclude acute joint infection, as untreated bacterial infections are rapidly destructive. The emergency assessment considers:
- Single or multiple joint involvement
- Level of pain
- Generalized illness

- Trauma
- Recent coincident surgery
- Previous history of arthritis
- Co-existent diabetes mellitus
- Diuretics
- Drug abuse/drug related immune suppression
- Genital or gastro-intestinal infection.

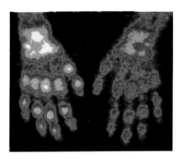

Arthritic joints are seen as the brightest areas on this false-colour gamma camera scan.

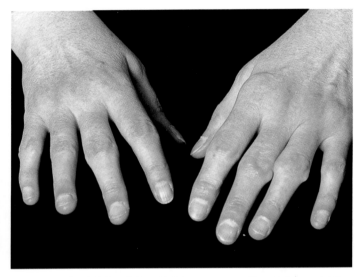

Swollen and painful peripheral joints are suggestive of rheumatoid arthritis. In acute cases, early diagnosis may prevent the disease from progressing.

Common causes of arthritis

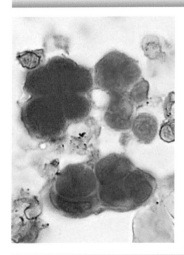

By following the checklist above, the doctor can consider the most common causes of acute arthritis. These include:

■ Infective arthritis
Acute joint infections by skin bacteria, such as *Staphylococcus aureus*, or blood-borne bacteria, such as *Streptococcus*, may occur by spreading from other sites of infection, following dental surgery, for example.

Streptococcus bacteria, here stained purple on a light micrograph, can cause arthritis. Gonorrhoea and meningitis are other known infective causes.

■ Reactive arthritis
When large joints, such as the knees, are acutely involved, the condition may be reactive arthritis following a recent bacterial infection, such as dysenteric food poisoning (caused by *Salmonella* or *Shigella*, for example).

■ Auto-immune rheumatic disorders
Patients develop characteristic abnormalities of immune function leading to damage of 'self' tissue, hence auto-immunity. Systemic lupus erythematosus (SLE) is one of the most clinically challenging

of this group of diseases. If inflammation of peripheral joints, particularly the small joints of the fingers, is predominant and very symmetrical, then rheumatoid arthritis must be excluded.

■ Inflammatory joint disease
Osteo-arthritis is a common cause of joint pain, affecting up to 50 per cent of adults, and may present acutely.

■ Miscellaneous
Some drugs can cause allergic reactions, including arthritic symptoms. Episodes of arthritis may occur in sickle-cell disease.

Metabolic causes of acute arthritis

Historically, one of the most dramatic causes of acute arthritis was gout. Its characteristic symptom is a big toe joint that is excruciatingly painful, red, hot, and untouchable. It is caused by the deposition of uric acid crystals within the soft tissues and the joint. This attracts a marked inflammatory response from the white blood cells involved in clearing these crystals from the tissues.

Gout occurs in approximately two per 1000 of the population, and the incidence of the condition increases with age. Similar arthritic changes to gout occur with calcium pyrophosphate dihydrate (pseudogout) and calcium phosphate crystals.

Other metabolic disorders, such as over- or underactive thyroid glands or overactive pituitary glands, can lead to developmental changes in bones and joints, but these are generally chronic in nature.

When the patient is suffering from bone pain rather than joint pain, Paget's disease a chronic disorder of bone turnover), osteomalacia and rickets (vitamin D deficiency) should be considered.

Excessive uric acid in the body can crystallize in the joints, causing pain, swelling and joint destruction. Treatment for gout involves anti-inflammatory analgesics.

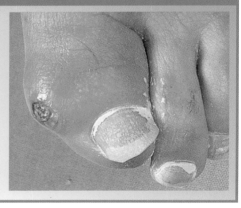

Investigations

Initially, the doctor carries out a full examination to determine the underlying cause of acute arthritis. If necessary, further tests will also be performed.

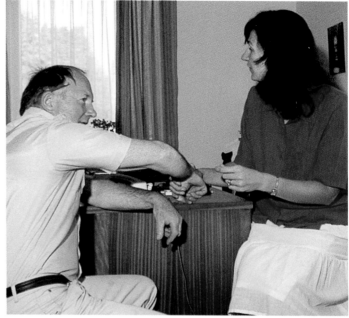

Examining the patient

Initially, the doctor will take a detailed clinical history, paying particular attention to the location and type of pain, the number of joints involved and the speed of the onset of the symptoms. This is because different types of joint disorders have different characteristics.

A full clinical examination then follows. Basic observations of the musculoskeletal system, such as posture, gait and simple movements, will indicate the distribution and occurrence of pain. Specific joints are then examined for:
■ Joint deformity – classified as fixed or reducible: fixed joints cannot normally be aligned during examination; reducible joints can be restored.

■ Range of movement – this is examined passively (the patient demonstrates the movements) and actively (the doctor examines range of movement and sensitivity)
■ Joint effusion – a collection of excess fluid in and around the joint secondary to inflammation may be palpated
■ Tenderness, increased temperature and swelling – these characteristic signs of arthritis are detected by palpation (manual examination).

Finally, the patient's extra-articular systems (skin, heart, lungs, abdomen) are examined for systemic signs and symptoms of disease.

The clinical history and examination allows the doctor to

exclude a number of rheumatic disorders from a provisional diagnosis. Specific tests will then be performed to allow for an accurate diagnosis and an appropriate course of treatment.

Basic observation of the patient's range of movement will inform the doctor about the distribution and severity of the pain. This helps to form the basis of a provisional diagnosis.

Specific investigations

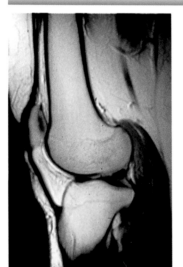

Although magnetic resonance (MR) imaging is not routinely used to diagnose rheumatic disorders, it is helpful for visualizing joint damage.

Laboratory investigations for arthritis include blood tests, joint fluid analysis and X-rays:

Haematology
■ A full blood count will be performed to exclude inflammatory processes, such as a raised white cell count. Other blood disorders may help with a specific diagnosis – normocytic anaemia, for example, can indicate rheumatoid arthritis
■ An erythrocyte sedimentation rate (ESR) test investigates the rate at which red blood cells settle out of suspension. The ESR

increases if levels of specific proteins rise, and may be indicative of rheumatic disease.

Blood chemistry
■ Liver and kidney function tests are carried out to assess the extra-articular complications of rheumatic disorders that may require treatment
■ High levels of uric acid in the blood may indicate gout.

Joint fluid analysis
■ Some changes in joint fluid will be obvious to the naked eye. The fluid is usually transparent and viscous – a thin, cloudy fluid will be symptomatic of an active synovial inflammation, for example
■ Microscopic analysis of joint fluid will also be diagnostic –

mononuclear cells will be high in cases of osteoarthritis, for example.

Immunopathology
■ A rheumatoid factor will be present in the serum of patients suffering from rheumatoid arthritis. A high level indicates an aggressive disease.

Imaging technology
■ Radiography may be used to visualize joint erosion, swelling of soft tissues, sclerosis (tissue hardening) and other rheumatic disorders
■ More rarely, MR imaging, CT scanning and ultrasound may be used to visualize physiological problems stemming from suspected rheumatic disorders.

Non-inflammatory joint disorder

Patients who present with pain but no damaging inflammation of the synovium, and therefore no long-term damage to the joints, are often suffering from a recent viral infection, such as glandular fever, mumps or measles. The recently defined viral infection, parvovirus-B19, is known to cause joint pain, fever, and skin rashes on young children's cheeks.

Although a very small proportion of children suffer from arthritis, parvovirus-B19 appears to be a definite risk-factor for transient

arthritis in adults who have not been exposed to the virus in childhood. Polymyalgia rheumatica, usually affecting people aged over 60, is an acute condition of pain and stiffness affecting the shoulder and the pelvic girdle muscles and is closely related to rheumatoid disease. However, the joints very rarely suffer permanent damage.

Viral infections, such as mumps (pictured), can give rheumatic symptoms, but joint inflammation does not occur.

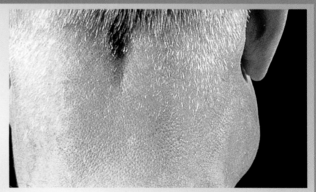

Rheumatoid arthritis

Rheumatoid arthritis is a chronic autoimmune inflammatory disease that affects the joints. The disease is difficult to diagnose and treat, as symptoms typically 'wax and wane' over time.

Rheumatoid arthritis is a common inflammatory condition affecting multiple joints. Estimates suggest that the condition affects one to two people in every 100 people worldwide and that around two to three times as many women are affected by rheumatoid arthritis as men.

MID-LIFE ONSET

Rheumatoid arthritis is a chronic disorder that tends to appear initially between the ages of 30 and 50. Children can develop a similar, but distinct, condition which is known as juvenile rheumatoid arthritis.

Typically, rheumatoid arthritis has an insidious onset: the symptoms of stiff, swollen, painful joints develop slowly over weeks or months. Swelling usually appears first in small joints, such as those of the hands and feet, before progressing to larger joints, such as those of the knees and hips.

Over time, the condition can lead to joint damage and deformities. The number of joints affected by rheumatoid arthritis is variable, but almost always involves more than five.

AUTOIMMUNE DISORDER

Rheumatoid arthritis is an autoimmune disorder, which means that the body fails to recognize its own tissues and produces antibodies to destroy them (autoantibodies). In this case, the synovial membrane (membrane enclosing a movable joint) is affected, resulting in inflammation and damage to joints. The antibodies can also target other body tissues, such as the heart and blood vessels.

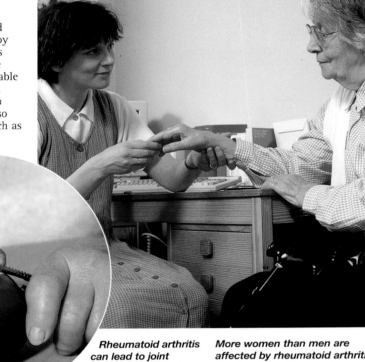

Rheumatoid arthritis can lead to joint damage and deformity. Even day-to-day activities can be severely curtailed.

More women than men are affected by rheumatoid arthritis. The hands and fingers in particular are affected, and become stiff and swollen.

What causes rheumatoid arthritis?

Although the cause of rheumatoid arthritis is currently unknown, the following factors have been implicated in the development of the condition:
■ **Rheumatoid factor**
High levels of an autoantibody in the blood called rheumatoid factor (Rf) occur in 75–80 per cent of affected people at some time during the course of the disease. However, there are other infectious and autoimmune diseases that produce high Rf levels, and so a positive result is not a true and reliable diagnostic indicator
■ **Cytokines**
Chemicals derived from macrophages (cells involved in the body's defence mechanism) and called cytokines (for example TNFalpha, IL-1) seem to be involved in the onset and progress of the chronic inflammatory process within the joints of affected people
■ **Infectious agents**
Many viral infections, such as parvovirus (virus that causes slapped cheek syndrome), rubella (German measles) and HIV, are associated with the development of acute polyarthritis (rheumatic disease affecting a number of the joints). Note that an association with rheumatoid arthritis, rather than a cause, has been shown for many of these infective agents
■ **Genetic susceptibility**
There is an increased incidence

A blood test may be done to measure a person's rheumatoid factor (Rf) levels. High Rf levels are present in most people affected by rheumatoid arthritis.

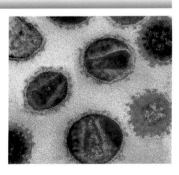

The human immunodeficiency virus (HIV) is seen here under the electron microscope. HIV is one of the viruses associated with acute polyarthritis.

of rheumatoid arthritis in people who have family members with the condition. Studies show that certain population groups are more susceptible than others, as they possess tiny proteins on the surface of some white blood cells, called human leucocyte antigens (HLAs).

Symptoms and complications

The symptoms of rheumatoid arthritis typically 'wax and wane', making it difficult to diagnose and treat. The main features are:
■ Pain on moving
■ Morning stiffness in joints
■ Swelling of the joints.

The joints are usually affected in a symmetrical pattern; thus if the left hand is affected, then so is the right hand.

Other features include fever, weight loss, malaise and fatigue, which can precede or accompany the joint symptoms.

COMPLICATIONS
Although the joints are the main focus of symptoms, other organs can be involved. In such cases, a person can experience clinical features, such as:
■ Nodules – firm, non-tender lumps that occur over pressure areas, such as the elbow, but can also develop on tendon sheaths in the lungs, heart and sclera (the outer covering of the eye)
■ Heart conditions – in about 10 per cent of people, the pericardium (membranous sac that surrounds the heart) becomes inflamed, a condition called pericarditis. Accelerated atherosclerosis (fatty plaques in the lining of the coronary arteries) is also associated with rheumatoid arthritis
■ Eye disease – mild, painless red eye (episcleritis) is common
■ Vasculitis – the most common manifestations of vasculitis are nail-fold infarcts (clots in tiny blood vessels to fingertips)

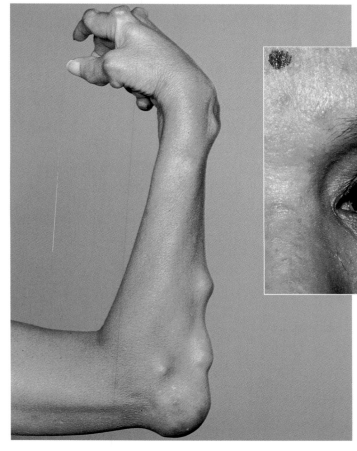

Episcleritis (painless red eye) is a common symptom of rheumatoid arthritis. If it becomes painful (scleritis), it can lead to complications.

Nodules are firm lumps that occur over pressure areas in the body. Nodules are present in about 25 per cent of people with rheumatoid arthritis.

■ Lung disease – fluid in the lungs (pleural effusions) can develop. Fibrosing alveolitis (inflammation of air sacs in the lungs) is a rare complication
■ Neurological complications – a loss of sensation in the lower extremities can occur, along with trapped nerves such as in carpal tunnel syndrome
■ Osteoporosis – increasingly, this is a recognized complication of both the disease and the steroid treatment used to treat it
■ Haematological conditions – the manufacture of red blood cells may be affected, thus causing anaemia. Thrombocytosis (raised platelet levels) may also be a feature
■ Sjogren's syndrome – about 10 per cent of patients develop this inflammatory disorder of the salivary and tear glands.

Identifying factors

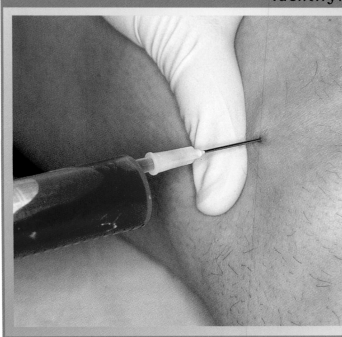

Synovial fluid may be aspirated (withdrawn) from an inflamed joint, in this case the knee. The fluid is then examined for evidence of inflammation.

Doctors will carry out investigations in any patient with joint pain, starting with a thorough review of the patient's medical history. This is followed by a physical examination, looking especially for identifying features, as set out by the American College of Rheumatology in 1987.

Diagnosis
The presence of four or more of the following criteria for at least six weeks indicates a diagnosis of rheumatoid arthritis:
■ Morning stiffness in and around the joints, lasting for at least one hour before maximal improvement

■ Soft-tissue swelling of three or more joint areas, as observed by a physician
■ Swelling of the finger or wrist joint
■ Symmetrical joint swelling
■ Rheumatoid nodules
■ The presence of rheumatoid factor in the blood
■ Erosions (defects in bone) and the loss of bone mass around the hand and wrist joints (osteopenia).

Some of these factors are revealed by X-ray examinations although, initially, X-rays may only highlight soft-tissue swelling or may even fail to show any disease involvement at all.

Doctors may also perform further tests on blood and synovial fluid.

As no single investigation is reliably indicative of a diagnosis of rheumatoid arthritis, doctors have to rely on a combination of the test results.

Managing rheumatoid arthritis

The management of rheumatoid arthritis is dependent on the pattern of disease in the individual. Treatment is typically offered by a multidisciplinary team of healthcare workers.

Rheumatoid arthritis is a chronic disease that necessitates long-term management. Individual treatment options vary, depending on the severity of the disease and the age and health of the affected person.

DISEASE PATTERNS

It is impossible to predict how rheumatoid arthritis will progress in any individual, but there are several common patterns of the disease, constituting what doctors call the 'clinical course'.

In some cases, there is a spontaneous remission within the first six months, particularly in patients without rheumatoid factor. Others may experience recurrent explosive attacks followed by quiet periods – this is known as relapsing and remitting disease. Finally, some patients may have a 'waxing and waning' of persistent and progressive symptoms.

Overall, 25 per cent of patients will remain fit and active, 40 per cent will develop moderate impairment, 25 per cent will become severely disabled and 10 per cent will become wheelchair-bound.

EARLY DIAGNOSIS

To limit potential disability, it is vital that the doctor diagnoses the condition as early as possible before damage has occurred, tries to predict the likely clinical course and then institutes appropriate therapy.

Looking after people with

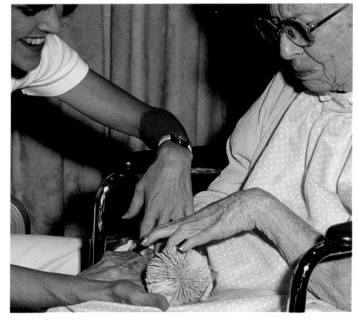

Hand therapy is particularly important in keeping joints flexible. Regular gentle exercise, such as squeezing a ball, helps to prevent stiffness.

Occupational therapists provide aids to simple tasks. This specially designed lever enables the tap to be turned.

rheumatoid arthritis involves many different healthcare professionals. A typical multi-disciplinary team consists of the consultant rheumatologist, surgeon, specialist nurses, physiotherapist, occupational therapist and social worker. Good communication between the patient and healthcare professionals is of paramount importance. Central to this are patient education programmes, which develop patients' knowledge of their disease and its implications.

Relieving joint stress

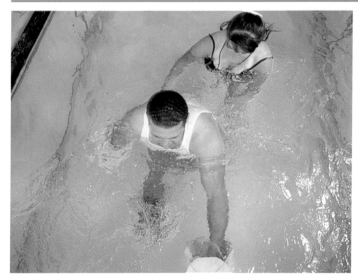

The reduction of joint stress is one of the first lines of therapy.

METHODS

Methods of reducing stress on the joints of an affected person include the following:
■ Maintaining a healthy weight. Being overweight or obese puts stress on what may be already inflamed joints, so losing a few pounds as directed by a doctor may prove very beneficial
■ Taking sufficient rest
■ Taking exercise – this is generally beneficial because it

Hydrotherapy involves exercising in water to improve joint mobility. The supporting effect of the water is beneficial to rheumatoid arthritis patients.

prevents the joints from becoming lax and also stops muscle-wasting. However, anyone with inflamed joints should not participate in vigorous physical activity until the pain and inflammation in the joints has eased, otherwise they risk causing themselves major damage
■ Using aids, such as a walking stick or walking frame
■ Working with physiotherapists and occupational therapists – this type of therapy helps to keep joints mobile and protects against further damage. Occupational therapists are also able to suggest the use of various devices to facilitate the activities of daily life for those with rheumatoid arthritis.

Drug therapies

There are three classes of drugs used to treat rheumatoid arthritis: non-steroidal anti-inflammatories (NSAIDs), corticosteroids and disease-modifying antirheumatic drugs (DMARDs).

NSAIDS

NSAIDs, usually aspirin or ibuprofen, relieve pain, reduce inflammation and prevent joint damage. They are usually used intermittently to quell flare-ups of the condition. They are very effective drugs and have a rapid onset of action. There may,

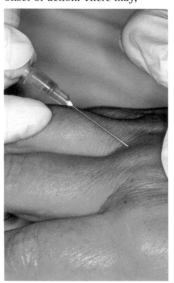

Synthetic corticosteroids can relieve pain and inflammation. Injections of the drug are frequently given directly into the joint itself.

however, be side effects, the most common being gastrointestinal upset. Occasionally, liver and kidney function are also impaired.

DMARDs

DMARDs, such as hydroxychloroquine and sulphasalazine, suppress the immune response, thereby reducing inflammation.

As doctors now know that erosions of the bone and cartilage within a joint can start within the first two years of the illness, medical professionals tend to start patients on a preventative course of one of the faster-acting DMARDs, such as methotrexate, early on in the course of the disease, especially as these drugs can take up to six months to become effective. Serious side effects of methotrexate are uncommon and include nausea, mouth ulcers, liver toxicity and gastrointestinal disturbances.

If symptoms become particularly severe, a patient will be prescribed a more powerful DMARD. These drugs include cytotoxic drugs such as

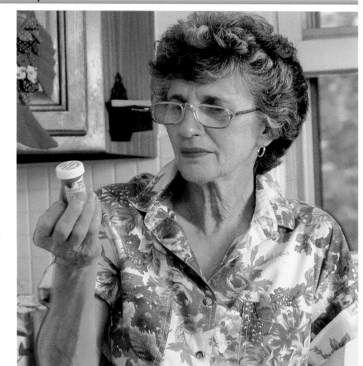

azathioprine, cyclophosphamide and cyclosporin A.

STEROIDS

Corticosteroids, such as prednisolone, have both immunoregulatory and anti-inflammatory actions. Injections of steroids directly into the joint are very effective at controlling

There are three classes of drugs used to treat rheumatoid arthritis. These drugs reduce pain and inflammation, and can prevent further joint damage.

flare-ups. It should be noted that, once started, steroid therapy is difficult to discontinue, even at low doses.

New developments

There have recently been some exciting advances in the understanding of rheumatoid arthritis, and these have led to the development of some new and extremely effective biological therapies.
Perhaps the best known of these new therapies is anti-TNFalpha treatment. TNFalpha, a cytokine, seems to play a central role in causing inflammation and in regulating other cytokines.
The last 10 years, in particular, have seen rapid progress in understanding many of the cytokine abnormalities that cause joint damage in rheumatoid arthritis.

Cytokine blocking
Studies have shown that, by blocking this particular cytokine, joint inflammation and the development of joint erosions can be ameliorated. A total of 100,000 patients worldwide are now taking this therapy.

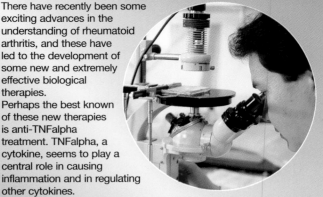

Research into new treatments is ongoing. Recently, scientists have made major advances in developing new biological therapies.

Further research is needed to look at the genetic factors of this disease, as well as to discover what initially triggers the disease and causes flare-ups. When this is known for certain, further progress towards finding a cure can then be made.

Surgery

Despite treatment, some patients will progress to end-stage joint disease and so may require joint replacement surgery.

Surgery can be extremely effective in relieving pain and improving function. Successful hip, knee, elbow, shoulder and knuckle joint replacements are now routine. Prostheses can also be made for younger patients.

SYNOVECTOMY

Synovectomy (the surgical removal of the synovial membrane) is useful in preventing large recurrent

effusions of the knee and tendon rupture at the wrist.

Osteotomy (surgery to cut a bone in two) and arthrodesis (surgical fusion of bones) may ease painful feet; spinal fusion may prevent cervical instability.

Carpal tunnel decompression (surgical release of pressure on median nerve as it passes through wrist) is often required.

The inflamed synovial membrane and tendons of the upper wrist are exposed prior to surgery. Removal of the synovial membrane is often beneficial.

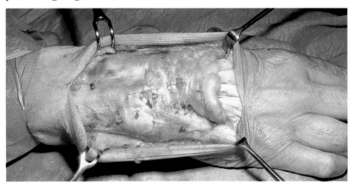

Osteoarthritis

Osteoarthritis is a common degenerative disease of the joints,
in which weakened cartilage exposes bone to direct friction. While
there is no cure, symptomatic treatment may be very effective.

The term osteoarthritis is used to describe joint disease that is characterized by loss of cartilage and signs of localized bony 'reaction'. However, there is no precise definition of osteoarthritis since many people may have evidence of the condition on X-rays and yet experience few or no symptoms, while others may have no X-ray changes but experience marked pain and physical impairment.

Osteoarthritis can affect most of the joints in the body and is the commonest joint disorder – it is estimated that one in seven

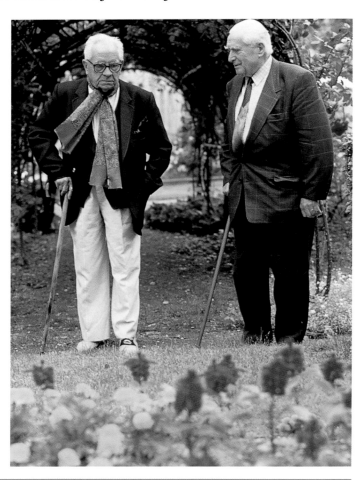

Osteoarthritis is a fact of daily life for many elderly people. Diseased hip joints can mean that even walking to the shops becomes an achievement.

people over 55 years of age have the condition, which is usually associated with ageing.

DEGENERATION
Normally, joints do not wear out unless they have been subjected to trauma or surgery, or are used excessively (as in professional sport). In osteoarthritis, the cartilage, which acts as a buffer between the bones in a joint, degenerates. As the cartilage weakens, it thins and becomes roughened.

DAMAGED BONE
Eventually, the cartilage wears away and the surfaces of the bone become exposed, causing friction and consequent damage.

It is this damage, together with swelling in the soft tissues around the affected joint, that causes pain and disability.

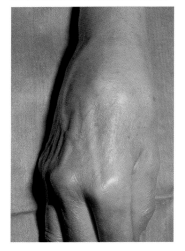

Osteoarthritis in the hand causes swelling, stiffness and pain. Moving the fingers and wrist becomes difficult, making everyday tasks impossible.

What causes osteoarthritis?

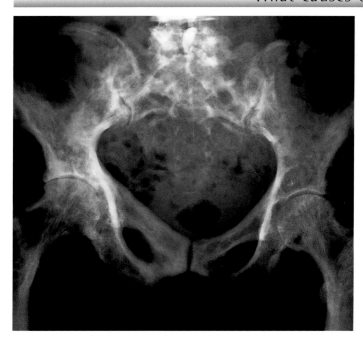

This X-ray shows a mottled appearance in the pelvic bones due to Paget's disease. This bone condition can predispose to osteoarthritis.

The actual cause of osteoarthritis is unclear although there do seem to be several factors that increase the risk of developing the condition. These include the following:

■ Increasing age – people under the age of 40 rarely develop osteoarthritis. It is thought that the condition may therefore simply be the result of natural wear-and-tear, although many physicians deny that this is the case.

■ Gender – osteoarthritis affects more women than men, especially in the knees.

■ Obesity – people who are overweight are more at risk, primarily because there is

increased strain on the weight-bearing joints.

■ Previous injury – a person who has experienced a direct injury to a joint in the past (such as a sporting injury) or who has had joint surgery (such as removal of a cartilage) is at greater risk.

■ Pre-existing musculo-skeletal conditions – disorders such as rheumatoid arthritis, Paget's disease (a non-malignant bone condition) or gout can predispose to osteoarthritis.

■ Occupational hazard – the risk of osteoarthritis developing in later life is increased in people whose occupations involve repetitive movements and abnormal stress on the joints – farming, for example.

■ Family history – a form of the condition called nodal osteoarthritis is known to run in families.

Types of osteoarthritis

Although osteoarthritis can affect almost every joint in the body, those most commonly involved are the hips and knees, hands and big toes.

There are several types of osteoarthritis, which are classified according to the affected joints.

LARGE-JOINT OSTEOARTHRITIS
The term large-joint arthritis is used to describe osteoarthritis in the hips and knees. People affected with large-joint osteoarthritis often experience severe difficulties with mobility, which is greatly reduced. Osteoarthritis of the hip tends to affect one side only, although often the second hip is affected at a later stage. Knee involvement affects more women than men and usually occurs in both legs. This

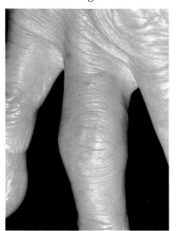

condition frequently results in a typical 'bow-leg' deformity, which can make walking extremely difficult.

NODAL OSTEOARTHRITIS
Nodal osteoarthritis most commonly develops in women, the joint inflammation often becoming obvious around the time of menopause. The condition affects the joints of the hands, which are usually affected one at a time over a long period.

After some years, the inflammation resolves and painless bony swellings, called Heberden's nodes, remain.

Despite these nodules, people with nodal osteoarthritis usually retain adequate movement in their hands and there are rarely long-term problems.

Nodal osteoarthritis is, however, a risk factor for developing osteoarthritis of the knee later in life.

CRYSTAL-ASSOCIATED OSTEOARTHRITIS
Crystal-associated osteoarthritis is so called because the damage to the cartilage is caused by deposits of calcium crystals (chondrocalcinosis) in the cartilage. Crystal-associated osteoarthritis mainly affects the knees and the wrists.

Nodal osteoarthritis affects the hands, causing inflammation. As the swelling recedes, nodules called Heberden's nodes appear on the finger joints.

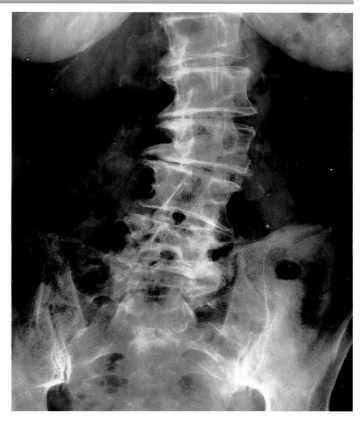

Long, thornlike projections of bone – osteophytes (circled) – can form on the vertebrae in osteoarthritis. These can press on the spinal nerves.

SPONDYLOSIS
Osteoarthritis can affect the cartilaginous discs between the bones of the spine (vertebrae). This condition is known as spondylosis and it can affect any of the vertebrae from the neck downwards. In some cases, bony spurs called osteophytes develop and can press on nerves.

This type of osteoarthritis often causes no symptoms at all until it is far advanced. In fact, X-rays show that the condition is very common in the elderly population.

Tissue degeneration in osteoarthritis

There are several types of joint that allow movement in different planes and directions; however, most of the joints in the body are synovial joints.

Synovial joints
In these joints, the bone surfaces are covered with cartilage that acts as a buffer against constant movement. The whole joint is surrounded by a membrane – the synovial membrane – which secretes fluid that nourishes and lubricates the cartilage. A fibrous capsule surrounds and protects the entire joint, and ligaments and tendons provide stability.

Degeneration
In osteoarthritis, the cartilage begins to degenerate and cracks appear, into which synovial fluid leaks. Plugs of fibrous tissue fill the gaps and if these break away, the bone surface is exposed

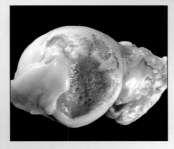

Osteoarthritis has caused severe damage to the head of this femur. The cartilage has completely eroded, exposing diseased bone.

completely. In addition, cysts can develop in the bone marrow, and small spurlike bone projections called osteophytes can form on the bone surface as the bone-producing cells attempt to produce new bone to repair the damage.

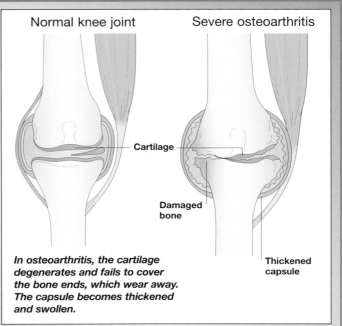

Normal knee joint   Severe osteoarthritis

Cartilage

Damaged bone

Thickened capsule

In osteoarthritis, the cartilage degenerates and fails to cover the bone ends, which wear away. The capsule becomes thickened and swollen.

Symptoms and signs of osteoarthritis

Symptoms develop slowly as osteoarthritis progresses over time. Analgesics, steroid injections, physiotherapy and some complementary therapies can often provide relief.

There is no well-defined set of symptoms in osteoarthritis as each individual has a different experience. Some people are symptom-free, while others have severe pain and immobility.

ONSET OF SYMPTOMS
As the disease progresses very slowly, the symptoms tend to be gradual at first and may not become obvious until years after the damage starts to occur.
Symptoms include:
■ Stiffness and pain in the joint, which becomes worse after using the joint and towards the end of the day
■ Difficulty in moving the affected limb
■ Creaking or grating noises on movement
■ Weakness in the muscles surrounding the joint
■ Swelling in the joint due to an increase in synovial fluid production or osteophyte formation
■ Back pain – the vertebrae and lower back are very often affected. Weakness in a limb can develop if bony overgrowths are pressing on a nerve.

DETERIORATION
Eventually, as symptoms worsen, a few people find that even basic activities, such as getting out of bed in the mornings and walking down stairs, become increasingly difficult and painful. It is at this stage that surgery may be considered.

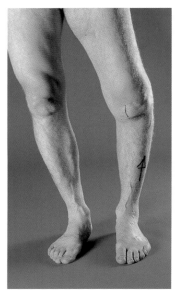

Severe osteoarthritis in the left knee has caused a typical 'bow-leg' appearance. When mobility is badly affected, as here, surgery is the only option.

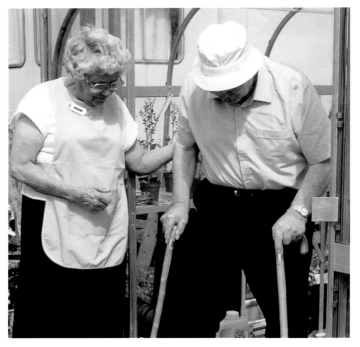

The symptoms of osteoarthritis develop slowly, causing a gradual loss of mobility. Joint stiffness, muscle weakness and pain prohibit movement.

Diagnosing osteoarthritis

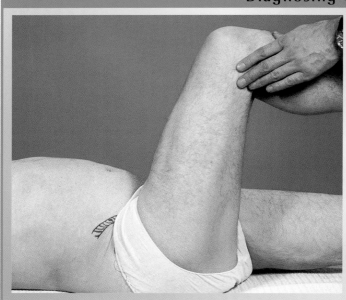

Osteoarthritis can affect many joints within the body. Here the doctor is testing ease of mobility in the hip and knee joints and feeling for fluid.

Most people with osteoarthritis seek help from their doctor when the symptoms of joint pain and stiffness become evident. A physical examination will then reveal which joints are affected and the extent of restricted movement. The doctor will be able to feel fluid collections and may hear creaking in the joint.

Blood tests
There is no specific blood test that can be used to diagnose osteoarthritis. However, the doctor may find it helpful to arrange blood tests that will exclude other disorders with similar symptoms, such as rheumatoid arthritis.

X-rays
X-rays of the affected joint sometimes reveal signs of joint damage, particularly if the disease is advanced. The space between the bones in the joint may appear narrowed and osteophytes or calcium deposits are likely to be visible.

Aspiration
Occasionally, if swelling around the joint is due to excessive production of synovial fluid, the doctor will remove a sample of fluid using a needle and syringe (aspiration). This can then be examined under a microscope for calcium crystals.

Managing osteoarthritis

There is no treatment available to reverse the degenerative processes in osteoarthritis. Instead, the medical team will concentrate on relieving the symptoms of pain and immobility and slowing down the progress of the disease.

Treatment may include:
■ Painkillers – analgesics such as paracetamol can help to relieve discomfort and, as a result, improve mobility. If the joint is inflamed, non-steroidal anti-inflammatories, such as ibuprofen, may help; these are available both as tablets and as creams or gels that can be rubbed

directly into the skin over the affected joint
■ Steroid injections – if the joint is very painful, the doctor may decide to administer a steroid injection directly into the joint itself. In some people, this relieves pain for a few weeks
■ Gentle physiotherapy – this can help to relieve joint stiffness. Exercises to strengthen the muscles surrounding the affected joint can also be helpful
■ Complementary therapies – osteopathy, chiropractic or acupuncture may help.

SURGERY
If all else fails, surgery may be an option. Joint replacements, particularly of the knee and hip, are extremely effective and new techniques are being developed all the time. The two main complications following surgery are infection and loosening of the artificial joint.

In severe osteoarthritis the joint can be replaced with a prosthesis. Here an artificial joint has replaced a diseased knee joint.

Although the risks are slight, it is for these reasons that surgery is carried out only when other treatment has failed to bring the patient relief.

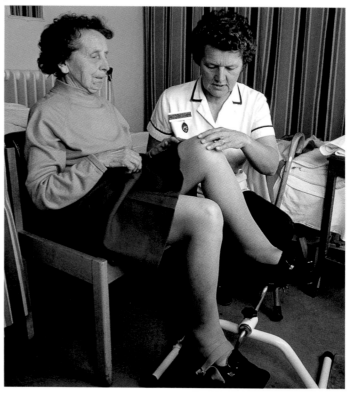

Physiotherapy can achieve good results in the treatment of osteoarthritis. Bicycling exercises can help to release stiffness within the knees.

Self-help measures

Many people with osteoarthritis are concerned about what the future holds, and whether they will become increasingly disabled.

In fact, osteoarthritis rarely spreads to other joints in the body and symptoms tend to be manageable with appropriate treatment. Many people's symptoms actually improve over time. As with any long-term condition, it is important to keep as fit and healthy as possible.

Diet
There is much ongoing research into possible links between diet and osteoarthritis, although there is currently no hard evidence that nutritional therapy has a positive effect. Some individuals, however, may find they benefit from adapting their diets or avoiding particular foods.

It is vital is to avoid putting on excess weight, as this can place added strain on the weight-bearing joints and increase the severity of the condition.

Exercise
People with osteoarthritis may be loathe to exercise, either because of anxiety about causing further

damage or because the exercise brings on the pain. Individuals should attempt to achieve a balance between complete rest and over-exercising. Experts advise a 'little and often' approach, so that joints are

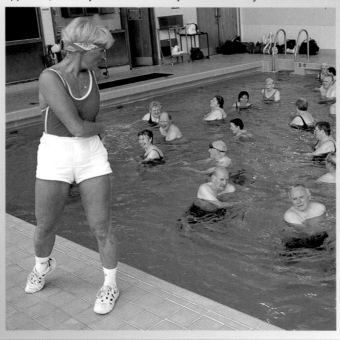

exercised in short bursts, but not for long enough to cause pain.

Swimming is an ideal activity because the water supports the body while the actions exercise the joints. People with severe joint disease may be advised

to have treatment in a hydrotherapy pool.

Strengthening the muscles around the joints is also vital; physiotherapists can provide advice about a suitable exercise regimen. For example, patients with an affected knee will be advised to build up the quadriceps muscles in the thigh.

Pain-relieving measures
As well as conventional painkilling drugs, many people with osteoarthritis apply localized heat to the joints, using an electric heat pad or a hot water bottle. Some pain-relieving creams work by causing a burning sensation in the skin. If a joint is inflamed, an ice pack may help.

Aids in the home
Many people find that even the most straightforward of practical tasks may become difficult, and aids such as jar-openers and bath seats can make life easier.

Swimming eases stiffness and pain. It is a gentle exercise, ideally suited to people with osteoarthritis, as the water supports the body's weight.

Osteoporosis

Osteoporosis is the most common metabolic bone disease.
It is associated with ageing, and affects women more than men,
especially after the time of the menopause.

Osteoporosis is caused by a generalized loss of bone from the skeleton, which is a natural part of the ageing process. The condition can be especially severe in post-menopausal women due to loss of the hormone oestrogen (manufactured within the ovaries), which helps maintain bone mass.

The skeleton, like all in body tissues, is a living structure. There is a continuous process of new bone forming and old bone being removed throughout life. The skeleton is at its strongest (peak bone mass) at the age of 30–35 years. After this time, there is a gradual decline in the amount of bone in the skeleton; that is, more material is removed than is replaced.

BONE STRUCTURE

Bone consists of a mixture of proteins, such as collagen, and inorganic minerals, predominantly calcium salts. About 40 per cent of bone is protein and 60 per cent is calcium salts. In osteoporosis, there is still the same mixture of protein and calcium salts, there is just less of it. With less bone in the skeleton, fractures occur more easily.

CLASSIFYING OSTEOPOROSIS

There are a number of types of osteoporosis:
■ Primary idiopathic

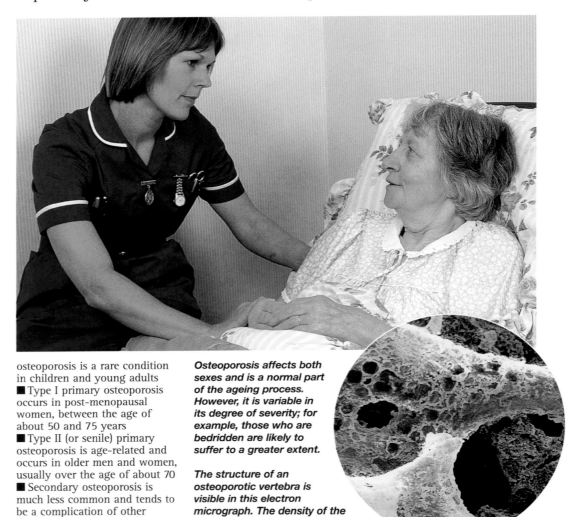

osteoporosis is a rare condition in children and young adults
■ Type I primary osteoporosis occurs in post-menopausal women, between the age of about 50 and 75 years
■ Type II (or senile) primary osteoporosis is age-related and occurs in older men and women, usually over the age of about 70
■ Secondary osteoporosis is much less common and tends to be a complication of other diseases or due to the effect of certain drugs.

Osteoporosis affects both sexes and is a normal part of the ageing process. However, it is variable in its degree of severity; for example, those who are bedridden are likely to suffer to a greater extent.

The structure of an osteoporotic vertebra is visible in this electron micrograph. The density of the cancellous (spongy) tissue within the bone is greatly reduced.

Clinical features

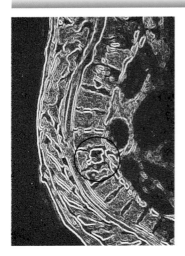

The commonest clinical feature of osteoporosis is a progressive loss of height occuring with age. This is a direct result of vertebral compression within the spine. During this process, the individual vertebral bodies begin to crumble, allowing the intervertebral discs, which lie between them, to protrude into what was previously hard bone.

If vertebral collapse occurs suddenly, or if compression is uneven, the patient may experience severe localized pain in the affected region, often the lower thoracic or lumbar spine. Often, deformities will develop. These include scoliosis, sideways deviation of the spine, and kyphosis, excessive outward curvature of the back, leading to a 'hunched' appearance.

People with osteoporosis are also more likely to suffer fractures of the wrist and hip.

This MR scan shows a sagittal section through the spine of an osteoporosis sufferer. One of the vertebrae (circled) has crumbled, painfully compressing nerves.

Kyphosis associated with osteoporosis can lead to severe deformity of the spine. The hunched back is sometimes referred to as a 'widow's hump'.

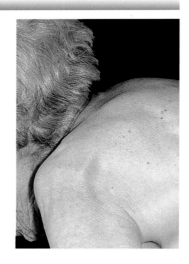

Causes of osteoporosis

Some degree of osteoporosis occurs in everyone after the age of 30. However, various types of the disorder occur under different circumstances.

In the general population, 20 per cent of women and 8 per cent of men are affected by osteoporosis of some kind.

Ninety-five per cent of cases are primary osteoporosis, which itself is subdivided into idiopathic (arising spontaneously), Type I and Type II – post-menopausal and age-related osteoporosis respectively. It is not known why the primary form of the condition arises, but various factors have been implicated which seem to predispose certain groups of people (see box below).

SECONDARY OSTEOPOROSIS
Secondary osteoporosis, which is much rarer and accounts for only five per cent of cases, may be due to one of a number of causes. These include the effect of drugs such as steroids on the bone formation process. It may also arise from the effect of hormones on the skeleton, as

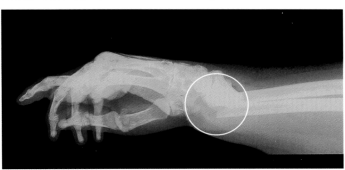

Hormone replacement therapy serves to replace oestrogen lost at the menopause. If HRT is not started at this time, osteoporosis is more likely to occur.

seen in endocrine diseases such as hyperthyroidism (when the thyroid gland is overproductive) and Cushing's syndrome.

If the skeleton is not used for long periods, as is the case with people who are immobilized during prolonged bed rest, then bone loss is accelerated. This even occurs in people who are healthy and otherwise not at risk from osteoporosis. Exercise is thus vitally important for maintaining healthy bones.

Osteoporosis is often present in people with other diseases affecting the bones, such as the disorder rheumatoid arthritis.

Risk factors

Although no specific causes are known for primary osteoporosis, a number of significant risk factors have been identified. These include:
- Being female
- Increased age
- Early menopause
- Amenorrhoea – lack or cessation of menstrual periods
- Lack of hormone replacement therapy in menopausal and post-menopausal women
- Being underweight
- Lack of physical exercise, especially when young
- Being Caucasian – people of African and Afro-Caribbean origin have a greater skeletal mass and therefore suffer less from osteoporosis than Caucasian and Asian people
- Cigarette smoking
- Pre-existing family history of osteoporosis (genetic factors)
- Alcoholism
- Long-term steroid use
- Rheumatoid arthritis.

Osteoporotic fractures

Osteoporosis on its own is asymptomatic (showing no symptoms of disease), and a person may well be affected without being at all aware of the presence of the condition. Symptoms develop only when the skeleton has been weakened enough to fracture. Although any bone can fracture after a fall, the most common osteoporotic fractures occur at the wrist (Colles' fracture), hip and spine. Other factors play a part in these fractures, such as general unsteadiness and a greater tendency to fall with increasing age.

VERTEBRAL COLLAPSE
Osteoporotic spinal fractures tend to result in chronic back pain, deformity of the spine (known as widow's or dowager's hump) and a loss of height.

The most common sites for fractures are the lumbar and thoracic vertebrae.

IMPLICATIONS OF FRACTURES
In the UK, some 60,000 hip, 50,000 wrist and 40,000 spinal fractures occur each year, the majority of them in elderly people. Hip and wrist fractures result in acute pain and deformity after the injury, and hip fractures are a major cause of disability.

It has been estimated that the overall cost to the National Health Service each year of osteoporotic fractures could be as much as £950 million, with a single hip fracture in one patient estimated as costing about £12,000. Therefore, if the numbers of fractures could be reduced, not only would this be beneficial for the health and welfare of elderly people in general, but it would also represent a significant cost saving to the NHS.

A Colles' fracture – when the radius and ulna of the forearm fracture (circled) – is common in osteoporosis. The increased brittleness of the bones makes them more likely to break under pressure.

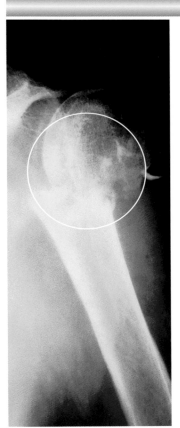

This coloured X-ray shows a fractured humerus in the shoulder of a patient with osteoporosis. The head of the humerus (circled) has broken away from the shaft and become dislocated to the right.

Diagnosing and treating osteoporosis

The earlier osteoporosis is diagnosed, the easier it is to treat.
Imaging techniques help to identify patients who are most at risk,
and various measures can be taken to manage the condition.

DIAGNOSING BONE LOSS

A clinical diagnosis of osteoporosis can be made only when the mineral density of bone is measured and is found to be reduced. Blood tests are not useful for diagnosis, as blood levels of calcium and phosphate both remain normal in osteoporosis.

X-RAY

Normal bone is a hard, dense structure that is clearly seen on X-ray. Because in osteoporosis there is less bone overall, there will also be less mineral contained within it; it is therefore less dense and will appear darker on an X-ray.

However, it is important to realize that approximately 25 per cent of the bone mineral has to be lost before X-rays become abnormal; it is therefore possible to for a patient to have osteoporosis and yet still have a normal X-ray.

SCANNING

Dual photon densitometry (also called dual energy X-ray absorptiometry, or DEXA) is an imaging technique used to measure the mineral density of bone. With a narrow beam of radiation, densitometry takes scans in 'slices' through critical areas of bone mass, such as the lumbar vertebrae or head of the

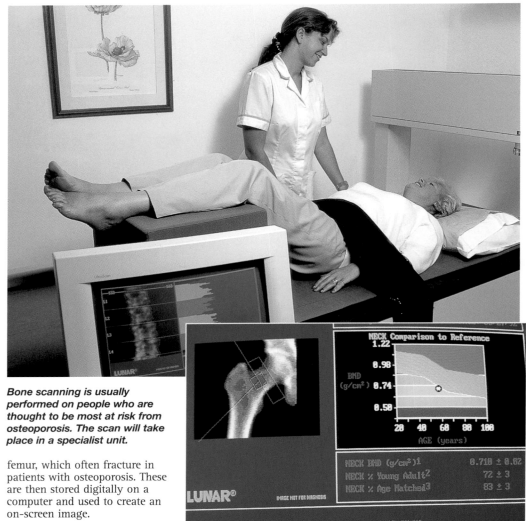

Bone scanning is usually performed on people who are thought to be most at risk from osteoporosis. The scan will take place in a specialist unit.

femur, which often fracture in patients with osteoporosis. These are then stored digitally on a computer and used to create an on-screen image.

BONE DENSITY

With densitometry, bone density is expressed as a value relating to standard reference data, so that a comparison can be made between each patient's score and the norm. Bone is defined as osteoporotic when its density is less than 0.8 g/cm². There is a

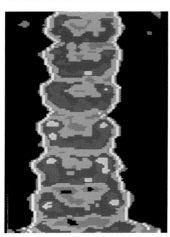

False-colour dual photon densitometry scan of part of the spine of a woman with mild osteoporosis. Bone mineral density varies from red (most dense) through yellow and blue to green (least dense).

margin of error of one per cent for the spine and two to three per cent for the neck of the femur (thighbone).

In the scan shown above, the area of bone scanned has a value of 0.71 g/cm². This value is 72 per cent of that of an average young adult and 83 per cent of the average for the patient's age. The graph shows the average age at which bone density has fallen to the level observed in this patient.

One of the major advantages of DEXA scanning is that it uses

This computer screen shows the result of a dual photon bone densitometry scan of the hip joint. The image on the left shows the direction of the scan through the neck of the femur.

very low doses of radiation. It is extremely useful for screening, so that treatment can be prioritized for those who need it most. In general, only those patients who are at risk from primary or secondary osteoporosis will be offered DEXA scanning.

Prevention

Once osteoporosis is established, it cannot be reversed, and so prevention is preferable. The aim of treatment is to diagnose early, before any fractures occur.

■ Remove possible cause

Stopping smoking is important; not only will this reduce the risks of developing osteoporosis, it will also have beneficial effects on general health. If possible, drugs that cause osteoporosis should also be stopped, in consultation with the doctors who have prescribed the drug. Associated conditions should be treated.

■ Exercise

Exercise is important both in childhood and adulthood. Exercise in childhood will increase the amount of calcium in the growing skeleton and this will have a lasting beneficial effect throughout life. In adulthood, exercise should continue to maintain as much

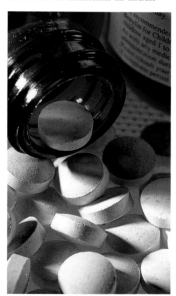

calcium in the skeleton; exercise is also of benefit to the cardiovascular system.

■ Diet

The National Osteoporosis Society has recommended the following daily intakes of calcium:

Young adults and women on HRT: 1000 mg

Pregnant women and breast-feeding mothers: 1500 mg

Men over 65: 1500 mg

Post-menopausal women NOT on HRT: 1500 mg

As well as an adequate intake of calcium, it is also important to reduce caffeine intake and moderate alcohol intake.

■ Hormone replacement therapy (HRT)

HRT is recommended to most women at the time of the menopause. HRT can be given as tablets or as patches and may be taken continuously or over 21 days followed by a seven-day break when there will be a menstrual period.

As well as protecting the skeleton from osteoporosis, HRT also protects against heart disease. The main disadvantage of being on HRT may be the return of monthly periods. Also, women on HRT are at increased risk of developing a deep vein thrombosis (DVT), and there may

An increased intake of calcium has been shown to be beneficial in reducing the effects of osteoporosis. They will often be subscribed in conjunction with other drugs.

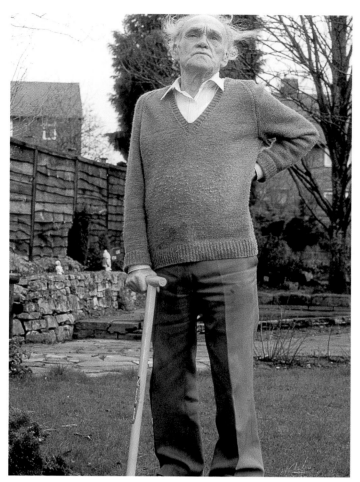

be a very small increase in the risk breast cancer.

Certain women should not take HRT. Pre-menopausal women, women with breast or uterine cancer, a history of a stroke or DVT, and women with severe cardiac, liver or renal disease should not take HRT. Currently, it is recommended that HRT is taken for 5–10 years.

■ Other drugs

Bisphosphonates (etidronate and alendronate) are drugs that act directly on bone to reduce the amount of calcium being

Backache is a frequent problem for patients who have symptomatic osteoporosis. Elderly men in particular should seek medical help before the problem worsens.

absorbed out of the skeleton. They are useful to prevent osteoporosis in elderly men and in women who are unable to take HRT, and can also be used to treat osteoporosis once it has resulted in a fracture. Generally, these drugs need to be taken for some years and are often given with calcium supplements.

Treating fractures

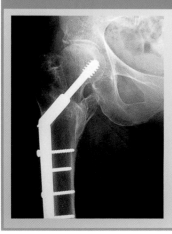

The treatment of osteoporotic fractures depends on the site of the fracture. Although any fracture may occur, the following are the most common:

■ Wrist fractures (Colles' fractures) are treated in a below elbow plaster of Paris cast. If the fracture is displaced, it may need to be manipulated into a better position under local anaesthetic. The cast is worn for about a

A hip fracture may be repaired by the 'pin and plate' method. This involves strengthening the femur with metal fittings.

month. Once the cast is off, the wrist and hand may be stiff and physiotherapy is recommended.

■ A hip fracture can occur after a very minor fall, often no more than a stumble. The fracture can occur at two sites and these are treated in a different way. It may be treated with a hemiarthroplasty or with a 'pin and plate'. Both forms of treatment require an operation.

■ Fractures of the spine are more difficult to treat. The aim of treatment is to provide pain relief; occasionally the spine may need to be supported with a brace. Surgery is not usually required.

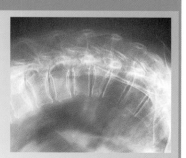

Compression fractures of the spine are a major cause of pain and disability in osteoporosis. Little can be done surgically, but medical treatment is very useful.

Paget's disease

Paget's disease (osteitis deformans) is a bone disorder that occurs in middle-aged and elderly people. The normal process of bone renewal becomes disrupted leading to weak, deformed bones.

Healthy bones undergo a constant process of renewal; old bone is continually broken down and replaced. In Paget's disease, this normal turnover of bone becomes excessive in one or more areas of the skeleton.

The structure of the new bone is disorganized, with the affected areas of bone becoming thickened, yet weak and more likely to fracture.

OCCURRENCE

Paget's disease is a condition of middle to old age and is very uncommon in young adults. The condition affects three to four per cent of people aged over 40 years in the UK, this figure increasing to 10 per cent by the age of 85 years.

For reasons that are unknown, the condition is most common in Europe, particularly the north of England; it is relatively rare in Africa and Asia.

AFFECTED BONES

Paget's disease can develop in any bone, including the femur (thigh bone), tibia (shin bone), scapula (shoulder blade), and skull, but it most commonly affects the bones of the pelvis and spinal column. Paget's disease of the small bones in the hands and feet is rare.

POSSIBLE CAUSES

The cause of Paget's disease is not yet understood, but there are several possible underlying reasons for the condition:

■ **Genetic component**
The marked geographical distribution of the disease and the fact that it can run in families suggests that there is a genetic component involved in its development.

■ **Viral infection**
Some evidence has implicated the involvement of a viral infection, possibly canine distemper virus or measles. It is thought that the so-called slow-virus may be contracted early in life and cause Paget's disease to develop many years later.

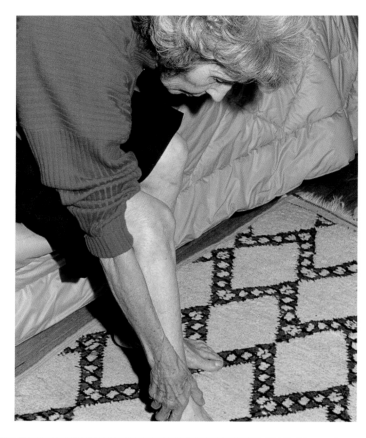

Paget's disease causes weakened and sometimes painful bones. Any bone in the body can be affected, including the tibia (shin bone).

Symptoms and complications of Paget's disease

Many people with Paget's disease have no symptoms. Indeed, patients are often diagnosed with the condition only after it is discovered on an X-ray that has been taken to investigate another disorder. In other people, the disease will become apparent following a bone fracture.

COMMON SYMPTOMS

The most common symptom of Paget's disease is pain, which may be localized to the affected area of bone or felt in a nearby joint, especially if osteoarthritis (arthritis caused by wear and tear on the joints) has also developed in the joint.

Affected bones can become deformed – for example, there may be curvature of the spine.

OTHER COMPLICATIONS

In some areas of the body, the overgrowth of bone may lead to pressure on adjacent nerves. If the skull becomes enlarged, hearing impairment may develop as a result of pressure on the nerves supplying the ear.

If the vertebrae of the spine are affected, compression of the spinal cord may occur.

The blood flow through an affected bone may be increased, sometimes causing the skin overlying it to feel warm.

Elderly people with severe Paget's disease may develop heart failure, the symptoms of which include shortness of breath. This is a rare complication, which occurs if the heart struggles to maintain the increased blood flow to the affected areas of bone.

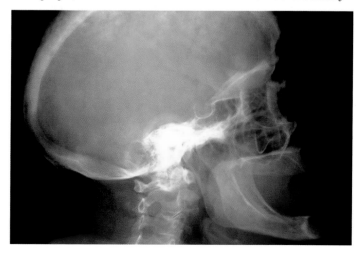

The X-ray shows the skull of a person with Paget's disease. Thickened bone (outer edge of white) can press on the nerve that supplies the inner ear.

As a result of Paget's disease, limbs can become deformed and bowed. This is particularly noticeable in the weight-bearing bones, such as the tibia.

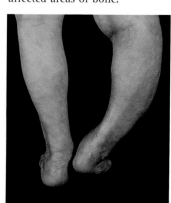

Diagnosing Paget's disease

The diagnosis of Paget's disease is often clear from a physical examination. An X-ray may be arranged to confirm the diagnosis and look for evidence of osteoarthritis in nearby joints.

BLOOD TESTS
Blood tests may be undertaken to measure alkaline phosphatase, an enzyme in the blood that indicates bone formation and which is markedly raised in Paget's disease.

BONE SCANS
An isotope bone scan may be recommended to assess the extent of the disease. Prior to the scan, a tiny amount of radioisotope is injected intravenously. This radioactive substance is absorbed by the bones, which are then clearly visible when the skeleton is scanned. Areas of bone affected by Paget's disease absorb the radioisotope to a much greater extent than normal bone.

Paget's disease can often be identified on X-rays. Affected areas will show characteristic thickening of bone tissue.

This bone scan shows bone mineral density in a patient with Paget's disease. The blue, green, yellow and red areas indicate increasing density.

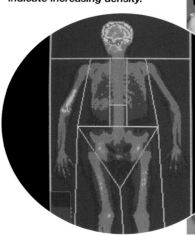

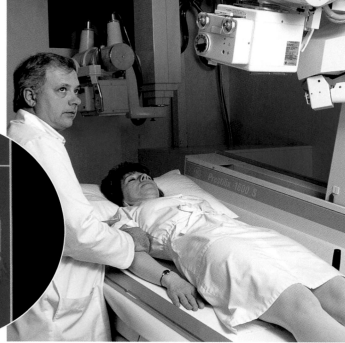

Treatment for Paget's disease

For many people with Paget's disease, simple painkillers or non-steroidal anti-inflammatory drugs are the only treatment that is needed.

SPECIFIC MEDICATION
In patients with persistent pain despite taking these medications and in those with problems related to the disease, such as deformity or nerve compression, medication that targets the disease itself may be appropriate.

This medication may also be recommended to younger people to delay its progression.

Although the drug treatments

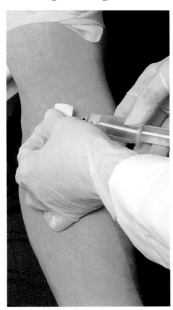

act primarily to prevent the breakdown of bone, this effect is also accompanied by a reduction in the deposition of new bone.

DRUG TREATMENTS
Drug therapies include:

■ **Biphosphonates**
These drugs are usually prescribed for up to six months and can reduce the excessive bone turnover that occurs in Paget's disease. Some are given orally; others must be given as a course of injections.

The effect of these medications may continue for some time after the end of treatment, in some cases for several years.

■ **Calcitonin**
Calcitonin is produced naturally in the body by the thyroid gland in the neck. It may be prescribed to reduce the excessive bone turnover and pain of Paget's disease. The treatment is given as a course of injections, lasting for up to three months.

The injections may be associated with nausea, and anti-nausea treatment may be prescribed if this occurs. Other possible side effects include facial flushing and diarrhoea.

Blood tests can be repeated at intervals to monitor the progress of the disease. These tests can also assess the response once treatment has been started.

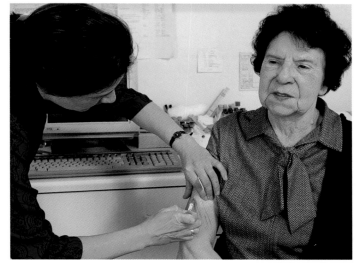

PHOSPHATASE LEVELS
In patients on drug treatment, alkaline phosphatase levels may be checked every few months. The aim of treatment is to bring these levels back to normal.

Patients with Paget's disease may receive calcitonin hormone injections to treat the condition. This synthetic form of calcitonin is used to relieve pain and reduces bone turnover.

Surgery

Surgery may be required to replace joints, such as hips or knees, that have been severely damaged by osteoarthritis.

Bone fractures
Bone fractures may also require surgery. Many people with Paget's disease who sustain fractures are elderly. In these people, bone healing may be prolonged, and doctors may decide to fix the fractures with internal pinning.

Prior drug treatment
Drugs may be required prior to surgery to reduce the activity of the disease, so reducing the blood flow in the affected area and the risk of excessive bleeding during the operation.

Post-operative hip and knee therapy

Procedures to replace damaged hip and knee joints
have major benefits for patients in terms of mobility and alleviation of pain.
Post-operative physiotherapy is vital in maximizing these benefits.

The first total hip replacements (THRs) were carried out in the 1950s, but most failed due to the lack of suitable materials and a secure method of fixation. However, in 1961, Sir John Charnley made a breakthrough with 'low friction arthroplasty', or joint replacement, combining a high-density polyethylene socket with a metal stem component (often stainless steel). With the addition of an acrylic cement to fix the stem part of the thigh component, total hip replacement became a successful and reliable procedure.

STRUCTURE
The hip is a ball-and-socket joint that combines free movement with stability for weight-bearing. Since the introduction of THR, there have been many different types and designs of components, but the 'Charnley' hip is still favoured for routine hip replacement in the elderly. For people with poor bone quality, the components are generally cemented into place.

An uncemented THR is an option for younger people, and there are two main types: a 'press-fit', which relies on bone to maintain a tight fit, and 'porous-coated', which has a small opening on the surface of the component, which encourages the growth of bone into the replacement.

PHYSIOTHERAPY
Before surgery, the patient will be evaluated by physiotherapists. Muscle strength and limb flexibility will be monitored, and a series of exercises and procedures will be demonstrated so that the patient is familiar with post-operative care. With both hip and knee replacements, it is important that the patient does not overstress the new joint, since this can lead to dislocation or damage, with obvious consequences to successful rehabilitation.

Pain is often a limiting factor to good recovery, so the patient

Muscle groups affected in a hip replacement

Depending on the surgical technique used, some muscles surrounding the prosthetic hip may be detached from and reattached to bone during the operation. The physiotherapist will also work on particular muscle groups to strengthen the joint post-operatively.

Gluteus maximus
The biggest muscle in the body; it is responsible for extending and rotating the hip joint away from the middle of the body

Sartorius
Flexes leg at knee joint and thigh at hip joint

Ball-and-socket joint of hip
Head of the femur (ball) fits into acetabulum (socket) of pelvic bone

Tensor fasciae latae
Extends the knee joint and steadies the trunk; it also rotates the hip joint away from the middle of the body

Rectus femoris
Extends the leg at the knee joint and flexes the thigh at the hip joint

Iliotibal tract
This muscle extends beyond the knee joint; its main function is to brace the knee, preventing the joint buckling when the other foot is raised during walking

will be taught breathing exercises and pain control as part of their post-operative care. Exercise is also a vital part of physiotherapy, because it promotes circulation and 'warms up' muscles. This is specially important before

The hip-joint socket, made of durable plastic, will accommodate the stainless steel 'ball' that has been set into the femur bone with cement.

commencing more vigorous exercises. This entire process is tailored to suit the individual needs of the patient, and the physiotherapist will often develop a close working relationship with each person, helping them to overcome their fear and pain.

Exercises help the patient to adapt to their new joint, and they may well have to relearn basic mobility skills. Simple, 'unconscious'

movements – such as getting out of bed or dressing – will also have to be considered. Ultimately, these considerations become second nature, and patients usually adapt well to their new mobility.

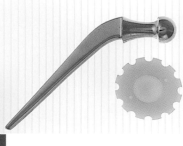

The relatively simple design of the prosthetic hip gives patients the chance of a pain-free, mobile joint, and has made a huge impact on orthopaedic surgery.

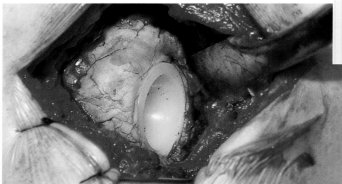

Hip replacement surgery

An incision is made at the side of the hip through the skin and muscle, exposing the entire joint. The hip joint is then dislocated and the 'ball' part – the top of the femur (thigh bone) – is removed. The socket area is deepened and shaped to afford a good fit for the new component. The new, metal thigh component replacing the worn 'ball' is positioned into place.

Depending on the type of replacement, these parts may be fixed in with cement. The joint is now put back into place and tested to ensure it is stable yet mobile, and the wound is closed over.

During the operation, the gluteus maximus muscle –

Joints that are frequently used or are weight-bearing, such as the hip, are more likely to degenerate over time. The hip is also susceptible to osteoarthritis, the incidence of which increases with age.

which rotates and extends the hip joint – is exposed. The fibres must be separated without damaging the associated nerve fibres and the underlying sciatic nerve – the major nerve of the leg. The origins of the muscles surrounding the socket may have to be detached during the operation, and the tendon connecting the gluteus maximus to the femur may be partially released.

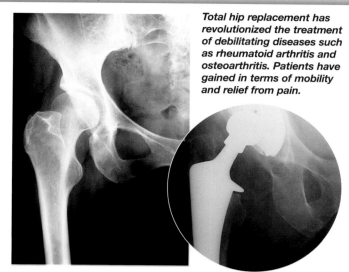

Total hip replacement has revolutionized the treatment of debilitating diseases such as rheumatoid arthritis and osteoarthritis. Patients have gained in terms of mobility and relief from pain.

Muscle groups affected in a knee replacement

Pain is usually a major limiting factor following knee replacement. Exercises to strengthen the gluteus and quadriceps muscles are begun soon after surgery. It may be necessary to completely immobilize the knee for a short period.

Rectus femoris muscle

Vastus medialis muscle

Vastus lateralis muscle

These muscles extend the leg at the knee joint; they represent three of the four muscles of the quadriceps

Position of prosthesis attached to femur

Patella
The knee-cap

Position of prosthesis attached to tibia

Patellar ligament
Joins the patella to the tibia – the larger of the two bones of the lower leg

Gastrocnemius muscle
Flexes both the ankle and the knee joints

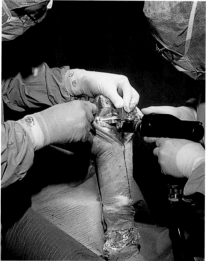

Surgeons use a hand-held power-saw to reshape sections of bone during knee replacement surgery. This will allow for the insertion of the prosthetic joint.

Knee replacement surgery

The surgeon makes an incision down the middle of the front of the knee. Depending on the type of deformity of the knee, the surgeon will release the tightened tissues and remove the ligaments that cross the inside of the knee joint (the posterior cruciate ligament is often retained if it is still viable) because they are not necessary for the function of a correctly aligned prosthetic joint.

Once the tissues are balanced, surgeons use a hand-held power-saw to remove the diseased area and reshape the

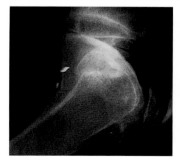

In this X-ray, severe degenerative changes in the structure of the knee can be observed.

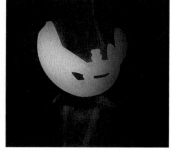

A prosthetic knee-joint is clearly visible in this X-ray. It is used when osteonecrosis (bone death) has eroded the natural joint.

surfaces ready for the new joint. The surgeons will aim to equalize the gap in the knee joint, so that the gap will be retained whether the knee is bent or straight.

The femoral and tibial components are inserted and their alignments checked, and the knee-cap is sometimes resurfaced using a polyethylene component. Once the wound is thoroughly cleansed and closed, a soft compression dressing is applied. The patient will be hospitalized for 10–14 days.

Physiotherapy after joint replacement

The role physiotherapy plays after joint replacement is vital. Without such rehabilitation, the patient cannot fully benefit from surgery. Physiotherapists also educate patients about how to avoid overstressing the artificial joint.

After surgery, the average length of stay as an in-patient is 7–14 days. A pre-operative medical assessment will have taken place at the orthopaedic clinic, and most units offer the prospective patient the chance to come to an informal meeting, which will give them the opportunity to discuss their hospital stay, the surgery and their rehabilitation.

The sessions are generally led by physiotherapists, nurses and occupational therapists. As well as giving the patient the chance to allay any fears about the operation, these sesssions also give the medical team time to prepare for that patient's individual needs, so that their hospital stay runs smoothly from admission to discharge.

POST-OPERATIVE EXERCISE

Following surgery, physiotherapy will aim to help the patient gain muscular control of the joint and to get them back on their feet as soon, and as independently, as possible. It is important to keep moving while in bed to aid circulation and to prevent pressure sores.

Specific knee exercises will be taught after total knee replacement on the first post-operative day, in order to regain control and strength in the thigh (quadriceps) muscle, which will help to both straighten the knee and prepare it for bearing weight. With osteoarthritis, the muscles around the knee often become very weak, and post-operatively the contraction of these muscles can become inhibited – due to swelling, pain and fear – so early exercise to overcome this is essential.

Generally, knee movement exercises are started on the second day after surgery, aiming to achieve 90° of flexion (bend) at the joint. This amount of movement in the knee is necessary to be able to perform most activities of daily life comfortably.

First days after surgery

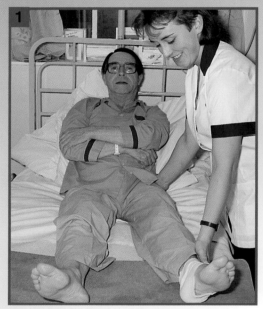

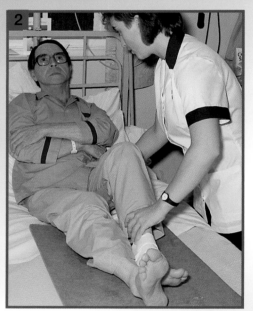

1 After surgery, it is important to maintain full range of movement of the knee joint as early as possible. The physiotherapist may begin exercises as early as the first day after surgery.

2 General bed exercises to strengthen the leg include moving the leg up and to the side to strengthen thigh muscles and the knee. Moving and massaging the feet also aids circulation.

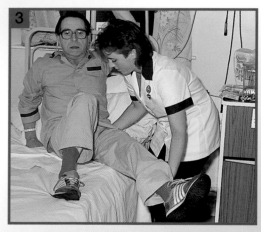

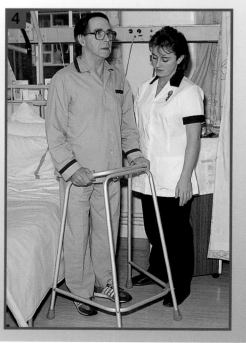

3 The patient is usually prepared for walking three days after surgery. Here, the physiotherapist assists the patient in getting out of bed.

4 The patient is now upright, and needs to support his leg while walking with a frame or elbow crutches. The physiotherapist advises on posture and weight bearing.

Stair climbing after joint replacement

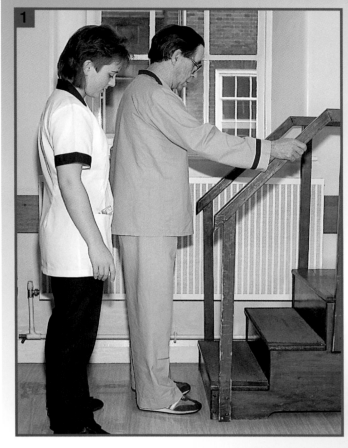

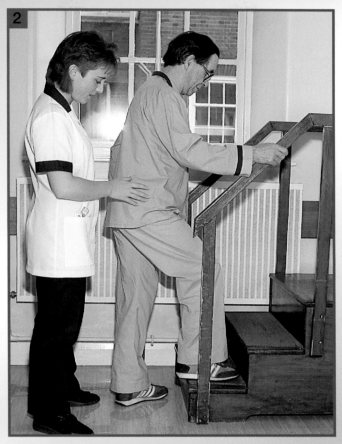

1 *Advice on climbing stairs is important in order not to over exert the new joint at this early stage. The majority of patients will need to be able to climb stairs before discharge from hospital.*

2 *Here, the patient is encouraged to put his 'good leg' on to a step, and then bring his other leg on to the same step. This is repeated for the flight of stairs, with the patient holding the banister for support.*

3 *The procedure is repeated for descending the stairs, but this time the operated leg is put down first, and the 'good leg' is then placed on to the same step. This is repeated down the entire flight of stairs.*

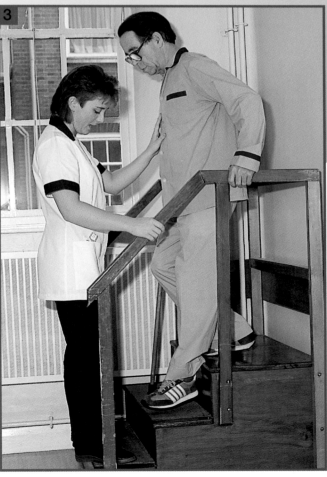

LEARNING TO WALK

On the second day after surgery, the patient will begin learning to walk with their new hip or knee joint. The physiotherapist will instruct the patient how to get in and out of bed safely, as well as encouraging their first steps.

A walking frame is most suitable for the early post-operative days, for improving balance and confidence as the patient adjusts to taking weight through a new joint. The amount of weight taken through the joint is determined by whether the joint replacement is cemented or uncemented.

WEIGHT BEARING

Cemented joints are able to sustain full weight, and the patient will be encouraged to take full weight through the leg, pain allowing. Uncemented joints need protecting for six weeks, and the patient will be advised to take up to half their weight only through the affected leg.

When independent walking is established (four to seven days after the operation), the physiotherapist will promote the type of walking aid to either two sticks for cemented joints or a pair of elbow crutches for uncemented joints. At this stage, providing there are no complications, preparations will be made for discharge, and functional activities, such as stair-climbing will be practised.

Most patients, on being discharged, will be able to continue their rehabilitation at home. Some, however, may require out-patient physiotherapy appointments.

Abnormal heart rhythms

The electrical activity in the heart that ensures a normal healthy heartbeat may become disrupted by a number of factors. As a result, the heart rhythm may become irregular, or abnormally rapid or slow.

The normal heart rhythm (sinus rhythm) is 60–80 beats per minute and is controlled by electrical activity within the heart. If the electrical conducting system becomes faulty, an arrhythmia (disrupted rhythm) can develop.

SLOW HEART RATES
Slow rhythms known as bradyarrhythmias may be due to:
■ **Sick sinus syndrome**
This is a condition of the elderly when the sinus node (the natural pacemaker of the heart) starts to fail, leading to slow activation of the heart, or even periods of a few seconds without a heartbeat. There may also be associated episodes of fast rhythm.
■ **Heart block**
In this condition, impulses from the sinus node intermittently fail to reach the ventricles due to interference in the normal conducting system of the heart. In its severest form, no impulses reach the ventricles, a rhythm called complete heart block.
■ **Drugs**
Some drugs slow down the rate of impulses from the sinus node. This is beneficial in the treatment of conditions such as angina, but if the drugs are taken in excess, heart block may result.
■ **Damaged conducting tissue**
Ischaemic heart disease, cardiac surgery and catheter ablation treatment for fast arrhythmias may also damage the conducting tissue and slow the heart.

■ Some rare diseases of the heart, and thyroid problems.

FAST HEART RHYTHMS
Inappropriately fast rhythms (tachyarrhythmias) are mainly caused by the abnormal transmission of electrical impulses through the heart, either as a result of malfunctioning heart muscle or a congenital abnormality.

Ischaemic heart disease, heart valve disorders, drugs, abnormal blood chemistry and thyroid problems can all interfere with the function of heart muscle and promote tachyarrhythmias. In susceptible individuals, an episode may be triggered by coffee or alcohol.

There are two main categories of tachyarrhythmia:
■ **Atrial tachyarrhythmias** – fast electrical impulses cause the atrium to contract at a rapid rate. Eventually, if the rate rises too high, the atria lose the ability to contract, a rhythm called atrial fibrillation. Some or all of the fast impulses generated within the atria are transmitted to the ventricle, which also beats faster.
■ **Ventricular tachycardia** – this is usually more serious since the ventricle may not be able to pump blood properly around the body, leading to circulatory shock. It can progress to cardiac arrest, either on its own or by precipitating ventricular fibrillation when the ventricles stop contracting completely.

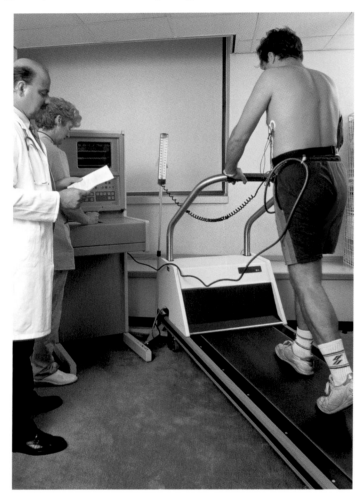

An electrocardiogram (ECG) examination is the most useful way of identifying abnormally rapid or slow heart rhythms. The electrical activity in the heart is shown on a monitor.

The heart rate in health

The normal beating heart responds rapidly to changes in activity, stress, anxiety and illness. This response is essential in order to increase the cardiac output, in response to the greater requirements for oxygen and other nutrients by the body tissues.

SINUS RHYTHMS
This increased heart rate is a normal response and is known as sinus tachycardia. Conversely, while asleep or when we are resting, the heart rate may slow

down dramatically, especially in young fit people, causing a sinus bradycardia. Heart rates of 40 beats per minute are not uncommon. The pulse rate can therefore vary enormously in health. An arrhythmia is by definition an inappropriately fast or slow heart rhythm.

At night or when at rest, the heart rate may slow down markedly – a sinus bradycardia. This is especially common in young, athletic people.

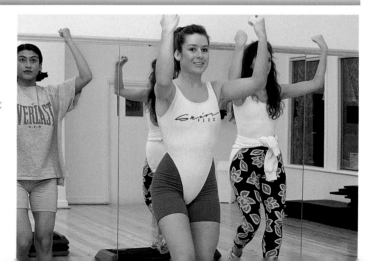

Arrhythmia symptoms

The heart may develop an arrhythmia in which the symptoms are continuous, or it may beat abnormally only intermittently, resulting in attacks or paroxysms.

People often tolerate arrhythmias and may not experience many symptoms. At the other extreme, a life-threatening arrhythmia may result in cardiac arrest or circulatory shock.

With continuous arrhythmia, the diagnosis is usually very simple. However, with an intermittent arrhythmia, problems can arise, not least because many of the associated symptoms are relatively non-specific and can occur in health.

Doctors should ask whether the symptoms occur at any particular time, and whether there has been any precipitating event, such as drinking alcohol. It can also be helpful to take the pulse during an episode, and to check whether or not the heart beats irregularly.

COMMON SYMPTOMS
Symptoms of arrhythmia include:

■ **Palpitations** – the experience of a fluttering or palpitation in the heart is the most usual symptom associated with tachyarrhythmias. Unfortunately, because the heart rate can respond rapidly to many normal stimuli, especially anxiety, palpitations are a common experience and do not necessarily mean that there is a problem. Features such as sudden onset when relaxing with equally fast resolution are more suggestive, especially if associated with other symptoms such as breathlessness.

■ **Dyspnoea** – shortness of breath in association with tachy- or bradyarrhythmias reflects the impaired ability of the heart to increase blood supply. Dyspnoea is usually first experienced during exercise. Later, if the arrhythmia severely impairs the function of the heart, the cardiac output may be insufficient even at rest. In these cases, other symptoms of heart failure may develop, such as waking in the middle of the night gasping for breath – paroxysmal nocturnal dyspnoea.

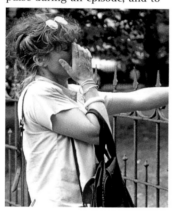

A common symptom of an arrhythmia is shortness of breath (dyspnoea). In severe cases, other symptoms of heart failure may develop.

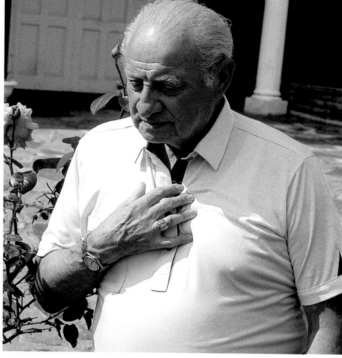

■ **Pre-syncope** – although dizziness is a common sensation not necessarily related to the heart, it can be a symptom of low blood pressure resulting from an arrhythmia. When it is very severe, blackouts (syncope) may occur.

■ **Chest pain** – may occur with arrhythmias, more usually tachyarrhythmias. The important pattern here is that chest pain only occurs during the arrhythmia. Chest pain occurring

Dizziness and blackouts may be due to low blood pressure resulting from an arrhythmia. Blackouts (syncope) can often occur without warning.

at other times, such as during exercise or following meals, is likely to have another cause.

Cardiac arrest is a consequence of an arrhythmia that severely affects heart function. Unless prompt treatment is given, cardiac arrest is fatal.

How arrhythmias occur

Arrhythmias occur if the normal electrical conducting system of the heart is interrupted, diseased or overridden by external factors.

Conducting system
In order for the heart chambers to contract in a coordinated fashion and pump blood to the body, a single electrical impulse is generated and transmitted through the heart by specialized conducting tissue.

Sino-atrial node
The sino-atrial node is the natural pacemaker of the heart and is located in the right atrium. The node governs the rate at which electrical impulses are initiated.

Normally the heart beats 60–80 times a minute, corresponding to our pulse. This rate is affected by stimulation by nerves and circulating hormones, allowing the amount of blood pumped by the heart to increase and decrease rapidly in response to demand, as during exercise.

Atrioventricular node
The electrical impulse travels through the atria to another small specialized area, the atrioventricular (AV) node. Here, the impulse is slowed down before passing into the conducting tissue of the ventricles. Finally, the impulse reaches the tips of the ventricles and spreads throughout the muscle which then contracts.

All parts of the conduction system in the heart can generate electrical impulses, but the rate of electrical discharge is less than that produced by the sinus node.

A wave of electrical impulses spreads through the heart, causing the muscle to contract. The sino-atrial node trigger initiates this process.

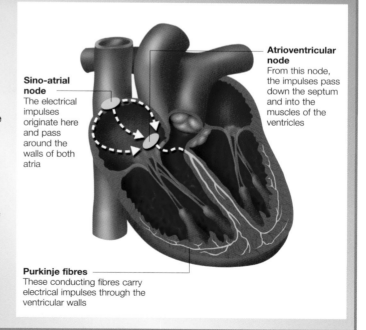

Sino-atrial node
The electrical impulses originate here and pass around the walls of both atria

Atrioventricular node
From this node, the impulses pass down the septum and into the muscles of the ventricles

Purkinje fibres
These conducting fibres carry electrical impulses through the ventricular walls

Identifying and treating arrhythmias

Recent technological advances have made the detection and treatment of arrhythmias more efficient. Once normal heart rhythm has been restored, attention focuses on avoiding recurrence.

The most useful way of identifying an arrhythmia is by examining an electrocardiogram (ECG). Electrocardiography records the pattern of the electrical impulse as it travels through the heart generating the heartbeat. In a continuous arrhythmia, this will be used to give the diagnosis.

In an intermittent (paroxysmal) arrhythmia, an ECG is diagnostic only if it is performed during an attack. If the bouts of abnormal rhythm are infrequent or short-lived, it is almost impossible to obtain the answer from a one-off recording and ambulatory techniques are required.

ELECTROPHYSIOLOGY

An alternative technique for diagnosing arrhythmias is electrophysiological study. This technique involves the delivery of impulses at different points in the heart using electrodes inserted into the heart via blood vessels, to precipitate and identify the arrhythmia. It can be used to diagnose a suspected arrhythmia in difficult cases and detects the area of abnormality within the heart that is responsible for generating the arrhythmia.

INVESTIGATING CAUSES

The second stage in the investigation of arrhythmias is identifying the underlying cause:
■ **Blood tests** – the levels of potassium, magnesium and calcium in the blood are measured – when abnormal these substances can cause arrhythmias. Measurements of thyroid function and cardiac enzymes may also elucidate the underlying cause
■ **Exercise testing** – an electrocardiogram performed as the patient is exercising is a useful technique for identifying ischaemic heart disease. It may also be used to provoke an arrhythmia. The patient is asked to walk on a treadmill during the procedure
■ **Echocardiography** – imaging of the heart using this ultrasound technique may uncover heart valve disease at the root of the problem
■ **Coronary angiography** – may be needed if ischaemic heart disease is thought to be present.

Coronary angiography is used to diagnose heart disease that may cause an arrhythmia. The blood supply to the heart is assessed and pressures are measured.

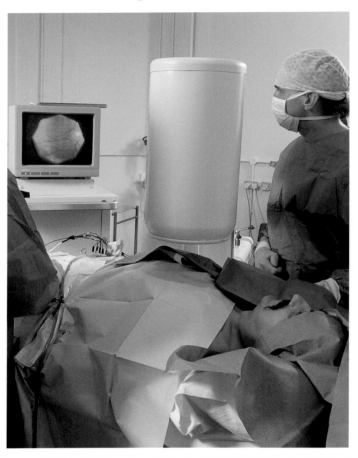

Detecting paroxysmal arrhythmias

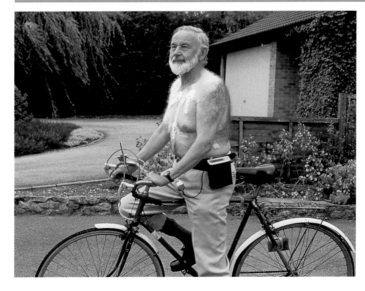

There are some useful techniques that allow identification of paroxysmal arrhythmias. Several different methods are available:
■ A continuous recording of the ECG can be made for a 24-hour period using electrodes which aree placed on the chest and connected to a cassette recorder worn on the belt
■ Other devices can be worn for longer periods, recording the ECG only when an abnormal rhythm is detected or when the device is triggered by the wearer during a bout of symptoms

Ambulatory ECG recordings are useful in identifying paroxysmal arrhythmias. This patient is wearing a 24-hour ECG recording device.

■ Even longer periods of monitoring are possible using devices that can be simply placed on the front of the chest during an attack of symptoms.

DATA ANALYSIS

The ECG at the time of an episode of arrhythmia is recorded and can be transmitted down a telephone line to the cardiac centre for immediate analysis. This depends upon the individual being capable of handling the machine during an attack.

It is also possible to implant a small recorder under the skin of the chest, which continuously monitors the ECG for up to 18 months and records any abnormal rhythms.

Treatment of arrhythmias

The treatment of arrhythmias depends on the type of the abnormality.

TREATING SLOW HEART RATES
Severe bradyarrhythmias can lower the blood pressure, so treatment is needed to prevent the development of shock.
■ If a drug is responsible for causing the bradyarrhythmia, withdrawing that agent is often the only treatment required
■ In severe cases, an injection of atropine or isoprenaline may speed up the heart
■ If drugs are not effective, a temporary pacemaker may be required to restore a normal heart rate and hence the blood pressure. Pacemakers replace the missing electrical impulses.

Intermittent bradyarrhythmias associated with age or disease may require a permanent pacemaker if they are severe or cause troublesome symptoms. Permanent pacemakers are implanted under the skin at the top of the chest, beneath the collarbone.

The small device delivers electrical impulses along a wire that is inserted into the heart muscle. It stimulates both ventricles to contract, and the rate of delivery of these impulses can be varied to restore the normal heart rate and blood pressure.

TACHYARRHYTHMIAS
The initial priority in the treatment of tachyarrhythmias

is to restore the heart back to its normal rhythm. This can be attempted by administering either drugs or an electric shock (cardioversion):

■ Drugs (such as oral digoxin, verapamil and beta-blockers) – may be used to delay the heart rate. In severe cases of ventricular tachycardia,

intravenous lignocaine or amiodarone may be effective
■ Cardioversion – can be used to treat tachycardias that do not respond to drugs (see below)
■ Catheter ablation – uses radiofrequency to treat abnormal areas of heart muscle

If treatment is effective at restoring sinus rhythm, a second concern is to prevent a

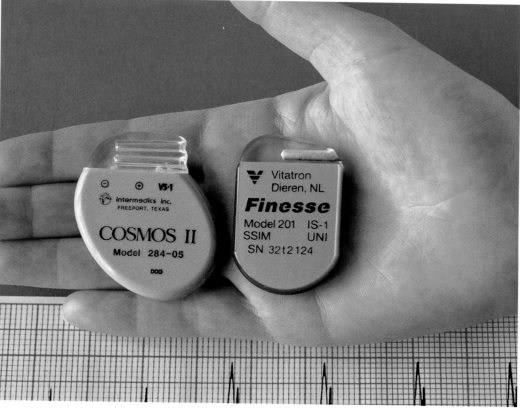

A pacemaker delivers electrical impulses along a wire to the heart. Most modern devices are of a very small size, as can be seen here.

recurrence of the arrhythmia. This may involve stopping any precipitating drug, or treating an underlying cause as well as administering drugs.

Cardioversion

Sometimes a ventricular tachycardia does not respond to drug therapy. In these cases, cardioversion may be an option. In this treatment, an electric shock is used to revert a rhythm to normal.

ATRIAL FIBRILLATION
An exception to this rule is atrial fibrillation, in which there is a risk of blood clot formation inside the heart chambers. If this

arrhythmia has been present for more than 24–48 hours, cardioversion using electricity is associated with an increased risk of stroke because it may dislodge the clot.

RESTORING RHYTHM
Under a light general anaesthetic, the doctor applies two paddles to the chest wall and delivers an electric current. The burst of high-voltage

electricity temporarily disrupts the abnormal electrical activity in the heart and restores a normal rhythm. This technique is also used as an emergency treatment to restart the heart following cardiac arrest.

IMPLANTABLE DEFIBRILLATOR
Recently, patients who have experienced episodes of ventricular tachycardia or fibrillation have been found to benefit from the implantation of a device under the skin, much like a pacemaker, called an implantable defibrillator. This can detect a tachyarrhythmia and deliver an electric shock to the heart automatically.

Cardioversion can be carried out to restore a normal heart rhythm in a case of ventricular tachycardia. It is often used if initial drug therapy fails to work.

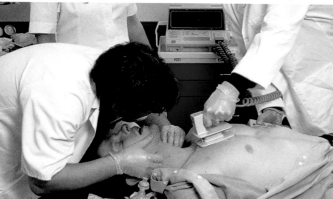

Catheter ablation

A recent technique known as catheter ablation often follows electrophysiological studies in the treatment of tachyarrhythmias.

If the abnormal area of muscle causing the arrhythmia can be identified, a special catheter can be passed into a vein or artery in the groin or arm and threaded up to the heart. The abnormal area is then ablated (tissue is destroyed) using radiofrequency.

Need for a permanent pacemaker
This technique can abolish the risk of further arrhythmias completely, although there is a small chance of disrupting the normal conducting tissue, causing heart block. If this happens, a patient may need to have a permanent pacemaker inserted.

Angina

Angina is normally experienced as a pain in the centre of the chest that has as its origin the heart muscle. Affected people frequently feel this pain after physical exercise.

The term angina describes the symptoms arising from an area of heart muscle that is being starved of oxygen, most commonly because of an inadequate blood supply (myocardial ischaemia).

TYPICAL SIGNS

Typically, angina is described as a crushing chest pain that often radiates down the left arm and is associated with breathlessness, sweating and nausea.

Many people with angina have symptoms that conform to this classical pattern, but for others the experience of myocardial ischaemia differs markedly. Chest pain may be mild or even absent and breathlessness may be dominant.

Some people may feel the pain only in areas other than the chest, such as in one or both arms, the neck, jaw or teeth. With such a range of symptoms, it can sometimes be difficult to be sure that the cause of a pain is angina, which means that further tests are necessary to establish a diagnosis.

CAUSAL TRIGGERS

Angina is usually precipitated by exertion, especially after food and in cold weather, and is often relieved by rest. Emotional stress can also bring on an attack.

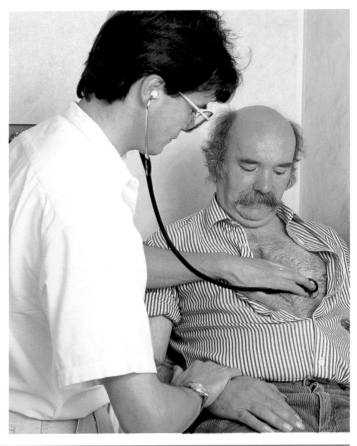

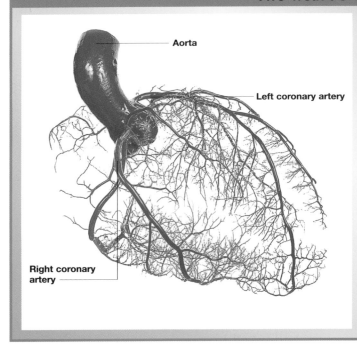

Angina occurs when there is an inadequate supply of blood to the heart. The heart muscle is therefore starved of oxygen, causing constrictive pain.

Symptoms of angina range from a mild ache to a severe pain in the chest. Doctors will first carry out a thorough examination using a stethoscope.

The heart's blood supply

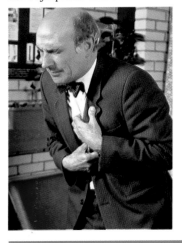

- Aorta
- Left coronary artery
- Right coronary artery

The heart muscle pumps approximately 1000 gallons of blood every day throughout life, beating on average 70 times every minute. To function efficiently, the heart requires its own blood supply to provide nourishment for the heart muscle.

Coronary arteries

Oxygen and nutrients are delivered to the muscle cells via the coronary arteries, so named because they appear to form a 'crown' around the upper part of the heart.

There are two coronary arteries, right and left, which branch off the aorta (the main artery in the body) just as it

The heart muscle is nourished by a supply of oxygen-rich blood from the coronary arteries. If an artery is blocked, the tiny vessels may take over.

leaves the left ventricle of the heart. Each time the ventricle beats, and oxygenated blood is forced out of the heart into the circulation, blood enters the coronary arteries.

The right coronary artery supplies the right side of the heart and branches into the marginal artery and the posterior interventricular artery. The left coronary artery runs towards the left side of the heart, where it divides into the anterior interventricular artery and the circumflex artery.

Collateral circulation

Between these main vessels runs a network of tiny vessels (collateral circulation). In many people, if one of the arteries becomes blocked, the collateral circulation takes over and it is not until an artery is completely blocked that heart muscle dies.

The cause of angina

Angina is an indicator that there may be a problem with the blood supply to the heart muscle.

NARROWED ARTERIES
The commonest cause of reduced blood supply is a condition called atherosclerosis, which causes progressive narrowing (stenosis) of an artery as a result of the build-up of atherosclerotic plaques in the arterial wall.

These plaques grow, and increasingly protrude into the lumen (cavity of a blood vessel);

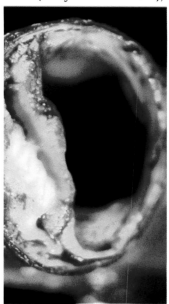

Angina is most commonly caused by atherosclerosis. In this condition, fatty deposits build up in the arterial wall, reducing the passage of blood.

eventually, the artery can become so obstructed that blood flow to parts of the heart muscle is compromised.

LACK OF BLOOD SUPPLY
As the heart pumps harder and faster to increase the blood supply to the working muscles, the greater demand for oxygen and nutrients by the heart muscle has to be met by an increased blood flow along the coronary arteries.

If the stenosis in a coronary artery is severe enough, this may limit the increase in blood flow. As a result, the heart muscle supplied by the artery will not receive the blood supply it requires. The muscle is then said to have become ischaemic, and symptoms may result.

DISEASE PROGRESSION
The artery has to be severely narrowed before ischaemia is encountered, usually to the extent of a reduction in the lumen of the vessel by 70 per cent or more. This is one of the reasons why coronary artery disease may be present for many years before any symptoms become apparent.

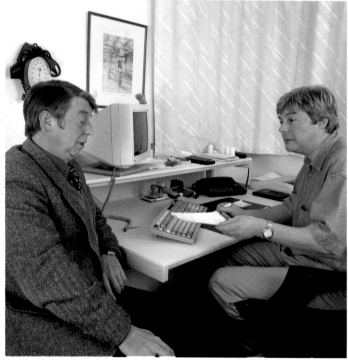

The atherosclerotic process can start in young men in their twenties, but it is often not for 20-30 years that the narrowing of the arteries is severe enough to compromise the blood supply.

As the atherosclerosis progresses and the arterial stenosis becomes more severe, the capacity to increase blood flow diminishes, and the level of

It is important for people with angina to be aware of disease progression. Regular check-ups are vital to monitor the condition and evaluate treatment.

exertion required to produce ischaemia falls. Eventually, symptoms of angina may develop even during simple tasks like dressing or washing.

Unstable angina

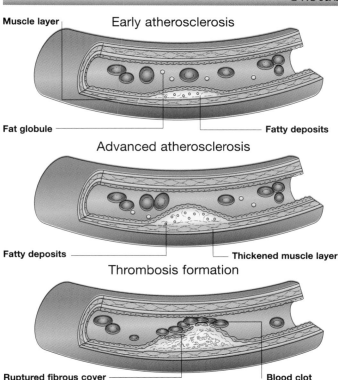

Early atherosclerosis
Muscle layer
Fat globule
Fatty deposits

Advanced atherosclerosis
Fatty deposits
Thickened muscle layer

Thrombosis formation
Ruptured fibrous cover
Blood clot

Occasionally, a sudden, severe episode of angina may occur which is out of keeping with previous symptoms. Rapidly worsening angina over several hours or days is another way in which people may experience the condition.

These worrying symptoms are collectively termed unstable angina, the causes of which are slightly different from those of stable angina.

PLAQUE SURFACE
Although the arteries are narrowed by atherosclerosis to some extent (also found in stable angina), this is not the cause of the rapid deterioration in symptoms. The factor responsible is a sudden and dramatic change in the nature of the surface of the atherosclerotic plaque.

Angina is caused by fatty deposits (atheroma) in the coronary arteries. If an atheroma plaque ruptures, a localized clot can form and block the artery.

The bulk of the plaque is made up of a cholesterol-rich core within the arterial wall, which is separated from the flow of blood by a fibrous layer, or cap, overlying it. When this cap splits, the underlying core is exposed to the bloodstream.

BLOOD CLOTS
Blood clots form on this roughened surface, creating a thrombus (blood clot). As the size of the thrombus grows, the space within the vessel narrows accordingly, and this produces ischaemic symptoms.

HEART ATTACK
If the vessel is blocked completely, a myocardial infarction (heart attack) may result. This is when death of part of the heart muscle occurs due to the supply of oxygenated blood being cut off by the narrowed artery.

If some blood flow persists in a severely stenosed artery, angina may be present on minimal activity or even at rest.

Investigating angina

To diagnose stable and unstable angina, specific tests and imaging techniques may need to be performed. Once the condition has been identified, treatment options can be explored.

In diagnosing angina, a doctor will have to rule out other conditions that have similar symptoms. These include gastro-oesophageal reflux disorder, in which stomach acids cause inflammation of the lower oesophagus, resulting in some discomfort.

If the features are thought to reflect a possibility of coronary artery disease (blocked coronary arteries), further investigation is required.

BLOOD TESTS
The blood pressure is recorded and blood tests are taken to exclude:
■ Anaemia, a disorder in which oxygen-carrying pigment in red blood cells, haemoglobin, is deficient (often a cause of worsening anginal chest pain)
■ Kidney disease (which may suggest atherosclerosis of the arteries supplying the kidneys)
■ Diabetes mellitus.
The cholesterol level is also measured.

ELECTROCARDIOGRAM
An electrical recording of the heart, or electrocardiogram (ECG), may show evidence that part of the heart muscle is being starved of blood.

Ischaemic myocardium conducts the electrical impulses stimulating heart contraction abnormally, and leads to changes in the ECG tracing.

In unstable angina, the ECG may show significant changes and provide the diagnosis, while excluding a myocardial infarction, which can present in a similar manner.

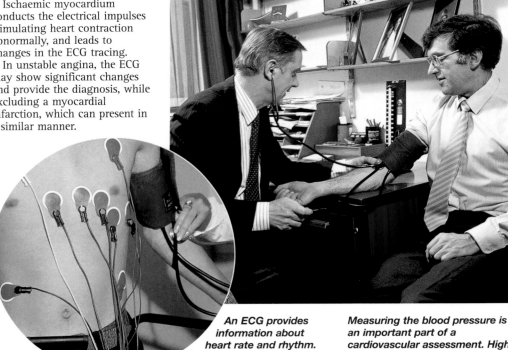

An ECG provides information about heart rate and rhythm. Electrodes pick up electrical signals, which are recorded.

Measuring the blood pressure is an important part of a cardiovascular assessment. High blood pressure is a risk factor for atherosclerosis and angina.

Provoking symptoms in patients with stable angina

In stable angina, the muscle is not usually ischaemic at rest, and the ECG is often normal although previous myocardial infarction may be detected.

Further tests to make the heart work harder to provoke ischaemia are then required.

EXERCISE TEST
An exercise treadmill test is the simplest to perform, allowing the ECG to be recorded when the heart is under exertional stress from walking on a treadmill.

In people who cannot manage the treadmill, an alternative method is to administer a drug to make the heart work harder. The presence of ischaemia can then be detected using ECG or imaging techniques.

IMAGING TECHNIQUES
Echocardiography uses ultrasound to provide an image of the heart muscle. During the procedure, ischaemic myocardium will appear not to contract as well as heart muscle with a healthy blood supply.

In another technique, radioactive dye is injected into the bloodstream. Using a special camera, the heart muscle can then be visualized. The greater the blood flow to an area of heart muscle, the more radiation is detected. The camera is then able to construct an image of the heart based upon the relative blood flow to different regions. Repeating the image when the heart is made to work harder can uncover areas with a deficient blood flow.

If any of these tests have positive results, it is usually necessary to proceed to coronary angiography to visualize the coronary arteries directly.

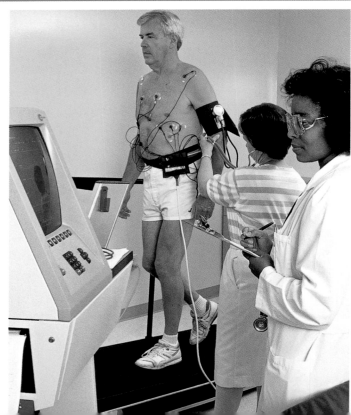

In stable angina, ECG tracings are often normal. Carefully monitored exercise may bring on the symptoms and help to diagnose heart ischaemia.

Treatment of angina

In unstable angina, emergency admission to hospital is necessary. Without treatment, unstable angina may progress to myocardial infarction.

TREATING UNSTABLE ANGINA

The initial treatment involves anticoagulation (thinning the blood) to slow down the development of the blood clot in the artery. Heparin or heparin-like drugs are administered by intravenous infusion or subcutaneous injection.

Chest pain may require morphine-like drugs in addition to an intravenous infusion of a nitrate drug, which has a direct action on the muscle of the wall of the artery, causing it to dilate and thereby maximizing blood flow. A medication called a beta-blocker is frequently given, since this reduces the work, and consequently the demand for blood, of the heart.

If the chest pain continues despite these measures, emergency coronary angiography may be necessary.

Depending on the severity and pattern of the coronary artery disease, treatment may involve either angioplasty (inserting a balloon into the narrowed artery to dilate it) or coronary artery bypass surgery.

TREATING STABLE ANGINA

The treatment of stable angina centres on controlling the symptoms, treating risk factors and reducing the likelihood of complications such as myocardial infarction.

Symptoms of stable angina are treated with four groups of drugs. The first drug to be given is usually a beta-blocker, since this reduces the workload on the heart. Other drugs, generically termed calcium channel antagonists, nitrates and a newer agent nicorandil can be added. All of these medications work by dilating the coronary arteries.

Treatment of risk factors can reduce disease progression and complications and involves managing hypertension, diabetes and high cholesterol, when present, usually with drugs.

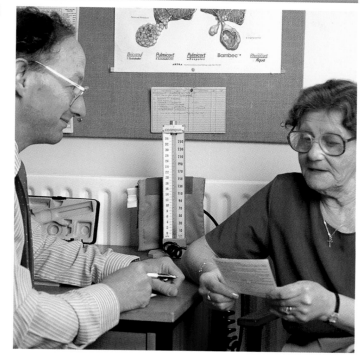

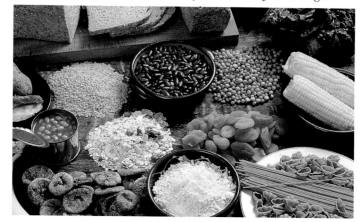

Management of angina involves a healthy diet. It is thought that the risk of heart disease is reduced by cutting down on foods that are high in fat.

To further prevent the risk of complications, a junior aspirin should be given daily, unless there is a history of stomach ulcers, since aspirin has been shown to improve the outlook.

LIFESTYLE CHANGES

Improving diet and increasing the level of exercise can prevent angina from worsening. A healthy diet must be encouraged, with minimal fat and cholesterol intake, and plenty of fresh fruit and vegetables.

Patients with stable angina are often prescribed nitrate drug therapy in tablet form. This treatment works by dilating the coronary arteries.

Cessation of smoking is essential because this has the greatest impact on the disease process.

It has been suggested that various vitamins and herbal preparation are able to reduce heart disease. However, it should be remembered that the claims of these products are often based upon anecdotal report and have little sound research behind them. Studies are on-going and will eventually give experts more accurate information.

Identifying those at risk

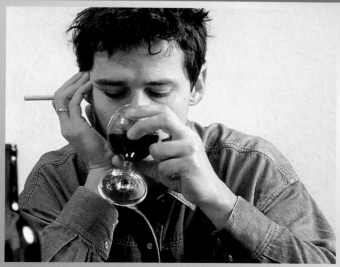

Some people are more at risk of developing complications of angina than others. Those who smoke, and drink alcohol to excess are at higher risk.

Another aspect in the treatment of stable angina is to identify the group of people who are at greater risk of complications such as myocardial infarction, and thus enable them to undergo screening in the form of coronary angiography.

Risk factors
Certain factors are taken into consideration when identifying people at high risk, such as:
■ Age – generally the risk of angina increases with age

■ Quality of life – factors such as a person's smoking habit, alcohol intake, high-fat diet and lack of exercise
■ Anginal severity
■ Family history – relatives with coronary artery disease
■ Results of tests, such as the exercise test.

Treatment options
Once the pattern of the coronary artery disease is known from angiography, a more formal decision about treatment can be made. The options include:
■ Simply continuing drug treatment
■ More invasive therapies such as angioplasty or coronary artery bypass surgery.

Arteriosclerosis

Symptoms

Arteriosclerosis (also known as atherosclerosis) is an accumulation of cholesterol and fatty streaks in the artery walls, causing them to narrow. The streaks develop into plaques that may grow large enough to impede blood flow.

BLOOD CLOTS
In some cases, the plaque disintegrates and a blood clot (thrombus) forms on its surface. The clot may cause a local blockage in the artery or break off into the circulation and block a smaller blood vessel some distance away. In other cases, the plaque weakens the artery wall, which may balloon out (an aneurysm) and rupture.

Arteriosclerosis usually develops over many years, and is the underlying cause of many heart attacks, strokes and other arterial disorders.

SIGNS
Arteriosclerosis often causes no symptoms, but can lead to:

■ Chest pain – narrowed or blocked coronary arteries can cause pain that is brought on by exertion and relieved by rest (angina), or a heart attack (myocardial infarction)
■ Leg pain – a blockage in the aorta (the main artery of the body) or in an artery in the pelvis or limbs can lead to leg pain
■ Abdominal pain – a blockage in the blood supply to the small intestine can cause chronic pain after meals (intestinal angina) or diarrhoea and vomiting
■ Signs of stroke – these include facial weakness, limb paralysis, difficulty in swallowing or speaking, headache and vomiting
■ Severe back pain – this may be due to blood leaking from a swelling in the wall of the aorta (aortic aneurysm).

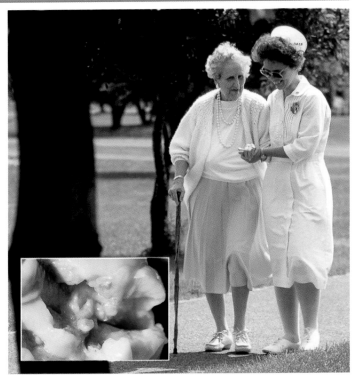

Signs of arteriosclerosis may include leg pain and limb paralysis. Arteriosclerosis is caused by fat deposition in the artery walls (shown in inset).

Causes

Atheromatous plaques consist of a core of fatty (lipid) material, encapsulated in fibrous tissue. They are common in areas of high pressure, such as the points where blood vessels divide or pass through a narrow canal.

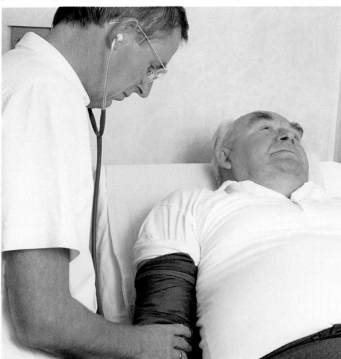

RISK FACTORS
Known risk factors for arteriosclerosis include:
■ Increasing age – the conditon does not usually cause symptoms until middle age, but the first changes may occur in childhood

■ Male sex – middle-aged men are up to four times more likely to develop arteriosclerosis than women of the same age; this gap narrows after menopause
■ Raised arterial blood pressure (hypertension) – in middle-aged men, an increase of more than 20mmHg systolic pressure (the upper figure in a blood pressure reading) increases death rates from cardiovascular disease by 60 per cent
■ Smoking – a major risk factor for ischaemic heart disease (IHD) arterial disease; the risk of IHD increases with the number of cigarettes smoked
■ Race – in the UK, immigrants from the Indian subcontinent have higher than average rates of IHD, while black immigrants from the Caribbean have lower rates
■ High blood fat levels – cholesterol is present in the blood in several forms, and high levels (hypercholesterolaemia) increase the risk
■ Genetic abnormalities – people affected by familial

Arteriosclerosis is more likely to develop in individuals with high blood pressure. The risk is increased still further in men, and after middle age.

hypercholesterolaemia may develop atheroma at an abnormally young age
■ Overweight – an increased amount of fat around the waist is related to a high risk of IHD
■ Diabetes – this can be associated with a high cholesterol level
■ Diet – a diet low in fibre (which is found in barley, oats, lentils, chickpeas, fruit and vegetables) and high in red meat content increases the risk of developing IHD
■ Early environment – poor growth in the early years of life increases the risk of IHD
■ Lack of exercise – regular exercise protects against IHD
■ Excess alcohol consumption – moderate alcohol consumption has been shown to protect against IHD, but heavy drinking increases blood pressure and the risk of IHD and stroke
■ Socio-economic deprivation – poor groups in wealthy countries are most at risk. However, poor countries in general have a lower incidence of IHD than wealthy countries
■ Water hardness – soft water is associated with a higher death rate from IHD.

Diagnosis

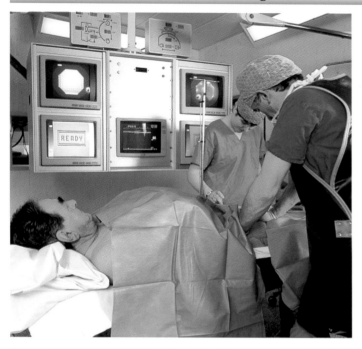

Raised blood pressure in a middle-aged person, angina or pain in the legs on exertion may suggest the presence of arteriosclerosis. Clinical examination can reveal the absence of normal pulses, abnormal sounds over larger arteries near the heart, and cold skin in poor condition.

TESTS
Investigations may include:
- Electrocardiogram (ECG)
- Ultrasound examination
- Echocardiography
- Doppler echocardiography
- Radionuclide studies
- Magnetic resonance imaging
- Angiography (X-ray examination of blood vessels).

Coronary angiography may be performed to assess the extent of arteriosclerosis. This X-ray technique visualizes the blood flow in the coronary arteries.

Incidence

Arteriosclerosis is a factor for many cases of ill health and causes many deaths. It is the prime cause of IHD, which causes 30 per cent of deaths among men and 22 per cent among women in England and Wales. The highest UK death rates from IHD occur in Northern Ireland, Scotland and the North of England.

Environment
Environmental factors are important in the development of arteriosclerosis. For example, in Finland, middle-aged men are about 13 times more likely to develop IHD than men of the same age in Japan.

However, Japanese people who migrate to a higher risk area, such as the United States, tend to develop increased rates of IHD.

Prevention

The implementation of lifestyle changes are vital factors in the prevention and treatment of arteriosclerosis.

Preventive measures
Lifestyle changes include:
- Eating a diet rich in fresh fruit, vegetables and oily fish, and low in animal fat
- Exercising
- Losing excess weight
- Stopping smoking
- Consuming only a moderate amount of alcohol.

If an arterial blockage is detected, an endarterectomy may be carried out. This removes the inner part of the artery wall to restore blood flow.

Treatment

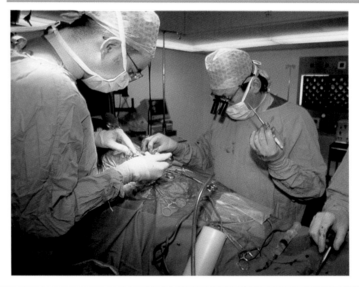

Hypertension and blood sugar levels must be carefully controlled, if necessary with antihypertensive drugs and insulin respectively. Patients with persistently high cholesterol levels may benefit from lipid-lowering drugs, such as statins.

REMOVING BLOCKAGES
Where a localized blockage is detected, possible treatments include:
- Angioplasty – the stretching of a narrowed vessel by balloon inflation across its lumen
- Endarterectomy – the surgical 're-boring' of an artery that has become obstructed
- By-pass grafting – the bypassing of part of a narrowed artery by a healthy vein.

Prognosis

Following treatment, the outlook for most patients with arteriosclerosis is much improved. The successful treatment of hypertension appears to reduce the risk of IHD by 14 per cent or more; some lipid-lowering drugs can considerably reduce the risk of heart attacks in some groups of patients. The risk of IHD falls in ex-smokers.

Most patients with claudication (cramping leg pain) benefit from stopping smoking, lifestyle changes and exercise.

In cases of severe atheroma, surgical procedures such as angioplasty may save limbs that would otherwise have become gangrenous and require amputation.

DIABETES
People with diabetes are at a greater risk of losing a limb as a result of impaired circulation and arterial disease. It is therefore important that individuals control their blood sugar levels. It is also important that they regularly see their doctor for check-ups to prevent any long-term health problems.

Even patients with existing arteriosclerosis can benefit from regular exercise. Half an hour of aerobic exercise, three times a week, can help maintain health.

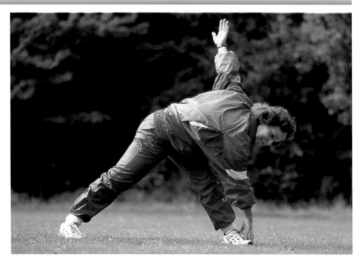

Heart attack

Heart attack, known as myocardial infarction (MI), is the term used to describe a condition that leads to the death of heart muscle. The condition is one of the commonest causes of death in the Western world.

A heart attack results from an acute occlusion (blockage) either in the main coronary arteries or one of their major branches supplying blood to heart tissue. This sudden disruption to the flow of blood within the coronary artery causes heart muscle to die.

The amount of damage caused to the heart muscle is dependent on the location of the occlusion, the speed of occlusion and the number of extra arteries supplying blood to the affected area of the heart. The most serious scenario is a blockage near the origin of an artery that occurs over a short space of time, in a region of the heart that has very poor additional blood supply from other arteries.

The most common cause of an occlusion is a clot forming on top of a ruptured or ulcerated atherosclerotic plaque. Atherosclerosis is a pathological process in which fatty and fibrous material (plaque) is deposited within the wall of the artery, thus weakening it and rendering it liable to a rupture.

When such a rupture occurs, the body's response is to repair the affected area. It achieves this by depositing blood cells called platelets, which form a clot. The disadvantage of this process is that the clot itself may end up occluding a blood vessel that has already been significantly narrowed by the atherosclerotic plaque in the first instance.

Structure of the heart

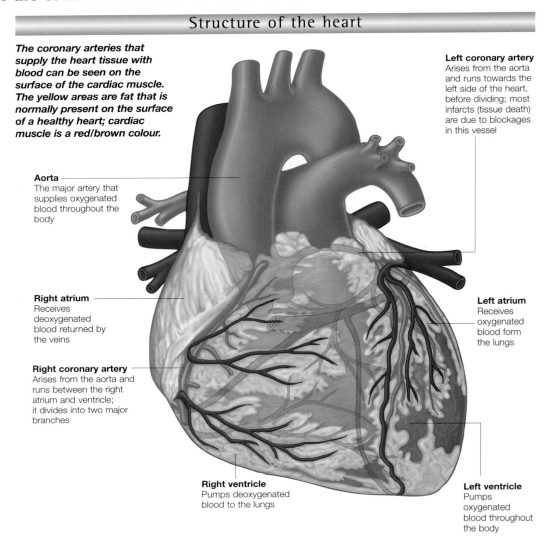

The coronary arteries that supply the heart tissue with blood can be seen on the surface of the cardiac muscle. The yellow areas are fat that is normally present on the surface of a healthy heart; cardiac muscle is a red/brown colour.

Aorta
The major artery that supplies oxygenated blood throughout the body

Right atrium
Receives deoxygenated blood returned by the veins

Right coronary artery
Arises from the aorta and runs between the right atrium and ventricle; it divides into two major branches

Right ventricle
Pumps deoxygenated blood to the lungs

Left coronary artery
Arises from the aorta and runs towards the left side of the heart, before dividing; most infarcts (tissue death) are due to blockages in this vessel

Left atrium
Receives oxygenated blood form the lungs

Left ventricle
Pumps oxygenated blood throughout the body

Signs of a heart attack

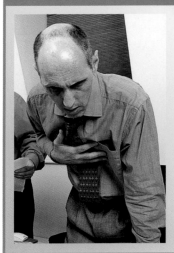

A heart attack occurs when the blood supply to part of the heart muscle is stopped because of a blockage in one of the coronary arteries. The result is the death of a section of the heart muscle (myocardial infarction), causing the symptoms of an intense, crushing pain in the chest and breathlessness.

A person having a heart attack is usually very distressed, and

Heart attacks vary in their severity, depending on the site and size of the infarction. The prognosis varies similarly, with the patient's age and general health being important factors.

may not be able to communicate. The skin is pale, cold and clammy, and the pulse is often rapid, weak and may be irregular.

The blood pressure can be either high or low, the latter being more common. If a significant amount of the heart muscle has been destroyed, the patient may display the signs associated with a failing heart and circulation, such as shortness of breath or cyanosis (a bluish discolouration of the skin due to a lack of oxygen). Shortness of breath is caused by the heart failing to pump blood effectively, resulting in the accumulation of fluid within the lungs.

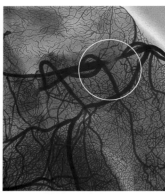

Angiography is performed by injecting a radio-opaque medium into the heart, which can then be visualized on X-ray. This can reveal obstructions in vessels (above, circled), which can result in a heart attack.

What causes a heart attack?

Heart attacks are caused by a build up of plaque on the inside of the arterial wall. The composition of this fat is complex, but includes deposits of calcium salts, blood components, cholesterol crystals, and a class of compounds called mucopolysaccharides.

There are a number of known risk factors which contribute to heart attacks which include:

- Family history of ischaemic heart disease – disease caused by inadequate blood flow
- History of smoking, current or previous
- Hypertension (high blood pressure)
- Diabetes mellitus
- Hyperlipidaemia – high concentrations of fat circulating in the blood stream

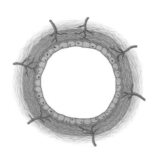

1 *Normally, blood flows through arteries to the heart without obstruction. However, a poor diet and smoking can cause a build up of plaque on the arterial wall.*

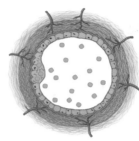

2 *High levels of lipoproteins (a complex of protein and fat) are taken up by cells called atherocytes. These burst and release their contents, attracting cells of the immune system.*

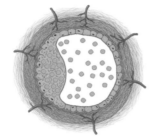

3 *This creates a vicious circle and causes the immune cells, along with migrating muscle cells, to accumulate in the arterial wall.*

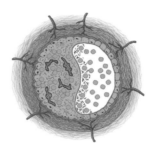

4 *Additional tissue continues to be produced and calcium and fat accumulate. When this significantly prevents blood flow, a heart attack may occur.*

Symptoms of a heart attack

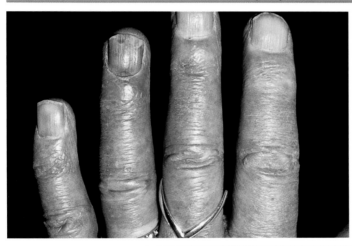

The classic symptom of a heart attack is a central chest pain that is often described as crushing, heavy or vicelike in nature. This sensation may radiate up the neck to the jaw or down the left arm, or sometimes both arms. The pain is similar to angina, but, unlike the latter, it is usually of greater severity, longer duration and

Cyanosis is a common indicator of a heart attack. The bluish coloration and slight swelling occurs when blood becomes starved of oxygen, which will happen when the heart is not beating effectively.

often resistant to simple alleviating measures, such as rest and deep breathing.

Difficulty in breathing, nausea, vomiting and profuse sweating are commonly associated with the pain. Not surprisingly, a patient having a heart attack can be extremely distressed and agitated during the whole episode.

The majority of the patients display one or all of the classic symptoms described, but painless, silent myocardial infarction can occur, and this is an increasingly recognized symptom of a heart attack, particularly in the elderly.

Natural history of a heart attack

The most important fact to emphasize about a heart attack is that it is a potentially fatal condition. Up to a third of patients who suffer a heart

attack die within the first hour, and nearly half of the patients die within the first month due to an acute (immediate) or chronic (late) complications. Even for

those patients who receive the appropriate treatment, up to one in ten patients may still die.

There are other investigations (see overleaf) that are performed

to investigate a heart attack, many of which are carried out in specialized cardiac centres. It is important to recognize that these investigations are 'first phase investigations' that form the basis of the diagnosis and initial assessment of a patient who has had a heart attack. 'Second phase investigations', such as treadmill exercise tests, coronary angiography and blood lipid measurements are designed to provide the clinician with a more detailed assessment of the patient's underlying coronary artery disease, which will be investigated after the patient has been stabilized.

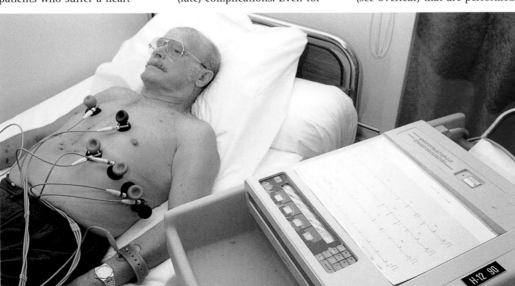

This man has already undergone surgery as a result of suffering a heart attack. The chest electrodes monitor the health of his heart, which is displayed on an ECG machine.

Treating a heart attack

A patient needs to be carefully monitored after a heart attack since recovery is often slow. After a patient has been stabilized, specialists can investigate the factors that caused the attack in an effort to prevent a recurrence.

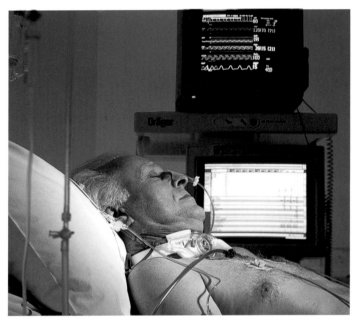

Monitoring the patient

After a person has suffered a heart attack, the first priority is to relieve pain and anxiety. Patients are therefore given powerful pain killers intravenously, such as diamorphine (heroin). All patients are confined to bed and placed on a cardiac monitor that continuously records and displays the electrical activity of the heart. Oxygen is also

Following a heart attack, the patient will undergo intensive cardiovascular monitoring. The top screen displays various vital signs: heart rate (green), arterial blood pressure (red, yellow), central venous pressure (light blue), blood oxygen (dark blue) and respiratory rate (white).

usually administered through a face mask.

The key aspect of the first line management is to try and break down the occlusion within the coronary artery and thus prevent or limit the damage to the heart muscle. This is achieved by the administration of thrombolytic, fibrinolytic and antiplatelet drugs. Commonly used thrombolytic agents are streptokinase, recombinant DNA tissue plasminogen activator, antistreplase and urokinase. These, in combination with an antiplatelet (blood-thinning) drug – aspirin is the most widely used – have been shown to reduce mortality in acute myocardial infarction by up to 40 per cent.

Surgical treatment of a heart attack

In specialized cardiac centres, more invasive and direct procedures are undertaken to open up a blocked artery, using a technique known as angioplasty and stenting. The procedure involves passing a balloon into the affected artery, and inflating it to open it up.

The balloon can be inflated with air or liquid to eight times atmospheric pressure for up to 60 seconds. This causes the plaque to split, allowing blood to flow normally. Then, a wire stent is positioned across the affected segment to maintain the open pathway within the artery.

This surgical procedure is brief, and the patient needs only a short period of convalescence. Afterwards, a coronary angiograph image, whereby a radio-opaque dye is injected into the arteries and its progress monitored using X-ray imaging, may be taken. This will reveal the success of the balloon angioplasty procedure.

Another, similar technique uses a laser catheter. This is

A cardioangiogram uses a contrast medium to detect obstructions or weakness in the blood vessels of the heart, either before or after a heart attack.

introduced into the artery and guided to the blockage using a fibre-optic channel. When it reaches the plaque build-up, a small balloon is inflated to temporarily stop blood flow, and a laser pulse is emitted. This breaks up the plaque, which is then removed from the artery using a vacuum device. Again, a coronary angiogram may be performed to check that the blood is flowing normally.

Angioplasty can be performed on any blocked blood vessel in the body. Leg arteries, as seen here, are a common site for this procedure.

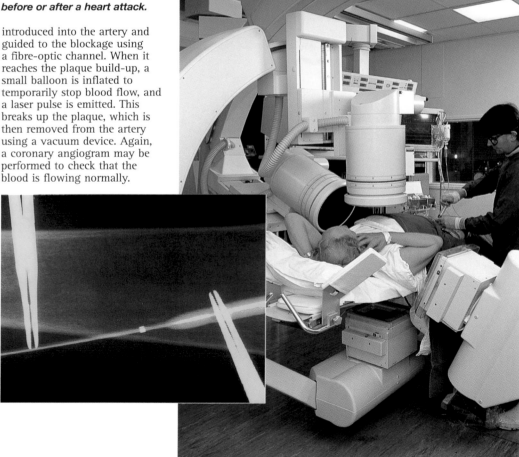

Second-phase management

The first and most important investigation in any patient suspected of having a heart attack is electrocardiography (ECG). This records the electrical activity of the heart that is obtained by placing electrodes on the chest and limbs of the patient. The ECG reading in a patient who's had an acute heart attack displays a characteristic trace, and confirms the diagnosis. In addition, the ECG gives valuable information about the area of the heart that has been damaged. The ECG changes evolve over a period of time, and it is not uncommon to find that, in a particular patient, the first ECG is normal. It is therefore common practice to perform several ECGs in series.

BLOOD ANALYSIS

The second important investigation relies on the knowledge that damaged or dying muscle releases a variety of substances or markers, such as enzymes and proteins, into the bloodstream. Some of these markers are unique to heart muscle.

The markers can be measured by taking blood samples from the patient, and once again, the samples are taken over time to enable the doctor to establish whether there is ongoing destruction of the heart muscle. Blood samples are also taken to assess other body systems, such as kidney function, which can be adversely affected when the circulation is inadequate, resulting from a failing heart.

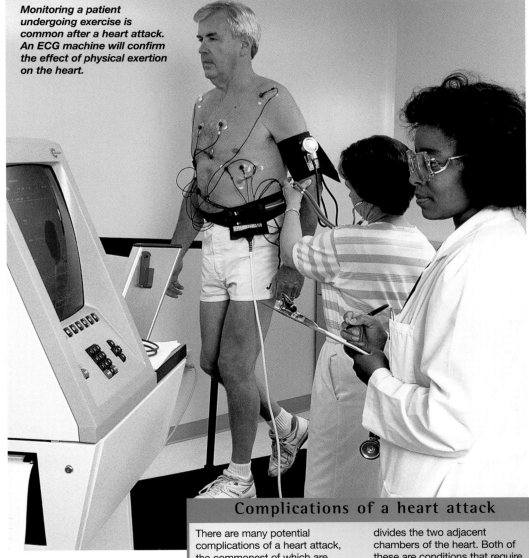

Monitoring a patient undergoing exercise is common after a heart attack. An ECG machine will confirm the effect of physical exertion on the heart.

Investigating a heart attack

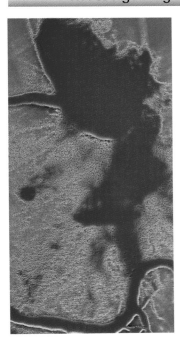

Other routine investigations include chest X-rays and echocardiography. The former gives the doctor static information of the heart and lungs. The latter is an ultrasound examination that gives dynamic or functional information, enabling the doctor to quantify the extent of the heart attack, the function of the non-damaged portion of the heart and the presence or absence of some of the complications of a heart attack. These include the accumulation of fluid around the heart and associated damage to structures within the heart, such as the cardiac valves.

Angiograms will often be taken after a heart attack. These are used to monitor blood flow around the heart after surgery, especially after coronary angioplasty.

Complications of a heart attack

There are many potential complications of a heart attack, the commonest of which are abnormalities of the heart rhythm. These are most likely to occur when the heart muscle is at its most vulnerable, namely at the onset of symptoms.

Another common complication is damage to structures within the heart itself, such as the heart valves or the septum (wall) that divides the two adjacent chambers of the heart. Both of these are conditions that require surgical correction.

This incompetent mitral (bicuspid) valve was damaged by a heart attack. It did not close completely, which led to a backward flow of blood into the atrium, and had to be replaced with a prosthetic valve.

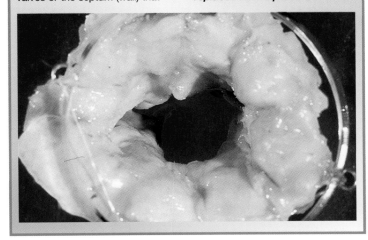

Heart failure

Heart failure is a major cause of ill health and mortality in the UK. Its incidence is estimated at nine per 1000 of the population, with almost 10 per cent of people over the age of 75 years being affected.

Heart failure occurs when the heart is unable to pump sufficient blood around the body to supply it with adequate amounts of oxygen, despite the presence of a normal circulating blood volume. This is in contrast to 'hypovolaemic shock', when cardiac function is compromised by massive traumatic blood loss.

Heart failure can occur in one of two clinical settings:

■ Primary pump failure
This is when the problem lies intrinsically within the heart

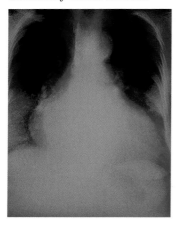

itself, as a result of disease of the endocardium (the internal lining of the heart), heart valves, myocardium (heart muscle) or pericardium (the sac that surrounds the heart).

As a result, the heart is unable to pump out all the blood returned to it from the veins. This causes a rise in the blood pressure in the veins as well as a build-up of fluid (oedema) in the tissues.

■ High cardiac output failure
This occurs as the result of certain pathological conditions such as prolonged anaemia, thyrotoxicosis or beriberi. Under these circumstances, the heart's cardiac output fails to increase sufficiently to ensure the normal oxygenation of all the body's tissues.

Patients with chronic heart failure may become seriously ill, requiring urgent attention. Many patients will be transferred to a specialist coronary care unit.

This false-colour X-ray of an elderly woman's chest shows an enlarged heart (centre) due to failure of the mitral valve.

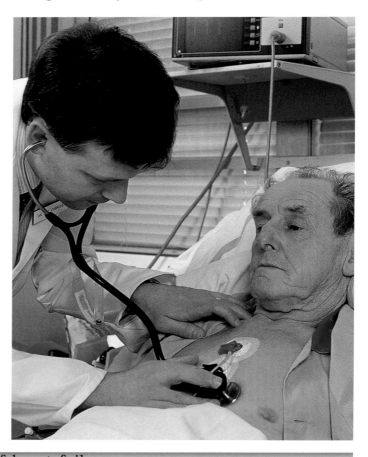

Physiology of heart failure

Ejection of blood from the ventricles

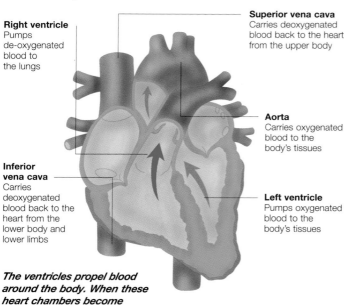

Right ventricle
Pumps de-oxygenated blood to the lungs

Superior vena cava
Carries deoxygenated blood back to the heart from the upper body

Aorta
Carries oxygenated blood to the body's tissues

Inferior vena cava
Carries deoxygenated blood back to the heart from the lower body and lower limbs

Left ventricle
Pumps oxygenated blood to the body's tissues

The ventricles propel blood around the body. When these heart chambers become diseased, circulatory efficiency is compromised.

The heart beats around 70 times every minute in a healthy adult at rest. During each beat, about 80ml (2¾fl oz) of blood are ejected by each ventricle as it contracts (this is called the 'stroke volume'). Thus the heart pumps out about 5.5l (11½ US pints) of blood every minute, an index called the 'cardiac output'.

EJECTION FRACTION
However, the ventricles do not pump out every drop of blood contained within them. Rather, in a healthy person each

ventricle fills with about 130ml (4¼fl oz)of blood, of which 80ml (2 ¾fl oz) are ejected, leaving 50ml (1½ fl oz) in the ventricle at the end of each beat.

The ratio of ejected blood to the initial filling volume is called the ejection fraction. In heart failure, this falls from about 0.6 to as low as 0.2.

Patients with heart failure have reduced cardiac output for the same filling volume or cannot increase cardiac output with an increasing filling volume.

The heart's resilience

The heart is normally a very resilient organ and is able to continue to function even in the most extreme situations.

For example, the heart rate can double and the cardiac output (the amount of blood that the heart pumps out each minute)

quadruple for short periods of time without a person feeling any major ill-effect.

Indeed, perhaps the most remarkable fact is that in the majority of people the heart manages to last a lifetime without causing any major problems.

Causes of primary heart failure

Heart failure may result from any condition that reduces the efficiency of the heart. The main causes are:

■ Ischaemic heart disease
This is a very common condition in which narrowing of the coronary arteries results in an inadequate blood supply to the heart muscle. This can cause impairment of cardiac function, particularly when a person tries to exert him/herself, giving rise to a condition known as angina.

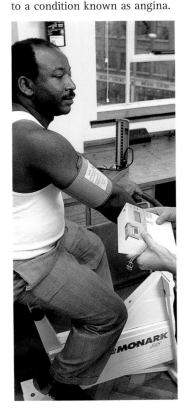

■ Hypertension
The resistance of the peripheral circulation increases in patients with high blood pressure, and as a result the heart has to generate a higher pressure to maintain adequate perfusion (passage of fluid). The heart can do this for a considerable period of time, but eventually it will fail due to the strain on the myocardial muscle caused by the sustained increase in workload.

■ Valvular heart disease
The heart's valves can become diseased, causing them to become leaky (regurgitant) or narrowed (stenosed). This increases the workload of the myocardial muscle, which initially can be compensated for by the muscle fibres increasing in size, but once the heart reaches its maximum compensatory capacity, it will eventually start to fail.

■ Abnormalities of rhythm
Any condition that causes an abnormal or disturbed rhythm can affect overall cardiac function. Furthermore, as with many other disease processes within the body, it is rare for disorders to occur in isolation. It is therefore not uncommon to find that a patient who has already sustained a heart attack is subsequently more prone to disturbances of rhythm.

Patients with hypertension are more susceptible to heart failure owing to the heart's increased workload. However, preventative measures can be taken.

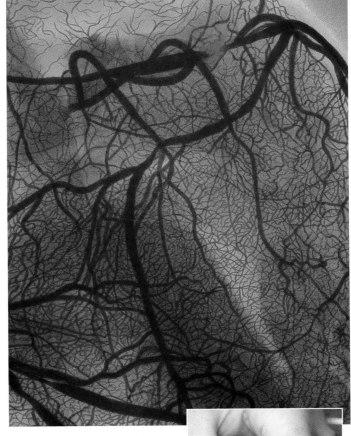

This coloured angiogram of the heart shows stenosis, or obstruction (circled), in a major coronary artery that supplies the heart muscle with blood.

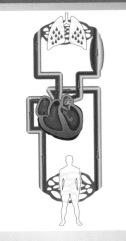

Valvular heart disease occurs when a valve malfunctions, altering the flow of blood. Replacing diseased valves may prolong the life of the recipient.

Left and right ventricular failure

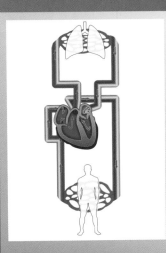

In a healthy person, the return of deoxygenated blood to the heart is matched by the ejection of oxygenated blood from the heart to the body's tissues.

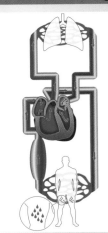

If the right side of the heart fails, blood pools in the venous side of the systemic circulation, leading to oedema, especially around the legs and ankles.

If the left side of the heart fails, oxygenated blood returning from the lungs pools in the pulmonary circulation, leading to oedema in the lungs.

The effect of heart failure may vary, depending on whether the right or left ventricle is affected:

Left ventricular failure
Blood pools in the pulmonary circulation, resulting in a condition known as pulmonary oedema, commonly referred to as fluid on the lungs. Classic symptoms include breathlessness, wheeziness, cough with frothy sputum (which can be pink in the most extreme cases) and lethargy.

Right ventricular failure
Blood pools in the venous side of the circulation, causing swelling of the lower limbs, nausea, vomiting, abdominal distension, lethargy and wasting. There may be signs of liver enlargement and cyanosis (lack of oxygen in the tissues).

Identifying and treating heart failure

The early symptoms of heart failure may initially alert the patient or the doctor to the condition. Once the condition is identified and has been investigated, treatment can be started.

The symptoms and signs of heart failure vary according to which ventricle is affected.

LEFT VENTRICULAR FAILURE
Symptoms include:
- Breathlessness, wheezing
- Cough
- Lethargy
- Tachypnoea (fast breathing)
- Dyspnoea (difficulty breathing)

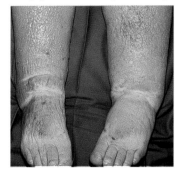

- Frothy sputum (may be pink).
  Signs include:
- Pulmonary oedema
- Displaced apex beat (heart enlargement)
- Peripheral cyanosis
- Signs of pleural effusion.

RIGHT VENTRICULAR FAILURE
Symptoms include:
- Abdominal discomfort
- Wasting
- Raised neck veins
- Enlarged, tender liver.
  Signs include:
- Peripheral oedema
- Peripheral pitting oedema
- Peripheral cyanosis
- Enlarged right ventricle.

Fluid can accumulate in the extremities in patients with right heart failure. In this condition, blood pools in the venous systemic circulation.

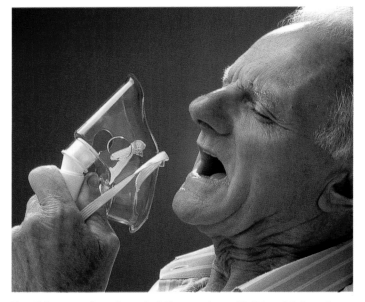

Breathlessness is a characteristic symptom of left heart failure, in which there is a fluid build-up within the lungs.

Investigating heart failure

Diagnostic tests include those used to assess the patient's general condition and those that are specifically directed towards the investigation and assessment of the patient's cardiac failure.

■ **Chest X-ray**
This gives important information on the size of the heart and the state of the lungs. It is particularly important in assessing the presence and extent of pulmonary oedema and/or effusions (the latter occur when fluid collects within the thoracic cavity).

■ **Electrocardiography (ECG)**
An ECG gives important information about the heart rate and rhythm. In addition, it can reveal evidence of previous myocardial infarction and confirm the presence of hypertension.

■ **Echocardiography**
This video technique allows a functional assessment of cardiac and valvular movements, and is crucial if cardiac failure as a result of valvular disease is suspected.

■ **Coronary angiography**
This defines the presence or absence of coronary artery disease. It can also be important in assessing valvular disease.

■ **Blood tests**
As adequate cardiac function is a prerequisite for tissue perfusion and oxygenation, evidence of secondary organ dysfunction (for example, kidney impairment) can be uncovered by general blood tests. More specifically, the degree of anaemia and thyrotoxicosis can be assessed by measuring specific markers within the blood.

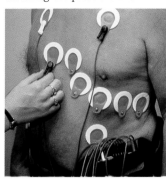

An electrocardiogram (ECG) gives information on the heart's electrical activity. A number of leads are placed around the heart to provide a signal.

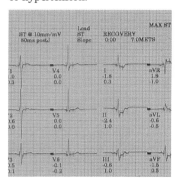

This ECG shows traces recorded from a patient undergoing an exercise test. Such testing is useful in diagnosing early heart failure.

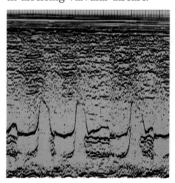

Echocardiography is used to investigate valvular heart disease. This echocardiogram shows mitral valve prolapse (between left ventricle and atrium).

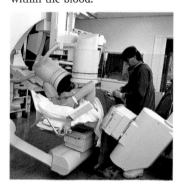

Coronary angiography enables blood vessels to be seen on X-ray or on a monitor following injection of a contrast medium into the coronary arteries.

Treating heart failure

Therapy for heart failure is directed at controlling the patient's symptoms and treating the underlying causes of the condition. Treatment can include lifestyle changes, drug treatments and, in certain cases, surgery.

When treating a patient for heart failure, drugs are often the first line of defence. In recent years, there have been major advances in the management of heart failure by the use of drugs.

DRUG TYPES

There are four main categories of drugs in use today. Within each category, there are a vast array of drugs available, with the final choice depending not only on the pharmacological effects of the medication but on the preference of the clinician. In most cases, more than one agent is required to obtain fine control of failure. Drugs include:

■ Diuretics – these are drugs that increase the amount of fluid lost through the kidneys. They are beneficial because they cause the body to get rid of the excess fluid that is a feature of cardiac failure. These drugs are also used in the treatment of hypertension (high blood pressure).

■ Angiotensin-converting enzyme (ACE) inhibitors – these drugs are of particular importance in the treatment of heart failure because they

control symptoms, improve exercise tolerance and reduce both acute exacerbations and mortality. In some patients, they can significantly and profoundly lower blood pressure and ACE inhibitor therapy is therefore often commenced in hospital.

■ Vasodilators – these act by dilating blood vessels. This has the effect of 'off-loading' the heart by reducing the amount of blood entering the ventricles (the so-called preload), lowering the heart's workload. In addition, a group of vasodilators act predominantly on the arterial system, thus reducing the afterload – that is to say, they reduce the resistance against which the heart has to eject blood.

■ Inotropes – these drugs have the effect of increasing the heart's force of contraction therefore increasing cardiac output. Drugs include digoxin and other cardiac glycosides.

Vasodilators such as oxpentifylline (shown here) are used in the treatment of vascular disease, which often contributes to heart failure.

Captopril is a widely used ACE inhibitor that is commonly prescribed for heart failure, often in combination with diuretic treatment.

Other therapies

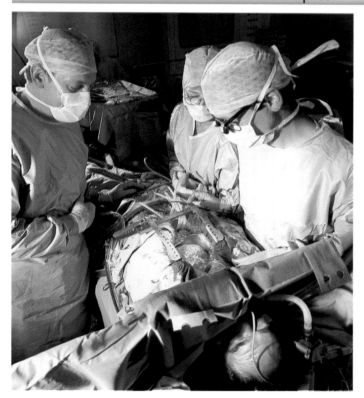

Lifestyle changes have an important role to play in all patients with cardiac disease, and involve measures such as taking regular exercise, losing weight and dietary changes (low-salt, fat-free diet).

HEART SURGERY

Despite other treatment, there are patients who continue to deteriorate both symptomatically and functionally. For a small proportion, the only viable option remaining is a 'new heart'. Providing they fulfil the criteria, cardiac transplantation may be considered for such patients.

However, considering the scarcity of donors and the risks involved in major surgery of this kind, the prognosis for patients for whom other therapies have failed is poor.

For a small number of patients, a heart transplant offers the best hope of survival. However, it can take time to find a compatible donor organ.

Assessing failure

Various systems have been devised in an attempt to standardize the functional severity of heart failure in a patient. The most commonly used classification is the New York Heart Association classification, which has four categories into which a patient can be placed. These diagnostic categories help to determine both the type of heart failure and the urgency of treatment:

Class I. No symptoms or any limitation of ordinary physical activity.

Class II. Symptoms leading to slight limitation of activity; for example, shortness of breath (or dyspnoea) when walking up an inclined plane.

Class III. Marked limitation of activity; for example, dyspnoea while getting dressed.

Class IV. Inability to perform any activity without becoming symptomatic, or experiencing symptoms at rest.

Cardiomyopathy

Cardiomyopathy refers to any disorder affecting the heart muscle. It can be divided into three categories, of which dilated cardiomyopathy is the most common type, accounting for four out of five cases.

The term cardiomyopathy refers to a group of diseases in which the primary abnormality lies within the heart muscle, rather than being a result of damage caused by failure of the heart valves or coronary artery circulation, for example.

Healthy heart muscle is very important in enabling the heart to pump blood around the body efficiently. If the muscle becomes damaged, the pumping efficiency of the heart decreases, causing a gradual worsening of symptoms.

RARE DISORDER

Cardiomyopathy is a relatively rare disease, affecting approximately 50 to 60 per 100,000 of the population, However, with increased awareness among doctors, and more effective investigation techniques, an increasing number of cases of cardiomyopathy are now being recognized.

CLASSIFICATION

As cardiomyopathy encompasses a diverse group of conditions, with some overlap between the types, it is a difficult disorder to classify. The most useful classification scheme is based on a description of the effects of the disease on the heart muscle, namely dilation, hypertrophy and restriction.

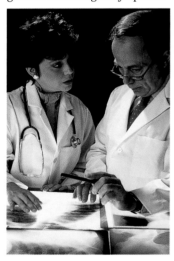

A simple chest X-ray can be very helpful in diagnosing cardiomyopathy. A visibly enlarged heart may indicate an abnormality in the heart muscle.

Cardiomyopathy is a serious disease in which the heart muscle becomes damaged. The disorder can lead to heart failure and, if not treated, can be fatal.

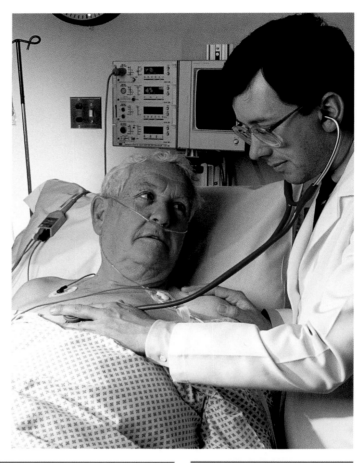

Types of cardiomyopathy

Type	Clinical features	Causes
Dilated cardiomyopathy (DCM)	■ Moderate enlargement of the heart (visible on chest X-ray) ■ Echocardiography: dilation and reduced function of left ventricle	■ Mostly unknown ■ Some chemotherapy drugs ■ Excessive alcohol consumption ■ Acquired immunodeficiency syndrome ■ Possibly genetic
Hypertrophic cardiomyopathy	■ Mild enlargement of the heart ■ Echocardiography: asymmetrical thickening of the wall between the left and right ventricles	■ Genetic – runs in families
Restrictive cardiomyopathy	■ Mild to moderate enlargement of the heart ■ Echocardiography: increased thickness in the walls of a normally functioning left ventricle, pericardial effusion	■ Inherited disorders such as haemachromatosis ■ Endomyocardial disease, for example amyloidosis or Churg-Strauss syndrome ■ Carcinoid disease

Filling capacity

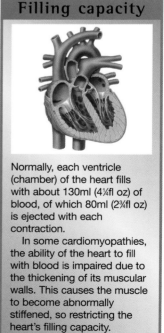

Normally, each ventricle (chamber) of the heart fills with about 130ml (4¼fl oz) of blood, of which 80ml (2¾fl oz) is ejected with each contraction.

In some cardiomyopathies, the ability of the heart to fill with blood is impaired due to the thickening of its muscular walls. This causes the muscle to become abnormally stiffened, so restricting the heart's filling capacity.

Dilated cardiomyopathy

Dilated cardiomyopathy is the most common form of cardiomyopathy, accounting for around 80 per cent of all cardiomyopathies. It is more common in males and those over the age of 45.

Dilated cardiomyopathy involves the enlargement of some or all of the chambers of the heart, causing their muscular contraction to become less efficient. This results in the symptoms of congestive heart failure, including breathlessness and fluid retention.

CAUSES
The causes of dilated cardiomyopathy include excessive alcohol consumption, chemotherapy treatment, AIDS, recent childbirth, neuromuscular diseases and prolonged abnormal fast heart rhythms.

One-fifth of patients with dilated cardiomyopathy have a

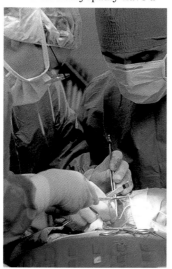

close relative who is affected and a variety of genes have been implicated in the disease.

DIAGNOSIS
Dilated cardiomyopathy can be diagnosed by:
■ A recording of the electrical activity in the heart (ECG) – this can show a wide variety of abnormalities and abnormal heart rhythms. It is important to recognize these since they may cause the cardiomyopathy or require specific treatment
■ Echocardiography – this uses ultrasound to study the size and function of the heart chambers and any valve abnormality
■ Cardiac catheterization with coronary angiography – this is often undertaken to exclude coronary artery disease, measure pressure within the heart and take a biopsy of the lining of the heart chambers to look for infiltrative diseases.

TREATMENT
If an underlying condition is found it should, if possible, be treated. If no cause is found, patients receive conventional treatment for heart failure.

This includes a combination of beta-blockers, angiotensin-converting enzyme inhibitors, anticoagulants in patients with very poor heart function to reduce the risk of blood clots forming within the dilated heart chambers and, occasionally, anti-arrhythmic drugs.

Severe cases of dilated cardiomyopathy require surgery. This may be done to treat leaky heart valves or to perform a heart transplant operation.

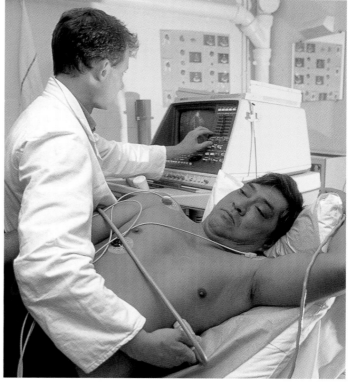

Some patients require pacemakers or implantable cardioverter defibrillators if there is abnormal conduction of impulses through the heart. Some individuals require surgery to reduce leaks through heart valves resulting from the heart's dilation and some will need heart transplantation.

RARE FORM
Arrhythmogenic right ventricular dysplasia is a rare form of cardiomyopathy. It mainly affects the right ventricle, in which the muscle

Dilated cardiomyopathy can be diagnosed by means of an echocardiogram. The heart can be viewed in detail on a screen and any abnormalities detected.

cells are replaced by fat or by fibrous tissue. It is assumed to be a genetic disease, and men are more commonly affected. The main feature is tachycardia (fast heart rate) arising in the abnormal right ventricle. Treatment is with anti-arrhythmic drugs and/or an implantable cardioverter defibrillator.

Alcoholic cardiomyopathy

Long-term excessive alcohol consumption (usually more than 10 years) can result in an individual developing dilated cardiomyopathy.

Alcohol can affect the heart directly, but damage to the heart can also result from the dietary deficiencies that are common in those who abuse alcohol.

Contaminants
Occasionally, damage to the heart may result from contaminants in the alcoholic drinks, such as cobalt, or excessive iron from the brewing of beer in oil drums.

Treating the disorder
Alcoholic cardiomyopathy is treated in the same way as heart

failure. Anticoagulation therapy carries risks, however, because of liver abnormality and the increased risk of head injury in alcoholics.

Alcohol avoidance
It is vital that affected individuals immediately cease all alcohol consumption. If this is done early enough in the disease, the heart can recover to almost normal. If heavy alcohol consumption continues, however, the outlook for the patient is poor.

Long-term alcohol abuse may cause cardiomyopathy. Those affected should avoid alcohol completely once a diagnosis has been made.

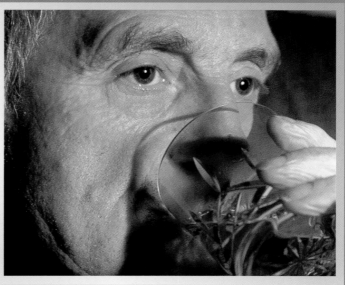

Endocarditis

Symptoms

Endocarditis, formerly known as subacute bacterial endocarditis (SBE), is a condition in which the heart valves or the endocardium (heart lining) become infected. Although usually a chronic illness, it may have a sudden onset. Virulent organisms such as *Staphylococcus aureus* may destroy the heart valves.

DISEASE PROCESS

Clumps of infecting organisms, fibrin and platelets, known collectively as 'vegetations', develop on an affected heart valve. These may destroy the valve cusps (flaps) and lead to regurgitation of blood flow if the valve becomes incompetent. The valve may become stenotic (narrowing of the orifice occurs). Endocarditis should be suspected in any patient with a fever in whom a heart murmur is heard.

CLINICAL FEATURES

Anaemia, flulike symptoms and weight loss are common, and a patient is often diagnosed with influenza or treated with antibiotics before endocarditis is confirmed. As the condition progresses, the following symptoms and signs may occur:
■ Vegetations may break off and circulate in the bloodstream, obstructing blood supply to an organ; this can cause myocardial infarction (death of part of the heart muscle) or a stroke
■ The walls of an artery may become weakened by an infected embolus, thus causing a haemorrhage
■ Vasculitis (inflammation of small blood vessels) produces small haemorrhages in the skin or mucosa, especially in the throat or the conjunctivae, retina (Roth's spots) or the nail beds (splinter haemorrhages); small red macules (spots) on the hands and painful swellings on the pads of the fingers and toes (known as Osler's nodes) may also occur
■ Haematuria (blood in the urine) due to glomerulonephritis, or infarction of the kidneys
■ In the late stages of the disease, finger-clubbing may occur.

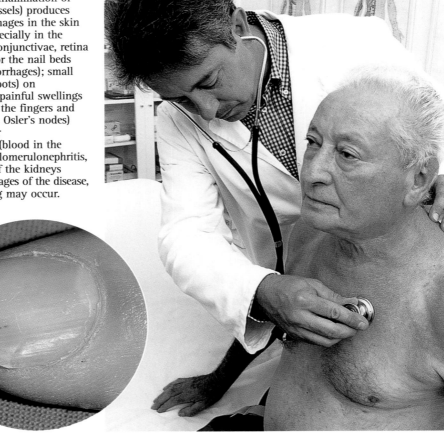

Inflammation of the blood vessels may occur as a result of endocarditis. This may be visible in the form of dark 'splinter haemorrhages' under the nails.

A heart murmur is a sign of an abnormal heart valve. A new murmur or a change in the character of a known murmur may indicate endocarditis.

Incidence

The prevalence is about 5–10 cases per 100,000 of the population in the UK. The incidence increases with age. Endocarditis is much more common in developing countries. It is now more common in older people with degenerative aortic or mitral valve disease.

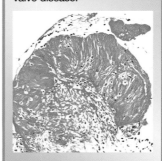

This micrograph shows a mitral valve affected by endocarditis. The red mass is a blood clot on the valve's upper surface.

Causes

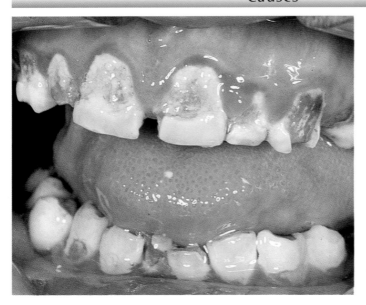

■ Endocarditis usually occurs on abnormal heart valves or on the low-pressure side of shunts such as ventricular septal defects; patients with prosthetic heart valves are vulnerable to infection
■ Patients with an internal pacemaker are susceptible to infective endocarditis
■ Staphylococcal infections from the skin and from conditions such as chronic eczema may cause the disease
■ Endocarditis may occur in patients with severe tooth decay or inflamed gums and after dental procedures or surgery.

Severe dental decay and gingivitis (gum inflammation) predispose patients to bacteria in the blood, and endocarditis may subsequently develop.

Diagnosis

Blood cultures are the key to investigating endocarditis. Three samples are usually taken over a 24-hour period before antibiotics are given in order to identify the infecting organism.

A range of blood tests will be performed. These may reveal typical complexes of immune system cells. Certain types of anaemia often develop.

OTHER TESTS
■ Chest X-rays may show evidence of heart failure, pulmonary emboli or abscess
■ Echocardiograms may identify vegetations; however, these need to be at least 2mm (¹/₁₆in) in size to be visualized; trans-oesophageal echocardiography is more sensitive in identifying vegetations
■ ECG readings are usually normal, but there may be a characteristic change, which indicates severe infection or possibly an aortic root abscess
■ Antibiotic sensitivities should be performed so that the organism can be targeted.

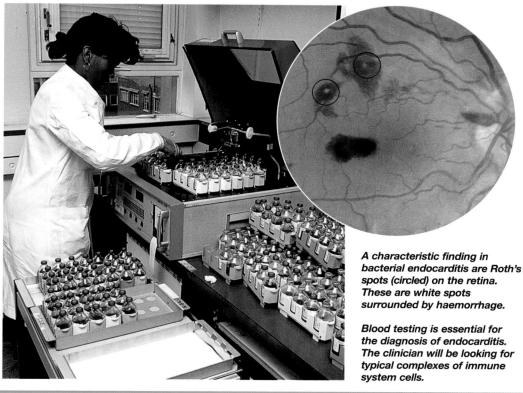

A characteristic finding in bacterial endocarditis are Roth's spots (circled) on the retina. These are white spots surrounded by haemorrhage.

Blood testing is essential for the diagnosis of endocarditis. The clinician will be looking for typical complexes of immune system cells.

Treatment

Any underlying source of infection must be sought. Dental radiographs, for example, may be taken to identify any dental root abscesses.

Antibiotics such as intravenous penicillin and gentamycin are usually started after taking blood cultures. Aminoglycosides will enhance the antibiotic effect. When the *Staphylococcus* bacterium is the cause, triple therapy using three different antibiotics may be given, as it is a very virulent organism. The drugs are usually administered intravenously for two weeks and then orally.

Surgery may be needed when any of the following are present:
■ Worsening heart failure
■ Uncontrolled infection
■ Prosthetic valves
■ Myocardial abscesses.

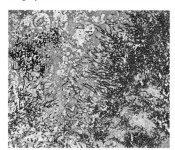

Cardiac surgery is often required when prosthetic heart valves are affected by endocarditis, as the infection is rarely treatable by antibiotics.

This micrograph shows Candida albicans, *which has caused fungal endocarditis on the patient's mitral valve. Antibiotics may help to ease the symptoms.*

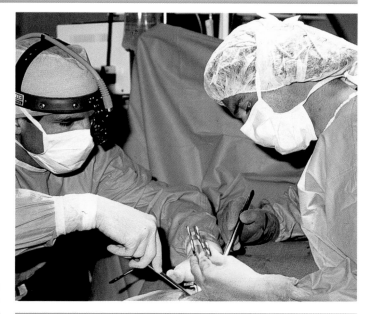

Prognosis

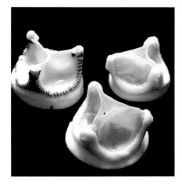

An early fall in the temperature and white blood cell count will accompany the patient's improvement. However, there is a high mortality rate of 20 per cent in the UK due to the high incidence of prosthetic valve endocarditis.

Patients with prosthetic heart valve endocarditis have a poor prognosis. This is because such infection does not respond well to antibiotics.

Prevention

Antibiotics are given prophylactically to dental patients who are known to suffer valvular heart disease or those about to undergo other potentially septic procedures.

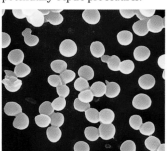

For dental treatment, amoxycillin by mouth is given before the start of treatment. Erythromycin may be used for those who are allergic to penicillin. Intravenous vancomycin is advised for those with prosthetic heart valves.

Staphylococcus aureus may cause severe cases of endocarditis. Drug therapy may prevent infection occurring in vulnerable patients.

Myocarditis

The heart is a muscular pump that circulates blood around the body. In myocarditis, the muscle of the heart becomes inflamed, and in rare cases this can lead to reduced pumping efficiency.

Myocarditis is a rare, but potentially serious, condition in which there is inflammation of the cells of the heart muscle (myocardium) called myocytes.

The condition is characterized by poor pumping action of the heart, disturbances of heart rhythm or changes in the electrical activity within the heart. Myocarditis can be difficult to diagnose since it has such non-specific symptoms.

Fortunately, the disease is short-lived and the outcome for most affected people is good. Myocarditis is often associated with a viral infection in adolescents and young adults, and is more common in men.

VIRAL CONNECTION
Mild myocarditis is thought to be a relatively common complication of diseases that affect the body's muscles – for example, a viral illness such as influenza. Only rarely would such a disease be severe enough to cause significant damage to the patient's heart function, and severe myocarditis is rare.

It is difficult to determine exactly how many people myocarditis afflicts because, in most cases, the symptoms of this condition are not specific or obvious, especially in the early stages of the illness.

Heart failure is a serious complication of myocarditis. In this condition, fluid can accumulate in the tissues, particularly around the ankles.

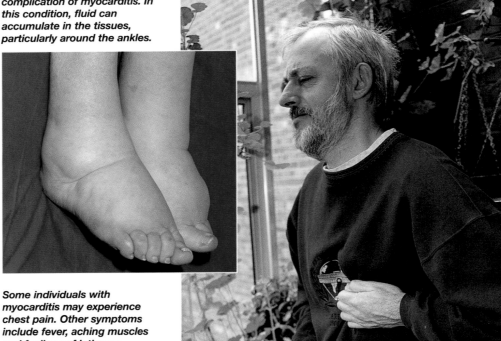

Some individuals with myocarditis may experience chest pain. Other symptoms include fever, aching muscles and feelings of lethargy.

SYMPTOMS
Most commonly, people with myocarditis experience flulike symptoms, such as:
■ fever
■ aching muscles
■ lethargy
■ chest pain.

Some patients develop palpitations originating in the upper (atria) or lower (ventricles) chambers of the heart.

The most serious symptoms of myocarditis result from damage to the myocardium itself, which may occur some time after the other symptoms have disappeared, and include signs of heart failure, such as breathlessness and swollen, oedematous ankles.

Causative factors

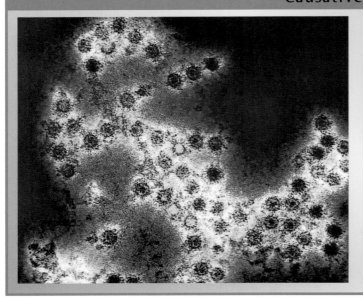

Myocarditis can be caused by the Coxsackie group of viruses (example shown here). These viruses are often responsible for the common cold.

In most cases, it is impossible to identify the cause of myocarditis. However, known causative factors include:
■ Viruses – in the West, the most common cause is thought to be viruses (especially Coxsackie B in Europe and North America), with myocarditis often developing after a viral respiratory or gastrointestinal infection
■ Bacteria – up to 25 per cent of cases are caused by the bacteria responsible for diphtheria (*Corynebacterium diphtheriae*), leptospirosis and Weil's disease

■ Fungi – for example, the fungus *Aspergillus*, which causes aspergillosis
■ Protozoa – the commonest cause of myocarditis in Central and South America is Chagas' disease, caused by *Trypanosoma* protozoa. *Toxoplasma gondii* can also cause myocarditis in people with inefficient immune systems
    Rarer causes include:
■ Toxins (for example, scorpion stings)
■ Radiation
■ Certain chemicals, such as lead
■ Allergic reactions to drugs (such as methyldopa, an older type of ood pressure-lowering drug)
■ Autoimmune diseases (such as systemic lupus erythematosus).

Investigating myocarditis

Because of the non-specific symptoms, many patients with mild myocarditis do not seek medical attention or, if they do, they are treated by their general practitioner.

Only patients with chest pain, palpitations or symptoms of heart failure are likely to be investigated further in a hospital setting. The diagnostic techniques on offer to doctors include:

■ Electrocardiography (ECG) – this records the electrical activity within the heart. Often, people with myocarditis have abnormal rhythms

■ Chest X-ray – the chest X-ray is usually normal unless there is overt heart failure, in which case there may be enlargement of the heart shadow, congestion in the lung fields and accumulation of fluid around the lungs (pleural effusions)

■ Echocardiography (cardiac ultrasound) – this investigation may show dilation of the heart chambers or reduced contraction in some or all areas; this test is useful to exclude other causes of heart failure. It may also detect any fluid collection around the heart (pericardial effusion), which is common in myocarditis

■ Blood tests – levels of cardiac enzymes (troponin proteins or

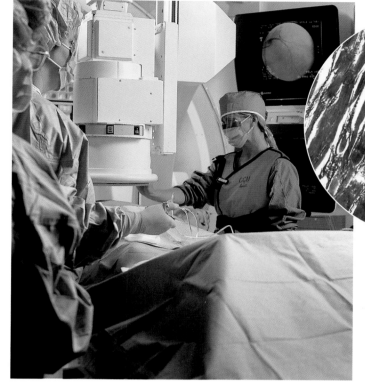

This greatly enlarged image shows heart muscle cells – myocytes. In myocarditis, these cells become damaged and fail to function adequately.

Coronary angiography enables visualization of the coronary arteries. This may help to exclude coronary artery disease as a cause of myocarditis.

creatine kinase) are usually elevated in the early phase of the illness as they are released from damaged heart muscle cells

■ Coronary angiography – investigation of the heart muscle's blood supply via the coronary arteries with coronary angiography is sometimes useful for excluding blocked vessels as a cause of the myocardial damage

■ Other imaging techniques – high-resolution techniques such

as magnetic resonance imaging are useful in certain situations

■ Biopsy – taking a small sample from the inner surface of the heart (endomyocardial biopsy) is seldom helpful and is now rarely performed.

Treatment options

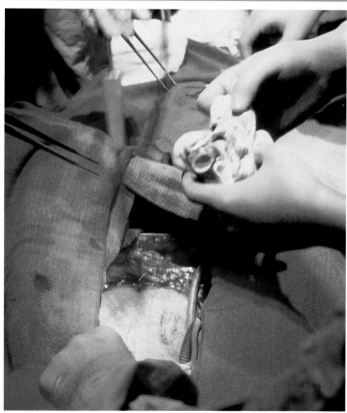

Myocarditis can cause enlargement of the heart. In a small percentage of people, a heart transplant may be required to treat severe heart failure.

Where a specific cause of myocarditis is found or is suspected, appropriate treatment is given. Otherwise, the treatment is supportive.

MEDICATION

Doctors may prescribe pain-killing drugs, such as non-steroidal anti-inflammatory drugs, or antibiotics for a bacterial infection. Diuretics and vasodilators (drugs to widen blood vessels) are used to relieve the symptoms of heart failure. Because of the heart damage, excessive exercise should be avoided in the early phase since this can worsen heart function and the long-term outcome.

As doctors understand more about myocarditis, it may be possible in the future to develop specific targeted treatments; at the moment, however, there is no good evidence for the use of either antiviral agents or

corticosteroids in most cases. Researchers are looking into the development of vaccines to certain viruses associated with myocarditis in the hope that vaccination will reduce the number of cases.

Prognosis

The long-term outcome of myocarditis is usually quite good, although babies under a year old and the elderly have a worse prognosis. More than half of patients make a good recovery, some regaining almost normal heart function. A proportion, however, progress to a condition in which the heart damage causes enlargement of the heart (severe dilated cardiomyopathy) and heart failure. Despite full medical treatment, these patients may need a heart transplant.

Surprisingly, those with a more severe illness in its early stages often do better in the long term than those with milder early disease.

Pericarditis

Causes

Pericarditis is inflammation of the pericardium (the three-layered membrane that surrounds the heart), which may result in pain in the chest.

The pericardium, or pericardial sac, contains fluid that lubricates the membranes, allowing them to move smoothly as the heart pumps. The pericardium also limits the distension of the heart and acts as a barrier to infection.

Pericarditis may be acute (sudden) or chronic (long-term) and is sometimes accompanied by inflammation of the muscle in the wall of the heart, known as myocarditis.

In the UK, the most common causes of acute pericarditis are:
■ Certain viral infections
■ Myocardial infarction
■ A bacterial infection carried to the pericardium in the bloodstream or directly from the lungs (relatively uncommon).

In developing countries, tuberculosis is a common cause.

Rare causes include:
■ Certain autoimmune disorders such as rheumatoid arthritis
■ Cancer – tumour cells may spread to the pericardium, typically from the lung or breast
■ Chest injury

■ Kidney failure.
In some cases of pericarditis, a cause is never found.

Pericarditis can result as a complication of other conditions. It commonly develops following a myocardial infarction (heart attack).

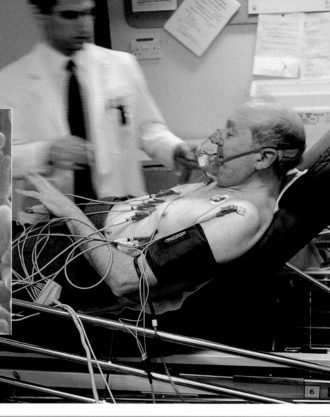

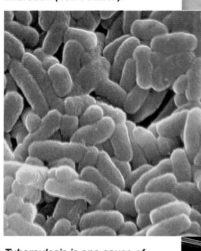

Tuberculosis is one cause of pericarditits. Mycobacterium tuberculosis is a rodlike bacterium that releases toxins which cause inflammation.

Symptoms

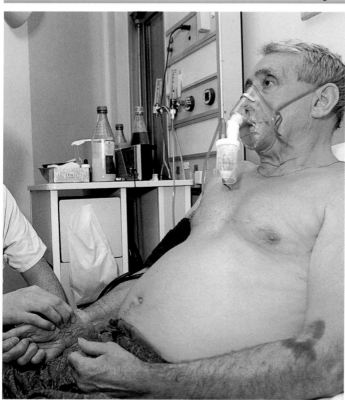

Symptoms can develop rapidly; in viral pericarditis, they can appear within hours.

ACUTE SYMPTOMS
The main symptoms of pericarditis are:
■ Pain in the centre of the chest behind the sternum (breastbone) that may spread to the shoulders and neck. The pain is typically made worse when taking a deep breath, lying down and swallowing, and improves when sitting forwards
■ A mild fever
■ Pericardial effusion, in which fluid accumulates within the pericardium and can stop the heart from pumping effectively. An effusion may cause a sensation of pressure behind the sternum. It can also lead to heart failure, which is typically associated with shortness of breath and ankle swelling.

Chronic pericarditis may develop following an infection. A fast, irregular pulse, known as atrial fibrillation, is an indication of the condition.

CHRONIC SYMPTOMS
In rare cases, persistent pericardial inflammation may follow pericarditis that is due to tuberculosis, a viral or bacterial infection or rheumatoid arthritis. The pericardium becomes thickened and scarred and tightens around the heart, preventing it from filling properly. Symptoms associated with this long-term condition, known as constrictive pericarditis, include:
■ Fatigue
■ Swelling of the ankles
■ Atrial fibrillation (fast and irregular heart beat).

Incidence

Pericarditis can occur at any age. Viral infections are the commonest cause of pericarditis in young adults. In older people, the condition is most often the result of a myocardial infarction. About 20 per cent of patients develop pericarditis shortly after a myocardial infarction.

Diagnosis

Suspected acute pericarditis may be investigated using a range of methods:
■ The cardinal sign of acute pericarditis is the 'pericardial rub', a characteristic rustling sound heard through a stethoscope as the inflamed pericardium moves
■ An electrocardiogram (ECG), a recording of the electrical activity in the heart, may show certain changes
■ A chest X-ray may be arranged, possibly followed by an echocardiogram. In echocardiography, an ultrasound scan is used to view the structure and movement of organs. In this case, the investigation is used to assess the thickness of the pericardium and to look for excess fluid around the heart
■ In addition, blood tests may be carried out to check for evidence of an autoimmune disease.

DETECTING AN EFFUSION
A pericardial effusion is often difficult to detect on clinical examination, although sometimes the heart sounds heard with a stethoscope are quieter than usual.

The ECG may show particular changes if an effusion is present, and serial chest X-rays may show rapid enlargement of the heart, occurring over days or even hours. Echocardiography may be used to confirm the diagnosis. Constrictive pericarditis may also be diagnosed by echocardiography.

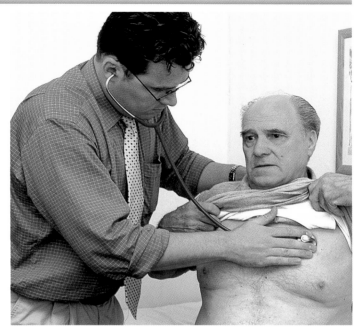

When listening to the heart through a stethoscope, a distinctive rustling sound may be heard. This 'pericardial rub' is a classic sign of pericarditis.

Treatment

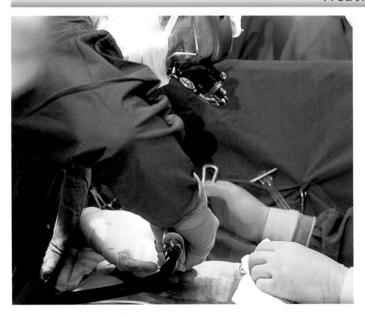

A persistent pericardial effusion may be treated with surgery. A small section of the pericardium can be removed to enable the fluid to drain away.

Pericarditis requires admission to hospital. Aspirin or stronger non-steroidal anti-inflammatory drugs may be given to relieve pain. Corticosteroids are sometimes prescribed to help relieve symptoms. In some cases, the underlying cause may require treatment. For example, pericarditis caused by a bacterial infection will require antibiotic therapy. It may also be necessary to drain the infected fluid from around the heart.

If a pericardial effusion is present, the accumulated fluid may be removed using a needle inserted through the chest wall.

The effusion may be drained completely; alternatively, a small sample of fluid may be withdrawn for diagnosis. If the fluid reaccumulates following drainage, the procedure may be repeated or a small piece of pericardium may be removed to allow continuous drainage.

In constrictive pericarditis, a large section of the pericardium may be surgically removed to restore normal heart function.

Prevention

There are no preventative measures for pericarditis. However, an early diagnosis is vital in order to avoid the occurrence of complications and to prevent the condition becoming life-threatening.

Prognosis

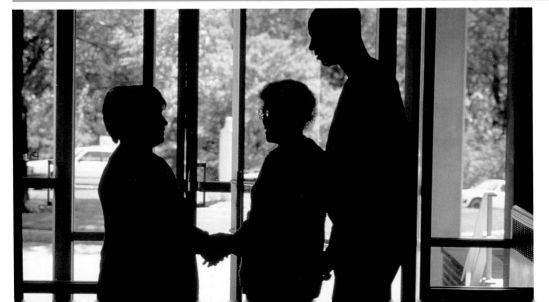

Viral pericarditis usually clears completely within days or weeks. In some people, however, the condition recurs after some months. Pericarditis caused by an autoimmune disorder can also recur.

Some types of pericarditis are particularly serious and, in rare cases, may be fatal. Acute bacterial pericarditis and constrictive pericarditis both fall into this category.

Most people with pericarditis recover fully and are discharged from hospital with no further problems. Patients are followed up on an outpatient basis.

Prevention of cardiovascular disease

Cardiovascular disease accounts for 30 per cent of all deaths worldwide, every year. Figures can be lowered by treatment on two fronts, at primary and secondary levels.

The cardiovascular disease epidemic affects millions of people across the world, killing around 15 million men and women each year. While it primarily affects developed countries, the problem is increasing worldwide.

TWO-PRONGED ATTACK
In order to reduce the number of premature deaths caused by cardiovascular disease, a two-fronted attack is necessary:
■ Primary prevention – to reduce the risk factors in the general population who do not yet have cardiovascular disease
■ Secondary prevention – to prevent the progression and consequences of cardiovascular disease where it already exists.

While primary prevention moderately reduces each individual's risk, it can be repeated across a whole population, and hugely reduces the total amount of disease.

Secondary prevention, however, greatly reduces the risks in an individual, but is only appropriate in a small number of individuals, so it has a lesser effect on the population as a whole.

Half of all those suffering myocardial infarction (heart attack) will die before reaching hospital. Many die within one hour of feeling the first symptom.

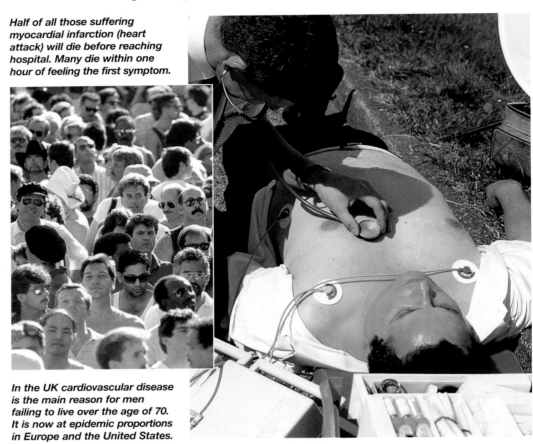

In the UK cardiovascular disease is the main reason for men failing to live over the age of 70. It is now at epidemic proportions in Europe and the United States.

The French paradox

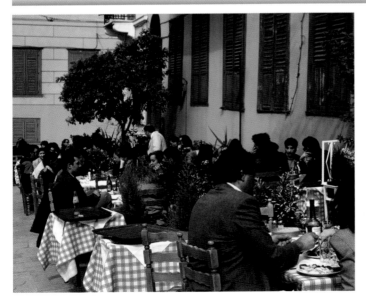

The French have about a quarter the risk of dying from coronary artery disease (CAD) as the British, despite similar risk factors.

Various explanations have been put forward for this:
■ The high consumption of red wine in France – moderate drinking certainly provides some protective effect, but this is due to the alcohol content rather than specifically to red wine
■ The frequent use of garlic and onions in France – this has not been confirmed in clinical trials
■ Lower smoker rates among French women – this may

The low rates of CAD in France have long puzzled UK doctors. However, recent changes in French diet (increasing fat intake) means the rate is rising.

explain their lower rates of CAD compared to French men, but does not explain the cross-channel divide
■ French doctors classify deaths from the complications of CAD as due to other factors – this accounts for part of the difference.

The real explanation is probably the 'time lag hypothesis'. CAD develops over many years, so risk factors in a person's life over the past decades are what determine the current risk. The French risk factor profile 30 years ago was much better than the UK's, largely because they ate much less animal fat.

They have now caught up with us in terms of animal fat consumption and are expected to catch up with our epidemic of CAD over the next decade.

The Big Three

The 'big three' modifiable risk factors for cardiovascular disease are smoking, high cholesterol and high blood pressure.

The vast majority of the epidemic can be explained by these factors alone. There is excellent evidence that they are involved in the development of cardiovascular disease and that reducing them greatly reduces the risks of the disease.

SMOKING

Smoking is the largest preventable cause of death in the developed world. It doubles the risks of coronary artery disease (CAD) in both men and women, the risks increasing with age and the number of cigarettes smoked.

Within two years of stopping smoking, the risk of dying of a heart attack halves; after 10 years, the risk falls to nearly that of a non-smoker. A 35-year-old smoker who gives up, adds an average of 3 years to his life.

There is good evidence that the various counselling and medical strategies to help people

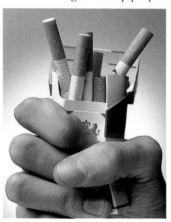

Many smokers are unaware of the risks of heart disease associated with smoking. It actually doubles the risk of suffering a CAD event.

stop smoking are successful in 20–40 per cent of cases and that this is highly cost-effective.

If we are to reduce the incidence of multiple smoking-related diseases in the future, we must help young people to see smoking as both dangerous and socially undesirable.

CHOLESTEROL

The epidemic of coronary disease is reflected in the epidemic of high cholesterol in the UK population. It is not appropriate to consider only those with 'above-average' cholesterol levels as being at risk. Even the average level of cholesterol in the developed world is far higher than the human body has evolved to cope with.

This results in progressive damage to every individual's arteries, and it is important that cholesterol levels are reduced by:
■ Primary prevention – a 10 per cent reduction in serum cholesterol, which can be achieved by good diet in most people, reduces the risk of dying of cardiovascular disease by 15 per cent
■ Secondary prevention – in individuals with metabolic abnormalities that result in excessively high cholesterol (such as familial hyper-lipidaemia) or an existing history of cardiovascular disease, treatment is necessary. In these people, a statin or other lipid-lowering agent may reduce the chance of dying from

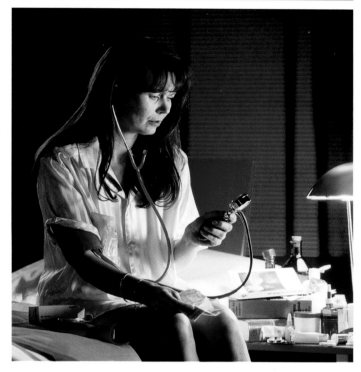

cardiovascular disease by up to 20 per cent. In assessing where treatment is appropriate, many authorities advocate a target serum cholesterol of less than 5mm for those with cardiovascular disease.

BLOOD PRESSURE

An increase in blood pressure of 7 mm Hg is associated with a 27 per cent increase in coronary heart disease and a 42 per cent increase in stroke. However, reducing blood pressure by 5–6 mm Hg cuts the risk of coronary heart disease by 15 per cent and of stroke by 42 per cent.

A number of life-style changes have been shown to

High blood pressure continues to be associated with a high risk of CAD. Where lifestyle changes fail to have effect, drug treatment will be necessary.

reduce blood pressure, including reducing weight, cutting down excessive alcohol consumption, reducing salt intake and increasing exercise.

Drug therapy may be used, depending on the level of blood pressure and the individual's risk of cardiovascular disease.

The ideal blood pressure is 130/80 or lower, and treatment may be given to those known to have cardiovascular disease or to be at high risk of developing it.

What is cholesterol?

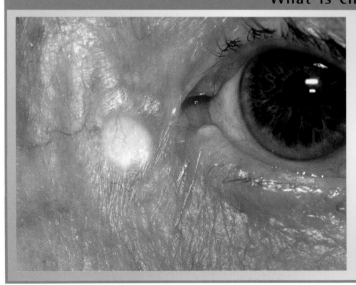

In people with inherited hyperlipidaemia, deposits of cholesterol can develop on the skin. These are known as xanthomas.

Fat is an essential component of every living cell in our bodies. There are three main types of lipid (fat) in the bloodstream: triglycerides (used for energy production); phospholipids (a cell membrane component) and cholesterol.

Fats are not soluble in water, and so have to be packaged in proteins (lipoproteins) to be transported around the body. The high-density lipoproteins (HDL) are high in protein, low in cholesterol and protect against

heart disease. The low-density lipoproteins (LDL) contain half as much protein and twice as much cholesterol; these are strongly associated with CAD.

Treatment
Reducing fat intake alone does not lower cholesterol sufficiently to reduce the risk of CAD. Treatment is through medication which targets the liver's control of lipids.

Familial hyperlipidaemia is a form of inherited lipid disorder, affecting 1 in 500 people in the UK. It causes very high LDL and visible deposits of cholesterol on the iris, skin and tendons. Without treatment, over half of those affected will show signs of CAD before the age of 60.

Reducing the risk of heart disease

Some people are more at risk of coronary artery disease
due to existing medical conditions, while others unwittingly
increase their risk through unhealthy lifestyle factors.

There are many other potential ways of reducing the risk of coronary artery disease (CAD).

HDL & TRIGLYCERIDES
Cholesterol is only one of the blood fats to be associated with coronary heart disease. A high level of triglycerides in the blood or a low level of high-density lipoprotein (HDL) is also associated with increased cardiovascular risks. Drug treatment may be necessary where these conditions exist alongside cardiovascular disease.

PHYSICAL ACTIVITY
The risk of CAD is almost halved by regular physical activity. This increases HDL, reduces total cholesterol and triglycerides, increases the body's sensitivity to insulin and reduces blood pressure.

OBESITY
The number of obese individuals (both adults and children) is steadily increasing in the developed world. Obesity can increase risk of developing CAD by up to 300 per cent.

HRT
It is well known that women have a lower risk of developing coronary heart disease than men until the menopause, when numbers tend to equalize. Studies are continuing into the possible effectiveness of hormone replacement therapy (HRT) to counteract this change.

ALCOHOL
Heavy alcohol consumption increases the risks of CAD, while those who drink one or two units per day are at lower risk than tee-totallers. The effects of alcohol depend mainly on its interactions with blood pressure, HDL levels and blood clotting.

DIET
Increasing our consumption of fresh fruit and vegetables reduces the risks of CAD. Studies into nutrients such as vitamin E, fish oils and folate are continuing.

Following a healthy diet is one of the main aspects of primary prevention of coronary disease. Fat intake should be lowered and vegetable content raised.

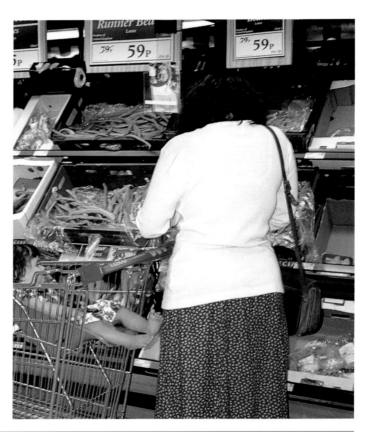

Diabetes

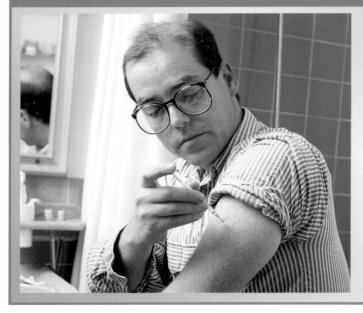

Hand in hand with the epidemic in CAD is an epidemic in diabetes, for very similar reasons. In over 90 per cent of cases, this is due to insulin resistance (type II diabetes) developing in older people rather than insulin deficiency (type I diabetes).

Although diabetes causes serious disorders by damaging small blood vessels, such as blindness and renal failure, most diabetics die from large blood vessel disease. Sixty per cent die of coronary disease, while 20 per cent die as a result of stroke and peripheral vascular disease.

The number of diabetics in the UK has increased dramatically as a result of modern dietary habits. Their risks of developing CAD is hugely increased.

Associated risks
Diabetes, particularly the insulin-resistant type, is strongly linked with all the known risk factors for CAD. When first diagnosed, over half of those affected have high blood pressure and over a third have high cholesterol. Many are also overweight, have a poor diet and take little exercise. In addition, they have high levels of glucose in the blood itself.

Treatment
Diabetes has been recognized in international treatment guidelines as a major risk factor. As a result, recommendations include:
- Firm control of blood glucose
- Low targets for blood pressure
- Statin treatment at lower cholesterol concentrations than in non-diabetics.

Drug treatment

Once an individual's risk factors have been assessed, certain drug treatments may be considered. In treating heart disease, there are three classes of drugs for which there is overwhelming evidence that their use save lives:
■ Aspirin (low-dose)
■ Beta-blockers
■ Angiotensin converting enzyme (ACE) inhibitors.

ASPIRIN
Originally, aspirin was used as an anti-inflammatory painkiller, but more recent research has shown its vital role in cardiovascular disease. This is due to its effects on the tiny platelet cells in our blood which are involved in the formation of blood clots.

Aspirin reduces the risk of dying from a heart attack by a quarter, and protects a wide range of people with vascular diseases against heart attack and stroke. It does, however, slightly increase the risks of bleeding.

The most recent studies have shown that aspirin can benefit not only those who have vascular disease but also those who are at a high risk of developing it. It has been proposed that anyone over 50 with one or more major cardiovascular risk factors should take regular aspirin.

BETA-BLOCKERS
This group of drugs has been widely used in cardiovascular medicine since the 1960s.

◀ Platelets (shown here in yellow) are cells in the blood responsible for clotting. Aspirin prevents these cells functioning and therefore 'thins' the blood.

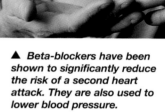

▲ Beta-blockers have been shown to significantly reduce the risk of a second heart attack. They are also used to lower blood pressure.

Beta-blockers are an excellent treatment for high blood pressure and in addition have been shown to reduce the risk of dying from a heart attack. When taken by those with CAD, they reduce the risk of further events by 18 per cent.

Beta-blockers act by blocking the effects of adrenaline on the body. The most widely used examples selectively affect the adrenaline receptors in the heart rather than those in the lungs, where it is possible they could exacerbate asthma.

These drugs also reduce the force of the heart's contraction, and for this reason they used to be avoided in patients with heart failure. However, exciting new evidence shows that this is exactly the group of patients who benefit most from this type of treatment. In these cases, it is essential that treatment is introduced gradually.

ACE inhibitors

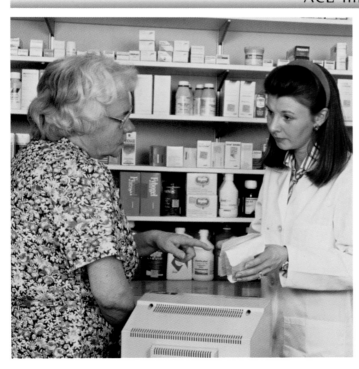

Over the past few years, there have been a number of reports in the press about 'miracle' drugs preventing cardiovascular disease. Most of these have focused on inhibitors of the angiotensin converting enzyme, or ACE inhibitors.

ORIGINAL USE
ACE inhibitors were originally used to treat high blood pressure. In the 1990s, they were also found to be extremely effective in treating heart failure, and they became the most important treatment in reducing the associated mortality rate.

It was then noticed that these drugs also lessened the number of other adverse effects, such as heart attacks.

A variety of drugs, used alone or in combinations, have proved successful in preventing heart disease. ACE inhibitors are often prescribed for 'at risk' people.

Studies have shown that in high-risk people who are not suffering from heart failure or uncontrolled high blood pressure, an ACE inhibitor called ramipril may reduce the rate of death, heart attack and stroke by over 20 per cent.

COMBINED TREATMENTS
ACE inhibitors may be used alone or in combination with other medicines in treating heart disease. It has been shown that the combination of another ACE inhibitor, perindopril, and a diuretic, indapamide, can cut the risk of a further stroke in someone who had already survived one by 25 per cent.

Treatment may combine any of the following: aspirin and other anti-platelet agents, anticoagulants, beta-blockers, heart rate-limiting calcium antagonists, cholesterol-lowering drugs (especially the statins) and ACE inhibitors.

Step-by-step pacemaker implantation

The electrical conduction system in the heart can sometimes become faulty. In these instances, it may be necessary to insert an artificial pacemaker to regulate the heartbeat.

An artificial pacemaker is a small device that is used to treat abnormally slow heart rhythms. In basic terms, the device is a computer with a battery attached to pacing leads that are implanted in or on the heart and provide electrical impulses when necessary. Normally, the heart has its own electrical conducting system and creates impulses that enable its chambers to contract in a precise order and with split-second timing. It is when this system fails in some way – due to a heart attack or fibrosis of the conducting system, for example – that a pacemaker may be required.

ADVANCES
The first pacemakers, which were approximately the size of a boiled-sweet tin, contained batteries that lasted for less than a year and simply stimulated the ventricles (lower chambers of the heart) at a fixed rate without any regard for the heart's underlying rhythm.

Modern devices are small, with batteries that last up to 10 years. They can sense activity in both the atria (upper chambers of the heart) and the ventricles, putting in impulses to coordinate the heart's contraction only when required. Some can increase the heart rate on exercise and decrease it at night, while others can adjust the delay between atrial and ventricular contraction to allow as many heartbeats as possible to be conducted down the normal pathway.

QUALITY OF LIFE
Although expensive (each pacemaker set costs £1000-£3500), pacemaker implantation is one of the most cost-effective treatments in modern medicine, improving quality of life for more than 15,000 new patients each year in the UK.

SPECIFIC SENSITIVITY
Pacemakers can sense activity from and stimulate: just the atria, if the sino-atrial node is affected and the atrio-ventricular node is functioning normally; just the ventricles if there is no organized atrial activity (atrial fibrillation); or both if the atrio-ventricular node is affected and there is loss of atrio-ventricular coordination.

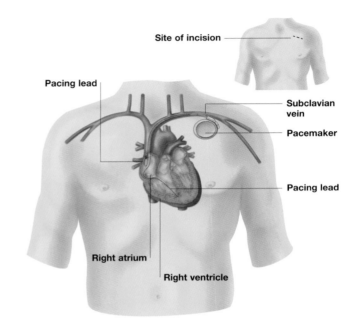

Site of incision

Pacing lead

Subclavian vein

Pacemaker

Pacing lead

Right atrium

Right ventricle

A pacemaker is a computerized device that sits under the skin. Leads are passed from the pacemaker down a blood vessel to one of the heart chambers.

Slow heart rhythms

Conducting system

Sino-atrial node

Electrical impulses

Atrioventricular node

In the healthy heart, the pulse rate is controlled by a group of specialized pacemaker cells in the right atrium, known as the sino-atrial (SA) node. An electrical impulse spreads from these cells across the atria, which contract, squeezing blood into the ventricles. The impulse then reaches another group of specialized cells, the atrioventricular (AV) node, which delays just long enough for the ventricles to fill, before transmitting the impulse down the specialized conduction tissue to the ventricles. The ventricular muscle contracts in a coordinated fashion, resulting in a normal heartbeat.

Safety mechanism
Every cell in the heart is capable of contracting spontaneously; the heart rate is controlled by the fastest-firing cells – usually the SA node. If the SA node fails, e AV node sets the heart rate; if this also fails, other cells in the heart muscle will take over. Malfunction of the SA node, the AV node or the specialized conducting system results in:
■ A very slow heart rate (bradycardia)
■ A heart rate that does not increase appropriately on exercise.

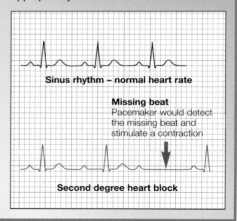

Sinus rhythm – normal heart rate

Missing beat
Pacemaker would detect the missing beat and stimulate a contraction

Second degree heart block

The heart contains specialized tissue that generates electrical impulses which cause the heart to contract. In the event of a faulty conducting system, a pacemaker will provide the necessary stimuli.

In some people, the heart beats too slowly (bradycardia). In heart block (a type of bradycardia – shown right), which can develop after a heart attack, a pacemaker is often required to stimulate contraction.

How pacemakers work

A pacemaker is a sophisticated computer attached to a battery, electronic sensors and a pulse-generator; all are housed within a small metal case. Pacemakers have either one lead (single-chamber pacemakers) or two leads (dual-chamber), which are inserted into the heart through veins. The pacemaker is able both to detect the electrical impulses that are naturally

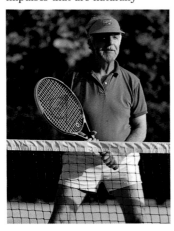

Modern-day pacemakers are constantly being adapted to allow normal activity. Some devices can increase the heart rate during physical exercise.

produced by the nodes in the heart wall, and to transmit impulses itself when needed.

SETTING THE PACE
The pacemaker senses the electrical signals from the heart generated with each heartbeat, and starts a programmable counter. If, for example, the pacemaker is set to maintain a heart rate of at least 60 beats per minute, the counter would be set to count for one second. If another heartbeat occurs during this time, the counter would start again from zero, but if no spontaneous heartbeat occurred, the pacemaker would deliver an impulse through the pacing lead to initiate a paced heartbeat. The counter is then re-started and the process is repeated.

INCREASED RATE
Some pacemakers can adjust the heart rate automatically so that the pulse rate increases on exercise. These pacemakers contain an accelerometer or other device used to detect movement. When this is vigorous, the counter parameter is changed to less than one second, resulting in a heart rate of at least 100 beats per minute.

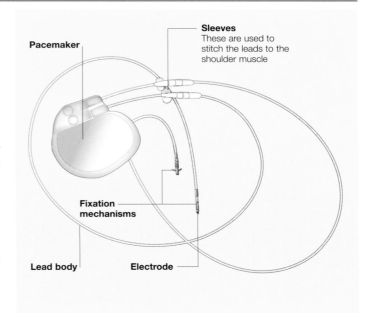

Pacemaker

Sleeves
These are used to stitch the leads to the shoulder muscle

Fixation mechanisms

Lead body

Electrode

MODIFICATIONS
Pacemakers are continually being modified. Many are now able to store large quantities of information and details of any abnormal rhythms over the months. This enables doctors to provide appropriate treatment.

Although pacemakers are used only to manage abnormally slow

The pacemaker is a computerized device containing a battery. The tips of the leads (electrodes) both detect and transmit impulses.

or irregular heartbeats, current developments include work on a pacemaker to help people with congestive heart failure.

Pacemaker technologies

The basic principles of pacemakers can be utilized to treat other rhythm abnormalities.

Some people with heart failure have incoordination not just between atrial and ventricular contraction but between different areas of the left ventricle, the heart's main pumping chamber. This can reduce the efficiency of the heart, leading to heart failure.

This type of incoordination can be re-synchronized by placing leads not only in the right atrium and ventricle, but also on the left ventricle via the coronary sinus (the main vein draining blood from the heart muscle back into the right atrium). Studies have shown dramatic improvements in some patients using this method.

Atrial fibrillation
The commonest disturbance of heart rhythm is atrial fibrillation, which affects some 5–10 per cent of people over the age of 65. In this condition, the atria have a chaotic electrical activity and blood flows passively into the ventricles rather than being actively pumped. This can reduce the volume of blood pumped in each heartbeat by up to 25 per cent and result in palpitations and breathlessness on exertion. Pacemakers have now been developed to reduce the occurrence of atrial fibrillation by preventing the types of pauses between heartbeats which can allow atrial fibrillation to start.

ICDs
Pacemakers can treat slow heart rhythms but cannot prevent the heart from beating too rapidly. Some people are at risk of dangerously fast heart rhythms (ventricular tachycardia and

During a cardiac arrest, a defibrillator can be used to restart the heart. 'At risk' patients can be fitted with an implantable defibrillator.

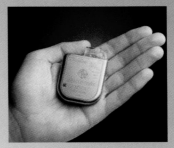

Implantable defibrillators are slightly larger than a pace-maker and provide an electrical shock if a life-threatening heart arrhythmia develops.

ventricular fibrillation), which can cause sudden death. Where someone has survived one of these dangerous rhythms or has been found to be at high risk of developing one, they can be fitted with an implantable cardioverter defibrillator (ICD) in the same way as a pacemaker.

This device can perform all the functions of a pacemaker but can also treat ventricular tachycardia or fibrillation with anti-tachycardia pacing or deliver an electrical current to shock the heart back into a normal rhythm.

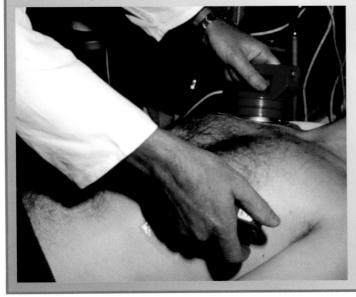

Hypertension

Hypertension – high blood pressure – is a symptomless condition
of unknown cause in most patients. It is a major contributory risk
factor for both coronary artery disease and stroke.

In a healthy person, blood pressure is tightly maintained at a level which ensures that the body's tissues receive an adequate supply of oxygen. This is primarily carried out by a region of the brain called the medulla, situated just above the spinal cord. Although it is quite normal for blood pressure to rise under certain circumstances – during periods of stress, for example – a persistent, raised blood pressure can be dangerous. This is because high blood pressure has been implicated in the development of circulatory disorders, such as coronary artery disease, stroke and peripheral vascular disease.

MEASURING
BLOOD PRESSURE

The most common method of measuring blood pressure is by sphygmomanometry, which can be done either manually or automatically. The technique involves wrapping a cuff containing a rubber balloon around the upper arm and inflating it to compress the brachial artery (found in front of the elbow) to such an extent that blood flow to the forearm ceases. The doctor or nurse then places a stethoscope over the artery 'downstream' from the cuff and slowly deflates the cuff. The pressure at which the blood can be heard flowing through the artery is then noted, as is the pressure at which the pressure sounds disappear.

This procedure gives the operator a value for the patient's blood pressure and this is expressed as a fraction, for example, 120/80 millimetres of mercury (mm Hg).

The upper value is an indicator of the 'peak' pressure generated within the artery as the heart pumps blood into the arterial circulation, and is termed the systolic blood pressure.

The lower value, known as the diastolic pressure, is the pressure present within the artery after the heart has completed the ejection phase.

Therefore, the blood pressure measurement is a reflection of the pressure required both to continue the forward flow of blood along the artery and to keep the arteries in an open, unobstructed state.

Modern blood pressure measuring machines can be programmed to repeat the cycle as often as required, and the the blood pressure value obtained can be displayed on a monitor.

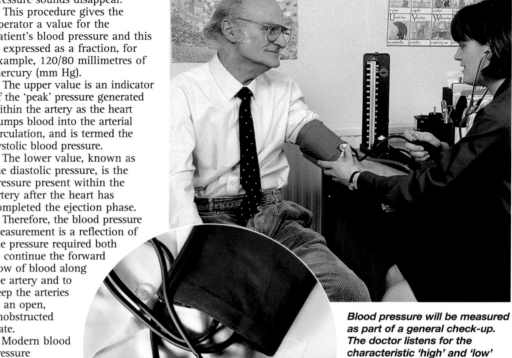

Blood pressure will be measured as part of a general check-up. The doctor listens for the characteristic 'high' and 'low' values relating to the blood pressure pulses.

The traditional method of blood pressure measurement uses a sphygmomanometer. It consists of a pump and a cuff linked to a pressure gauge, usually a column of mercury.

Where is blood pressure measured?

The brachial artery is the most commonly used artery from which to measure blood pressure. This is primarily because this artery is close to the surface of the skin in most people and, more importantly, it is easily compressed for a short period by placing a cuff around the upper arm.

This reading is a close approximation of the true arterial pressure. However, there are instances, such as in critically ill patients, when an accurate and continuous measurement is required. A true arterial pressure is therefore obtained by inserting a cannula directly into a peripheral artery.

A one-off measurement is virtually meaningless, since a large number of factors, such as emotional stimuli or physical activity, can affect the reading. It is important to recognize this because it explains why a doctor will often take several readings before making a diagnosis.

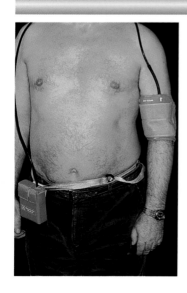

Ambulatory blood pressure equipment measures blood pressure at regular intervals, giving a more accurate picture of blood pressure over time.

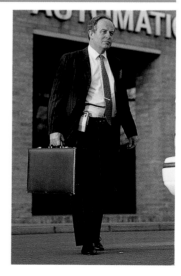

Ambulatory equipment can be worn throughout the day. This means that patients do not need to stop continually to measure their blood pressure.

Symptoms of hypertension

Long-term hypertension has a number of effects on the circulatory system and on important organs. It is a known risk factor for serious conditions such as stroke, heart disease and kidney failure.

High blood pressure is not, in itself, problematic, but the harmful effects that hypertension has on many organs of the body are significant.

The strain that hypertension places on arteries results in damage and weakening of the walls of these vessels, rendering them susceptible to plaque and thrombus (blood clot) formation. The arteries can also become blocked, often with disastrous consequences, such as in a patient who suffers a heart attack. In localized areas of weakness, it is not uncommon for arteries to bulge abnormally, forming an aneurysm (a balloon-like swelling), and occasionally these rupture, causing a fatal haemorrhage.

At tissue level, hypertension often results in the complete disruption of small blood vessels. It is now acknowledged that hypertension is a major risk factor for stroke, cardiac failure, ischaemic heart disease, kidney failure and peripheral vascular disease.

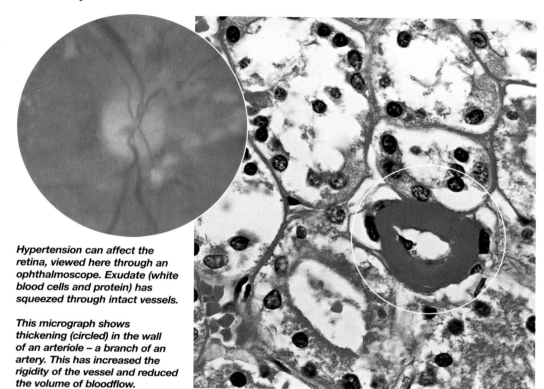

Hypertension can affect the retina, viewed here through an ophthalmoscope. Exudate (white blood cells and protein) has squeezed through intact vessels.

This micrograph shows thickening (circled) in the wall of an arteriole – a branch of an artery. This has increased the rigidity of the vessel and reduced the volume of bloodflow.

Factors in diagnosing hypertension

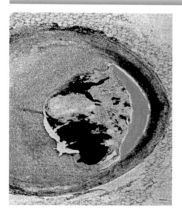

There is no such thing as 'normal' blood pressure, other than in the statistical sense of those who fall within a certain range of the average of the normal population. Equally, there is no blood pressure value above which a doctor must always treat.

Hypertension is damaging to blood vessels and encourages atherosclerosis (pictured). Such arterial blockages increase the problem, leading to even higher blood pressure.

Important factors in the decision-making process of whether or not to treat are:
- The patient's sex
- Age (generally blood pressure increases with age)
- Medical history
- Family history
- Lifestyle (such as smoking, alcohol intake and lipid [fat] and cholesterol status).

The presence of an elevated blood pressure level alone rarely requires immediate therapy unless patients show signs of hypertensive crisis.

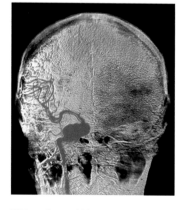

When should hypertension be treated?

There has been a great deal of research in attempting to define when a person's blood pressure is significant enough to warrant treatment. Amongst its recommendations, the British Hypertension Society suggests that treatment, in the form of medication, is recommended if the sustained diastolic blood pressure is greater than 100mm Hg on three or more readings taken a week apart (the average adult blood pressure is around 120/80mm Hg).

Treatment is also recommended if the sustained diastolic pressure is greater than 90mm Hg over six months, in the presence either of a systolic pressure greater than 100mm Hg or if there is evidence of organ damage. In addition, a sustained systolic pressure of greater than 200mm Hg should be treated.

Around a fifth of the UK population have a blood pressure of greater than 160/95. Many of these remain undiagnosed.

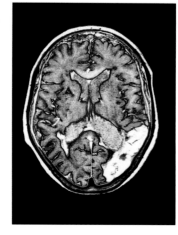

This coloured X-ray shows an aneurysm (swelling) in one of the carotid arteries, which supply blood from the heart to the neck and head. The incidence of brain aneurysms is greatly increased in patients with hypertension.

This coloured MR scan is a section through the brain of a 72-year-old woman. She has suffered a stroke, and internal bleeding has deprived parts of the brain of oxygen. These regions are shown in white. Strokes are much more common in people with hypertension.

Causes of hypertension

In the majority of cases of hypertension, a specific cause cannot be identified – treatment is based on the patient's symptoms. Some patients develop hypertension secondary to other conditions.

Despite years of research, there are no known causes for the high blood pressure seen in 95 per cent of hypertensive patients. Such patients are described as having 'essential', or 'primary', hypertension.

There are, however, a number of risk factors that are thought to be important, including a family history of high blood pressure, stress, alcohol intake and obesity. These risk factors may cause hypertension by acting to narrow the arteries themselves, or, alternatively, may affect the way that blood pressure is regulated by the brain.

Primary hypertension is diagnosed after eliminating the remaining five per cent of patients who have 'secondary' hypertension and in whom a causative factor is found. These patients often tend to be younger in age.

Causes of secondary hypertension include:
■ Inflammatory kidney diseases
■ Endocrine diseases, including Cushing's syndrome, Conn's syndrome, and acromegaly
■ Pre-eclampsia – hypertension caused by pregnancy
■ Congenital narrowing of a short section of the aorta (coarctation of the aorta)
■ Drug-related factors – for example, some oral contraceptives increase blood pressure in a small proportion of women.

Patients with hypertension are frequently either symptom-free or complain of what might at first appear to be non-specific symptoms, such as headache and lethargy. Unfortunately, in many patients hypertension is discovered only when one of the complications of the condition occurs, such as stroke, heart attack, renal failure or blindness.

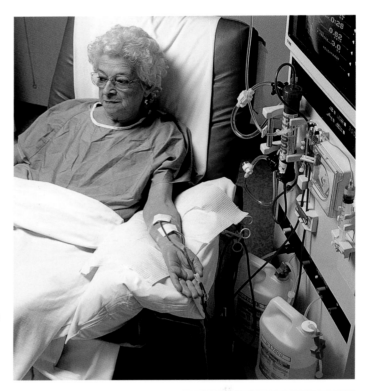

Patients with renal disease, such as this dialysis patient, are particularly prone to secondary hypertension. This occurs when the high blood pressure is the result of an existing condition.

Further investigations

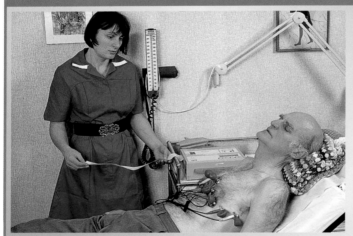

The extent to which a patient is investigated for the cause of their hypertension depends on a number of factors. These include the patient's age, the degree of the hypertension, the severity of the symptoms and the facilities available (some investigations must be carried out in a hospital setting only – for example, kidney scans and angiograms). As blood pressure increases with age, higher values are accepted in elderly patients with hypertension before either investigation or treatment is undertaken.

The heart may be visualized by ultrasound scanning. In this false-colour ultrasound scan, the patient's left ventricle (circled) is unusually large, as the heart is having to work too hard.

ECG examinations are carried out to assess cardiac function. This includes checking for any increases in the size of the heart and inadequate blood flow.

Routine investigations
In the first instance, the doctor will take time to obtain a thorough history from the patient and perform a full examination; this can often highlight a possible cause and thereby save the patient having to be subjected to a large number of investigations. However, there are certain routines that are performed principally to assess cardiac and renal function. These include:
■ Chest radiograph and electrocardiogram (ECG)
■ Measurement of blood urea and electrolytes
■ Examination of a sample of urine, together with a 24-hour collection of urine.

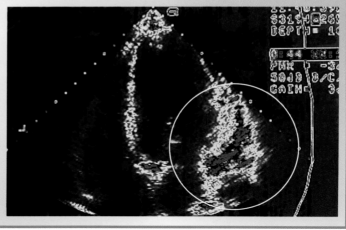

Treating hypertension

The management of hypertension is based on identifying a primary cause, long-term drug treatment and, if appropriate, modifying the patient's lifestyle.

The principles of hypertension treatment fall under three main categories:
■ Therapy directed specifically at those patients who have secondary hypertension; that is, those in whom a cause has been found. For example, surgery performed to alleviate hypertension due to renal artery stenosis
■ Non-drug treatment and lifestyle modification. These include stopping smoking, weight reduction, decreasing alcohol consumption, reducing dietary salt intake and reducing stress
■ Drug treatment; in most cases, this is for life. This emphasizes the need to establish a firm diagnosis prior to commencing therapy. There is a huge variety of so-called 'anti-hypertensive' drugs available on the market. Although these drugs lower the patient's blood pressure, they combat the symptoms rather than the cause of the disease.

Excessive alcohol consumption is a known risk factor in hypertension. Alcohol can also interfere with medication; its high calorific content can also make weight control difficult.

Smoking causes stiffening of the arteries (atherosclerosis). This can lead both to hypertension and coronary artery disease.

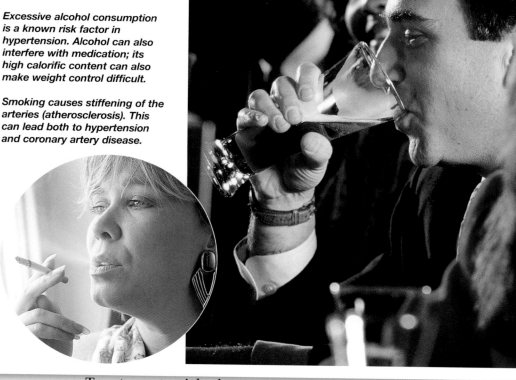

Treatment with drugs

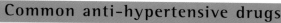

Most doctors have their personal preferences for treatment, both in terms of the drugs that are used and the regimen prescribed. However, most regimens begin with a single-agent treatment, escalating to multi-agent therapy if hypertension persists.

Tenormin is a trade name for the beta-blocker atenolol. These drugs block the action of adrenaline, causing blood vessels to widen and the heart to slow.

In the majority of cases, hypertension is controlled by oral medication, but a small percentage of patients require more powerful anti-hypertensive medication. In some cases, this must be given intravenously in a hospital environment.

HOW DO DRUG TREATMENTS WORK?
Blood pressure depends on three factors: the force with which the heart pumps out blood; the

Captopril is a member of the ACE-inhibitor group of drugs. It works by reducing the production of a protein that causes arteries to constrict.

diameter of the blood vessels (smaller vessels produce a larger pressure); and the volume of blood in the circulation. Thus, anti-hypertensive treatments act to reduce the strength of the heartbeat, to dilate the blood vessels or to reduce the blood's volume.

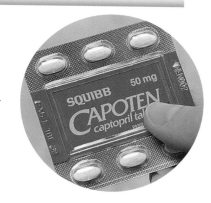

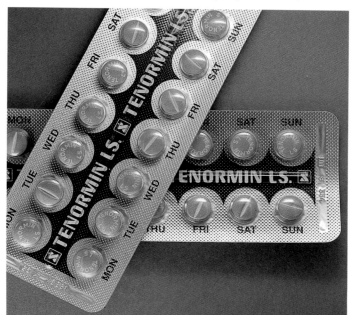

Common anti-hypertensive drugs

There are a number of anti-hypertensive drugs in use, and these include:
■ **ACE-inhibitors** (such as captopril). These drugs work by reducing the production of a protein (called angiotensin), which causes arteries to contract
■ **Beta blockers** (such as atenolol) reduce the force of contraction of the heart
■ **Vasodilators** (such as diltiazem) act on the muscles in the blood vessels to prevent them from constricting
■ **Centrally acting antihypertensives** (such as clonidine and methyldopa) act on the neurones in the brain that control blood vessel size
■ **Sympatholytics** (such as prazosin) block the nerve signals that trigger constriction of blood vessels
■ **Diuretics** (such as frusemide) act on the kidneys to increase water excretion and so reduce blood volume.

Most of these anti-hypertensive medications are associated with side effects, and it is important for patients to tell the doctor of any difficulties they may be experiencing.

Deep vein thrombosis

Symptoms

A deep vein thrombosis (DVT) is a blood clot (thrombus) that forms in a vein deep in the body, rather than one just beneath the skin. Some thrombi grow large enough to obstruct the blood flow and damage the valves of the vein.

RISK FACTORS
Veins in the legs and pelvis are the most common sites for deep vein thrombosis. Risk factors include conditions that damage vein walls, slow the flow of blood or increase the tendency of the blood to clot.

COMMON SYMPTOMS
Possible symptoms include:
- Pain – a deep vein thrombosis in the lower leg may cause pain and tenderness in the calf, worse when the foot is flexed, but most cause no symptoms; a thrombosis in the groin or pelvis may cause severe leg pain
- Swelling of the leg
- Blue discoloration (cyanosis) of the leg, due to lack of oxygen
- White leg – from spasm of the neighbouring arteries
- Feeling of heat in the leg
- Congested leg veins
- Slight fever.

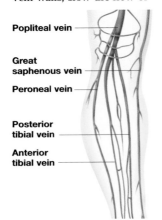

Popliteal vein

Great saphenous vein

Peroneal vein

Posterior tibial vein

Anterior tibial vein

◀ *Thrombi usually develop in the deep veins of the leg, shown here. A blood clot forms in a vein deep within the body rather than just under the skin.*

▶ *Swelling of this patient's left leg (right of picture) indicates a deep vein thrombosis. The leg appears red and inflamed and is warm to the touch.*

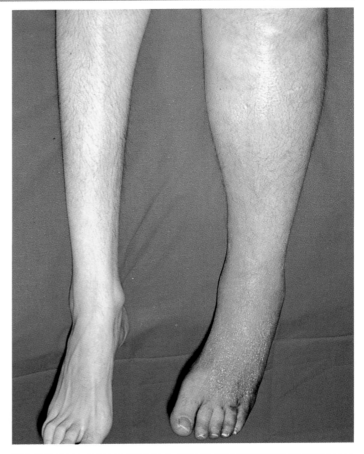

Pulmonary embolism

Pulmonary embolism is a highly dangerous complication of a deep vein thrombosis in the leg or pelvis. It occurs when a thrombus breaks free (forming an embolus) and travels through the bloodstream to the heart.

If an embolus is large enough, it may block the arteries leading from the right side of the heart to the lungs (pulmonary embolism), causing acute heart failure or sudden death. With smaller emboli, sections of the lung tissue may die (infarct), leading to acute pain on inspiration (pleuritic pain) or the coughing up of blood (haemoptysis).

Pulmonary emboli are rare with calf thromboses, which tend to be small. Thrombi formed higher in the leg and in the pelvis are more likely to produce pulmonary emboli.

In this image of lungs affected by pulmonary embolism, the patient's right lung is normal. The left lung (circled) shows infarction caused by an embolus blocking an artery.

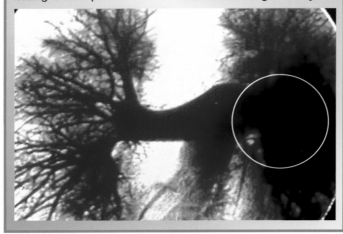

Incidence

Deep vein thromboses are common, with the incidence increasing with age:
- Each year, up to three people per 1000 aged 65–69 years develop a deep vein thrombosis
- The figure rises to eight per 1000 in those aged 85–89 years
- Deep vein thromboses occur in 50 per cent of patients after prostatectomy and in one-third of patients after a myocardial infarct (heart attack)
- Over 60 per cent of all people dying in hospital and examined post-mortem are found to have a thrombosis in a leg vein.

WOMEN AT RISK
Women are at greater risk of DVT than men as pregnancy, the combined (oestrogen-containing) Pill and hormone replacement therapy (HRT) drugs increase their risk. Each year in the USA, more women die from a pulmonary embolism following a DVT than from breast cancer.

Women are more likely than men to suffer from deep vein thrombosis. Taking hormone replacement therapy (HRT) drugs increases the risk.

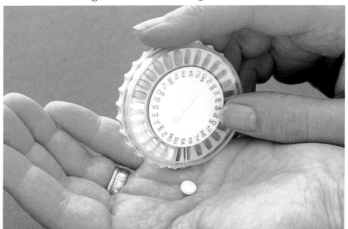

Causes

Deep vein thromboses sometimes occur for no apparent reason, but known risk factors include:

- Age over 40 years
- Obesity
- Immobility, bed rest for more than four days, inactive long-distance travel (particularly if associated with dehydration), recent stroke
- Medication with oestrogens (such as the combined oral contraceptive pill or HRT)
- Pregnancy and the puerperium (the period of up to six weeks after childbirth)
- Trauma – particularly to the pelvis, hips or legs
- Surgical procedures – especially orthopaedic, neurosurgical, urological and gynaecological procedures
- Personal or family history of deep vein thrombosis or pulmonary embolism
- Serious illness, such as heart failure, cancer, myocardial infarct, and inflammatory bowel disease, such as ulcerative colitis
- Severe varicose veins
- Hypercoagulability of the blood; for example, in polycythaemia, the haemoglobin concentration is abnormally high and the blood is thicker than normal; in thrombocythaemia, the number of platelets in the blood increases
- Inherited abnormalities of the blood – the most common is the factor V Leiden mutation, present in about five per cent of the population. This, and similar defects, increase the risk of thrombosis already present in women who are taking the contraceptive pill.

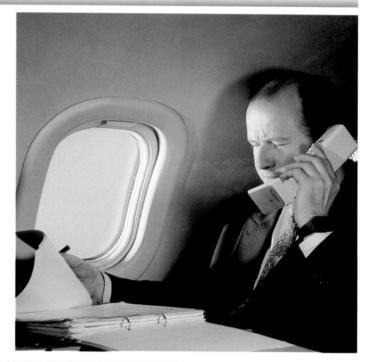

Inactive long-distance travel is a known risk factor. Flying in particular can cause deep vein thrombosis due to the likelihood of dehydration.

Treatment

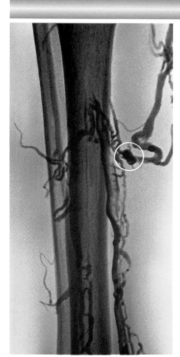

This venogram shows a large thrombus (dark red, circled) in the calf. A venogram is produced by injecting a radiopaque dye into a vein.

The main aim of treatment is to prevent pulmonary embolism by limiting the size of the thrombus. Treatments include:

Anticoagulant therapy
- Heparin

Intravenous heparin almost immediately reduces blood clotting and should be given as soon as possible. Treatment should continue for at least five days, either intravenously or with subcutaneous injections.

- Warfarin

Oral anticoagulation with warfarin is started on the first day of treatment, but is not effective for up to 72 hours. Once the effect of warfarin is established, heparin can usually be discontinued. The dose of warfarin must be carefully controlled with regular blood tests. It should be avoided in pregnancy because of risk to the fetus.

Thrombolytic therapy
- Clot-dissolving therapy – with streptokinase, for example – is occasionally used to dissolve large clots and may be effective in severe pulmonary embolism, although bleeding can occur.

Clot extraction
- Surgical removal of a clot or embolus may be attempted if there is a massive pulmonary embolus or very large thrombus in the groin or pelvis.

General measures
- Mobilization
- Leg elevation
- Compression bandaging.

Diagnosis

The symptoms of deep vein thrombosis are often mild, ill-defined or non-existent. Clinical examination is often an inaccurate way of making the diagnosis. Patients with suspected deep vein thrombosis should be referred urgently to hospital.

Investigations include:
- Doppler ultrasonography – ultrasound waves are used to study blood flow. It is now the investigation of choice, as it is reliable and non-invasive
- Venography – radiopaque liquid injected into a vein shows on X-ray as the liquid flows towards the heart. The procedure may be painful and technically difficult. Ultrasonography now usually makes venography unnecessary
- Blood tests – measuring circulating D-dimer concentrations may be used in addition to ultrasonography.

Prognosis

Up to 30 per cent of thromboses in calf veins disappear spontaneously; about 50 per cent remain for long periods; and 20–30 per cent of clots became detached and travel towards the heart, which can be life-threatening.

In the long term, about 60 per cent of deep vein thrombosis patients develop a chronic obstruction of the deep veins in the leg, which can give rise to pain and swelling.

Prevention

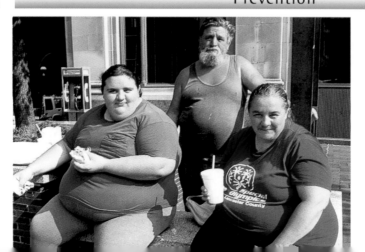

Exercise and weight control are important, and aspirin may provide some protection. Preventive anticoagulant treatment should be considered for high-risk patients. Intermittent pneumatic leg compression devices offer protection during surgery.

A known risk factor for DVT is obesity. A weight control programme can therefore significantly reduce the risk.

How ageing affects the brain

During the average person's lifetime, a small percentage of brain cells die and are never replaced. This cell loss hardly affects function, but degenerative disorders have more serious effects.

By the time people reach 80, their brains weigh about seven to eight per cent less than they did in their 20s. The reason for this is that brain cells, or neurons, are not replaced when they die.

LOSS OF BRAIN CELLS
The rate of loss varies between different areas of the cerebral cortex (grey matter). But since we are born with 100 billion neurons and a lifetime's loss represents only about three per cent of the total, this does not present a significant problem.

It has also been suggested that it is the number of interconnections between the cells, rather than the number of cells, which is important for cognitive function.

WASTE MATERIAL
Another change in the ageing brain is that granules of a yellowish-brown pigment called lipofuscin accumulate in the neuronal cell bodies. This material is thought to represent waste production. At around the age of 60, microscopic examination of the brain will reveal senile plaques of degenerated cells and other waste material scattered throughout the cortex.

At a day centre, carers can offer help and support to elderly people. They can help them to deal with everyday problems such as paying household bills.

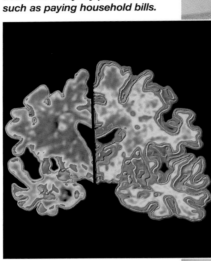

Alzheimer's disease can cause the death of brain cells and a reduction in brain size. These scans show an affected brain (left) and a normal brain (right).

DELAYED REACTIONS
Blood flow through the brain is reduced between the ages of 30 and 70. Nerve impulses travel at a slower speed with age. Conduction of impulses along nerve fibres is thought to be 15 per cent lower in a person of 80 than in someone of 30.

The result is that overall reaction times are longer in an older brain. This may be particularly significant when it comes to braking times when driving a car, or reaction times in order to break a fall.

DEMENTIA
Degenerative brain disorders occur in old age but are by no means an inevitable part of ageing. Dementia is a progressive loss of mental functioning, which can result in forgetfulness, impaired speech and mobility, an inability to carry out basic tasks, changes in behaviour and incontinence. It is estimated that dementia occurs

In elderly people, nerve impulses take longer to travel through the brain. This can make them slower to react in certain situations, such as driving a car.

in around 15 per cent of all people over the age of 65 and is the main cause of hospitalization and the fourth leading cause of death among the elderly.

Dementia is also caused by blood circulation problems. These include multiple small strokes, and arteriosclerosis (hardening of the arteries), which reduce the flow of blood to the brain. Dementia is also present in Huntington's chorea, an inherited progressive, degenerative brain disease.

ALZHEIMER'S
Alzheimer's disease is the leading cause of dementia and accounts for more than half of all cases of senility in the over-65 population. Alzheimer's rarely occurs before the age of 60, but has been known to affect people under 50 years old.

In Alzheimer's, the protein beta-amyloid accumulates in the tissues and cells of the patient's brain, causing them to die.

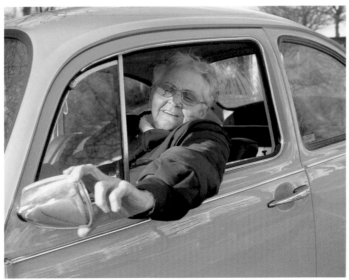

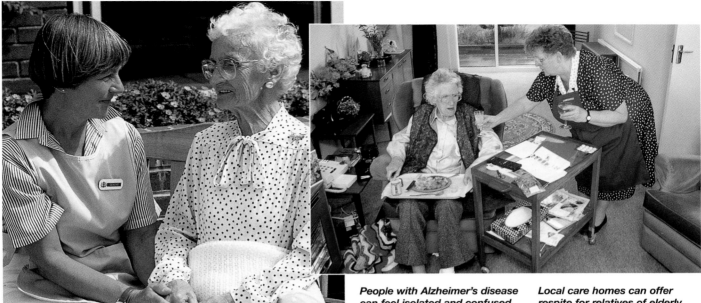

People with Alzheimer's disease can feel isolated and confused. Affected people may also appear to be suffering from severe depression.

Local care homes can offer respite for relatives of elderly people. However, close relatives may feel guilty that they are no longer the primary carers.

In normal, healthy people beta-amyloid is processed and rendered ineffective by the immune system. However, in people with Alzheimer's this protective sequence of events has started to break down.

SYMPTOMS OF ALZHEIMER'S

The first signs of Alzheimer's disease are failure of short-term memory and confusion about time and place.

In the later stages of Alzheimer's, affected people can develop forms of antisocial behaviour and, if the disease is severe, adopt obsessive rituals such as constant hand washing or touching of door knobs. Once these symptoms become obvious, the decline may be either slow or rapid, but it is always irreversible.

PERSONALITY CHANGES

Eventually, individuals can develop a change in personality and forget the names and faces of the most familiar friends and relatives.

In the declining stages of Alzheimer's disease, some elderly people may be unable to carry out a conversation or be no longer able to read a newspaper or listen to the radio or television. Some people can live for many years in this condition and eventually die not because of the Alzheimer's disease but due to a completely unrelated illness.

THE CARER'S ROLE

Dementia can be a burden for carers and loved ones. Throughout the illness, carers are faced with many difficult decisions. For example in the early stages of the condition, they have to decide whether or not they tell their loved one that he or she has Alzheimer's.

Carers live with the constant uncertainty of the illness. They can never be sure what the next stage will bring since everyone with dementia responds in a different way. For relatives, one of the saddest aspects of the disease is that their loved one

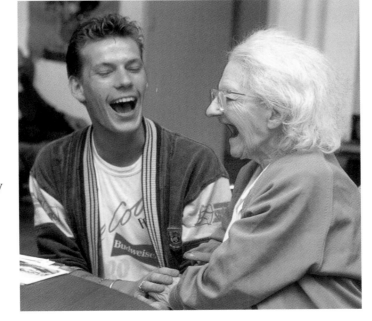

will not get better, but will only deteriorate further.

The structure of the household may change, with the healthy partner having to take on practical tasks, such as cooking or management of financial affairs, which were once the spouse's responsibility.

MAKING CARE DECISIONS

As the person becomes more confused, their ability to make important legal and financial decisions diminishes and it is usually necessary for the carer or other family members to assume these responsibilities on their behalf by gaining power of attorney. Later, when a relative needs round the clock attention,

a decision may have to be made about whether the individual would be more effectively cared for in a nursing home.

NURSING HOMES

Some people believe that permitting their loved one to go into a home is a mark of failure, and they may feel that they have let their relative down. On the other hand, it can be a relief to know that he or she is receiving the necessary care and attention. For these reasons, the experience is often an emotional one.

The financial burden of paying for a nursing home is an additional factor to consider. Local health authorities and support groups can offer advice, and financial assistance may be available in certain cases.

MAINTAINING MENTAL AGILITY

Although dementia does affect many elderly people, senility is not an inevitable consequence of ageing. Research has shown that the effects of ageing on the brain can be countered, to a certain extent, by keeping the brain active.

As with any muscle of the body, the brain needs to be exercised. Activities such as doing crosswords or reading combined with a healthy lifestyle (good diet, regular exercise and not smoking) help to maintain mental agility.

A residential home can offer elderly people happiness and security. However, they will probably experience mixed emotions as they settle in.

Alzheimer's disease

Alzheimer's disease is the most common cause of dementia in the UK. Although rare before the age of 45, its incidence increases with age, affecting up to 50 per cent of 90-year-olds.

Dementia is a clinical syndrome that is characterized by progressive loss of intellect and associated with a gradual deterioration in behaviour and personality. There is no reduction in consciousness nor impaired concentration.

The condition may be due to a number of causes of diffuse damage to the cerebral hemispheres. The commonest cause of dementia in the UK is Alzheimer's disease (AD), named after the German neurologist who first identified the disease. It is characterized by memory loss and an inability to reason.

WHO IS AFFECTED?

AD is a prominent problem of the elderly, increasing in incidence with age, but it is not due to the ageing process itself. The condition is rare in people under 45, but affects up to one person in 10 aged 65, one in five aged 80 and one in two aged 90. Its prevalence in the community is increasing due to greater longevity.

CAUSES OF AD

Over time, AD affects all of the higher brain functions (intellect) and progresses relentlessly to premature death. AD seems to result from an interplay between a number of genetic and acquired factors over a lifetime and appears as an illness when a critical number of neurones and their connections are lost.

The exact mechanisms causing the disease are unknown and the rate of loss of faculties varies. People with AD usually live, on average, for seven years after diagnosis.

The decline in mental capability in Alzheimer's disease leads to an increasing inability to perform activities of daily living, such as washing and dressing.

This coloured scanning electron micrograph of cortical neurones shows the branching interconnections between brain cells. These connections are destroyed in patients with AD.

Stages of dementia

Dementia varies in severity, but many patients follow a deteriorating course of:
1 Forgetfulness
2 Difficulty in performing at work and with speech and memory, although usually only detected by family or friends
3 Inability to count, spell, remember, recognize familiar faces, converse or travel alone
4 Assistance required to dress properly and needing to be accompanied as the patient becomes disoriented in time and place
5 Supervision required for going to the toilet, feeding, bathing and self-care
6 Severe loss of speech, with other severe physical symptoms and bladder and bowel incontinence
7 Death.

What is Alzheimer's disease?

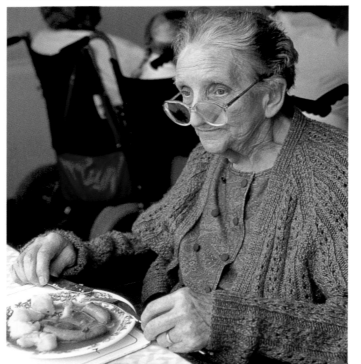

AD is a progressive degenerative brain disorder in which brain cells die more rapidly than normal. Symptoms and signs vary between individuals, but generally the patient suffers a gradual loss of memory and the ability to reason and to carry out tasks of everyday function. In the earliest stages of AD, differentiation from the effects of normal ageing can be difficult.

Following diagnosis, some 80 per cent of those who have AD continue to live with support in the community. It may only be in the last year of life that they lose the ability for self-care.

The progression of Alzheimer's disease is often gradual. Many people in the early stages of the condition are able to look after themselves to a large extent.

How AD affects the brain

The pathological findings in AD are characteristic, but the precise mechanisms behind brain changes are unclear.

PHYSICAL CHANGES

The physical changes to the brain are primarily a loss of brain tissue, with atrophy (wasting) of the brain substance and a progressive shrinkage of the brain over time. The brain of an AD sufferer weighs less than that of normal people.

The most marked loss of brain tissue occurs in the temporal lobes, including the area of the hippocampus, which is very important for memory function.

When the frontal lobe of the brain is affected, aspects of personality – such as the control and inhibition of behaviour – are disturbed. Parietal lobe damage results in the failure to process complex activities and the abnormal integration of information received by the

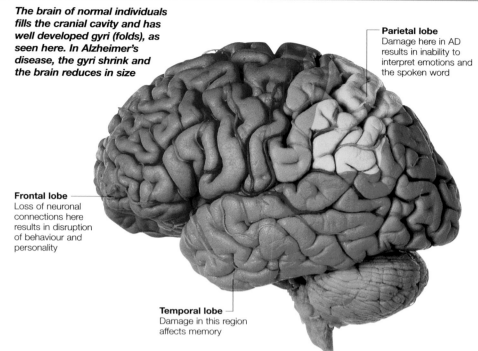

The brain of normal individuals fills the cranial cavity and has well developed gyri (folds), as seen here. In Alzheimer's disease, the gyri shrink and the brain reduces in size

Parietal lobe
Damage here in AD results in inability to interpret emotions and the spoken word

Frontal lobe
Loss of neuronal connections here results in disruption of behaviour and personality

Temporal lobe
Damage in this region affects memory

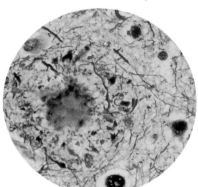

brain from the senses. This results in apraxia (inaccurate movements) and agnosia (the inability to interpret sensations).

There are three characteristic findings seen on microscopy of AD brain tissue at post mortem:

The characteristic pathological findings in the brain of Alzheimer's disease patients include senile plaques (circular lesions) and neurofibrillary tangles inside nerve cells.

■ The formation of disclike plaques of abnormal tissue (especially in cortical grey matter)
■ The collection of abnormal bundles of filaments – neurofibrillary tangles – inside nerve cells
■ Accumulation of an abnormal substance – amyloid.

These changes occur to a minor extent in all ageing brains but they are more widespread in cases of AD.

Risk factors

■ Advanced age
■ APO-E4 gene inheritance
■ Family history of dementia
■ Previous head trauma
■ Down's syndrome.

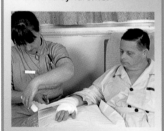

Some people are at higher risk of developing AD than others. People with Down's syndrome often develop AD, suggesting a genetic link.

Genes and AD

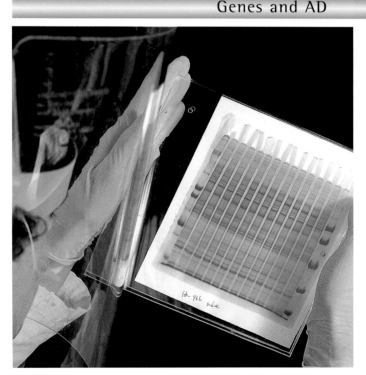

DNA fingerprinting, using gel electrophoresis to separate DNA fragments of identical length, has helped to identify genes implicated in development of AD.

AD is inherited in some families – usually in people who develop the disease at an early age. Abnormalities of the genes on chromosomes 1, 14 and 21 affect the inheritance of AD.

Other genetic factors influence the likelihood of a person developing AD. These genes do not cause the disease but increase the possibility that it may occur in the presence of other contributory factors. These are risk factor genes, the most prominent being the gene responsible for making a protein, apolipoprotein E (APO-E), which exists as APO-E2, APO-E3 and APO-E4. However, possession of a risk factor gene does not necessarily mean that a person will develop the disease.

Protective factors

■ APO-E2 or 3 inheritance
■ Use of oestrogen drugs
■ Use of anti-inflammatory drugs
■ High education attainment.

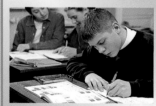

Academic achievement appears to afford an element of protection from AD.

Diagnosing Alzheimer's

Alzheimer's disease is gradual in progression and is initially difficult
to differentiate from the normal effects of ageing. Memory loss
is the predominant symptom, and this is often the first complaint.

Older people often suffer from benign senile forgetfulness, which 'takes the edge off' their memory. This condition is probably not associated with the later onset of AD, although medical opinion is still divided on this.

Memory loss is always associated with AD and is often, but not always, an early symptom. In the early stages of the disease, the sufferer is aware that memory and thinking processes are being eroded and that they are being slowly 'robbed' of their mental powers. This can cause anxiety and depression, which can make the diagnosis even more difficult.

This diagnostic complexity often slows the process whereby doctors confirm their own suspicions and inform the patient and their family or carer.

DIAGNOSTIC FACTORS

Diagnosis depends upon the identification of the following factors:
■ The presence of two or more deficits in cognition –

the mental process by which knowledge is attained and maintained, including perception, reasoning and intuition
■ Progressive loss of memory
■ Absence of any other medical disorder
■ Onset after at least 40, and usually 60, years of age
■ Decline in thinking function and intellectual capacity.

A firm diagnosis is made by excluding other conditions with similar symptoms. Early investigation has not been common in the past; however, the advent of new memory-enhancing drugs is changing attitudes towards making early diagnosis of this disease.

With AD, about one diagnosis in 10 is incorrect; in such cases, another condition is found to be the cause of the symptoms.

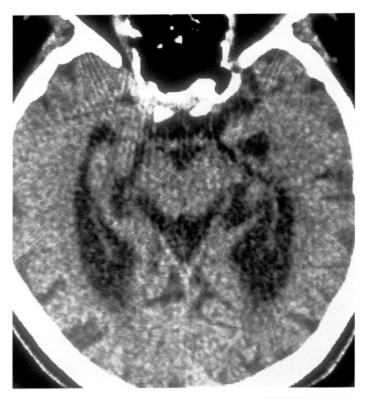

This CT scan of the brain of an Alzheimer's patient reveals enlarged ventricles (central dark areas). This indicates shrinking of the brain tissue.

Investigating AD

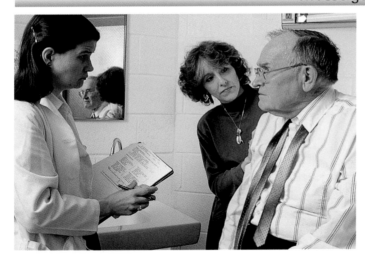

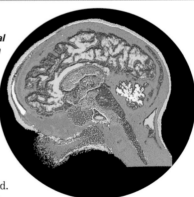

An investigating doctor will organize a full psychological, functional and social appraisal of the patient. This includes a variety of memory tests.

Investigations such as MR scanning (right) may be helpful in confirming a diagnosis. This enables damaged areas to be seen.

■ CT scan or MR scan if memory enhancement medication is being considered.

Management of a dementia patient should involve the extended primary care team and the social and community psychiatric nurse. They are usually delegated the task of checking for ability with functions of everyday living and social support using standardized assessment scales.

Differential diagnoses that can mimic dementia in the elderly include the following:
■ Depression
■ Acute confusion (delirium which can be due to infection or medication)
■ Thyroid over- and underactivity
■ Brain tumour
■ Vitamin B_{12} deficiency.

These conditions can be treated and once resolved, symptoms of dementia may disappear.

To identify true dementia and exclude other conditions, the GP should arrange for some simple investigations and procedures:
■ Blood tests
■ Memory tests
■ Depression tests
■ X-ray to exclude tumour

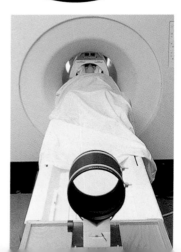

Diagnosis of Alzheimer's disease relies on being able to exclude other causes of dementia and brain damage. MR scanning is therefore a useful investigation.

Managing Alzheimer's disease

Managing Alzheimer's disease has concentrated on alleviating symptoms associated with dementia and providing quality care for those patients incapacitated by the disease. Some drugs are helpful but much treatment involves non-drug based therapies.

No current drug treatment can stop or slow the progression of Alzheimer's disease. Some drugs may, however, alleviate certain symptoms.

'MEMORY ENHANCERS'

One or two drugs – for example Exelon and Donepezil, which are acetylcholinesterase inhibitors – are now available on restricted NHS release. These drugs stop the neurotransmitter acetylcholine being destroyed in the brain and have been called memory enhancers. They appear to improve memory in the short-term for some patients who are in the earliest stages of AD.

OTHER PROBLEMS

Behavioural problems may occur in AD, and these include:
■ Aggression and shouting
■ Wandering
■ Sleep disturbance.

Antisocial responses can be treated with sedatives and antipsychotic medications. However, these drugs can cause the dementia and the behaviour to worsen and should be used in small doses in cases of very disturbed behaviour and subjected to frequent review.

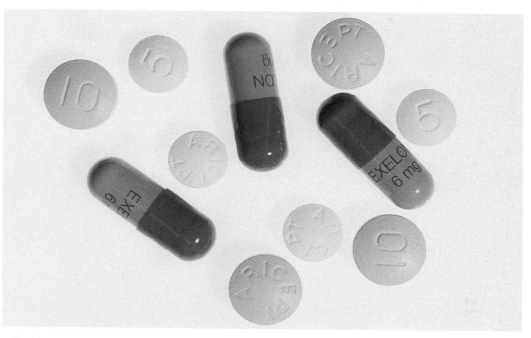

Antidepressants can be effective in improving the depression which some demented people also suffer. Treatment of depression will often improve other unpleasant symptoms of dementia and may encourage better sleep patterns.

Drug treatment should be used to treat the illnesses of old age which demented patients suffer just as others in their age group. Treatment of pain, constipation, inflammation and infection may improve behavioural problems caused by the dementia.

No medications have yet been developed that can slow or halt the progression of Alzheimer's disease. However, some drugs may help to alleviate symptoms associated with dementia, such as antidepressants and acetylcholinesterase inhibitors.

Non-drug treatments for AD

In the absence of appropriate curative therapy, non-drug interventions should be considered by the care team. These are often instituted by nurses and occupational therapists, but can also be carried out by the family carer.

These psychosocial or behavioural treatment strategies may involve:

■ Reality orientation – a technique that encourages verbal orientation and functioning and seeks to improve cognition
■ Reminiscence therapy – encourages patients to recall events from their past
■ Validation therapy – an empathetic approach that affirms the patient's personal reality.

Treatment plans for managing Alzheimer's disease should involve all members of the care team. This includes nurses and family carers.

PLANNING TREATMENT

Therapy will help some but not all patients, and may also be beneficial only at certain stages in the progression of dementia.

Irrespective of the treatment models adopted, every person with dementia should have a healthcare management plan developed by the primary care team involved. This should be agreed with the

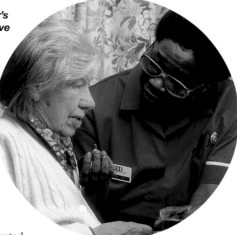

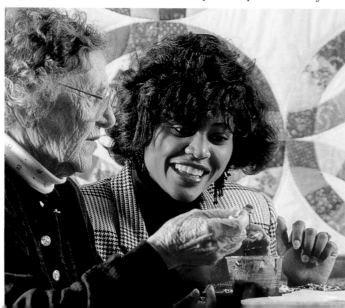

It is important to provide the highest quality care for patients with AD. Care plans need to be adapted for patients at regular intervals as AD progresses.

family carer – usually a spouse who will be caring at home.

A patient with AD requires highly organized support services to maintain them in the community and ensure that they have good healthcare and the best quality of life that a devastating terminal illness such as AD will allow.

Non-Alzheimer's dementias

Disease of the blood vessels of the brain is a major cause
of dementia in the elderly. The symptoms are similar to those of
Alzheimer's disease, but the treatment and management plans differ.

Over 70 different causes of dementia have been recognized. Alzheimer's disease is responsible for about half of all cases of dementia, with the majority of the rest caused by blood circulation-related problems. These are called the vascular dementias and have been referred to as 'preventable senility', as high blood pressure is often related to the condition.

Several types of vascular changes are involved, resulting in variations in the presenting symptoms of the dementia. It is now recognized that some people will have both Alzheimer's disease and vascular disease affecting the brain.

PATHOLOGY

Vascular dementia has been divided into three categories:
■ Acute onset
■ Multi-infarct
■ Subcortical.

The changes in the brain can be due to:
■ Multiple infarcts – death of brain tissue caused by an obstruction to blood flow
■ White matter ischaemia – when the white matter of the brain is starved of sufficient oxygen and nutrition.

■ Strategically placed infarcts – their position crucially affects brain function

CAUSES

Vascular dementia is related to the cause of the underlying circulatory problem, often atherosclerosis (hardening and thickening of the arteries). Restrictions of blood flow may result in high blood pressure.

When the condition affects the vessels of the brain, it is known as cerebrovascular thrombosis or ischaemia. Brain function can be affected by alteration of blood flow in or to brain arteries.

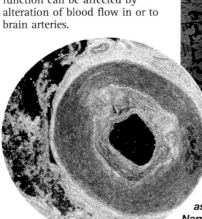

Vascular diseases such as atherosclerosis are associated with dementias. Narrowing of an artery may also cause high blood pressure.

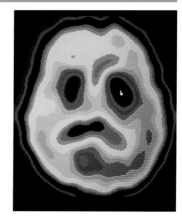

Alzheimer's disease is not the only cause of dementia in the elderly. Vascular disease is a common cause and can be prevented in some cases.

Patterns of cerebrovascular disease

Patterns of cerebrovascular disease that can result in dementia include:
■ Ischaemic cerebrovascular disease – a diffuse small vessel disease affecting the brain matter below the outer cortex. It is common in people with high blood pressure. There is a varying degree of brain cell death with loss of white matter of the brain. The person has difficulty walking and a progressive dementia. This is sometimes called Binswanger's encephalopathy.

■ Multiple brain cortex infarcts (death of outer tissue of the brain due to obstructed blood supply) – a major cause of dementia. This often occurs due to blood clots in the heart passing into the large blood vessels that supply the brain's circulation.

Multiple small infarcts are typically due to high blood pressure related to small vessel disease. Clinicians categorize vascular dementia into two groups: multi-infarct dementia and Lewy body dementia.

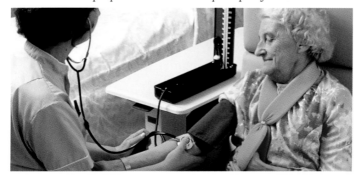

Blood pressure must be monitored in the elderly, as high blood pressure can damage small blood vessels in the brain, causing death of brain tissue.

The symptoms of dementia occur due to the loss of brain cells. This PET scan shows areas of atrophy in the cerebrum as darker patches.

Multi-infarct dementia

Multi-infarct dementia describes many, often tiny, infarcts in the cerebral cortex and the deeper areas of the brain. These cause brain damage that is patchy although extensive, and the total of all the tiny sites of damage correlates with the degree of intellectual impairment.

CLINICAL FINDINGS

People with the condition usually have generalized atherosclerosis throughout the body, but it is not the narrowing of vessels with reduced blood flow that damages the brain's nerve cells. In the cerebral cortex and deeper areas of the brain, many tiny areas of damage (infarcts) occur due to obstruction of the local blood supply by blockages such as thrombi (blood clots), otherwise termed strokes. The combination of many of these small strokes produces the dementia, as more and more brain areas lose their function in an irregular progression in symptoms.

Extensive areas of the brain will continue to work normally and the cause of death with this form of dementia is often a feature of generalized atherosclerosis, such as coronary artery thrombosis (a clot blocking blood flow to the heart).

An angiogram will determine if there are any blockages or narrowing of the blood vessels. The carotid artery is seen as the large orange vessel in the neck.

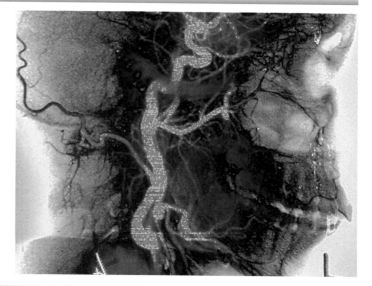

Lewy body dementia

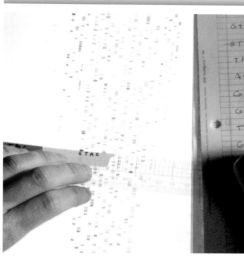
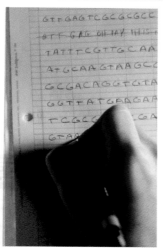

Diffuse Lewy body dementia has recently been recognized as a separate condition. The patients have senile plaques (lesions associated with brain cell loss) in their cerebral cortex, and 'Lewy bodies', which are seen in the cytoplasm of brain nerve cells as pink-staining structures.

GENETIC FINDINGS

Patients with Lewy body dementia produce even less of the neurotransmitter

Many patient's with Lewy body dementia have a defective apoE4 gene. This can be identified using genetic testing to determine risk of the disease.

acetylcholine than those with Alzheimer's disease.

Genetically, the gene apoE4 is over-represented in people with Lewy body dementia, and is associated with Parkinson's disease.

TREATMENT

It is important for doctors to differentiate the diagnosis of Alzheimer's disease from vascular disease and multi-infarct dementia from Lewy body dementia where possible, as drug management varies for the conditions. At present, there is no cure or preventative therapy for Alzheimer's disease or vascular dementias.

Symptoms of dementia

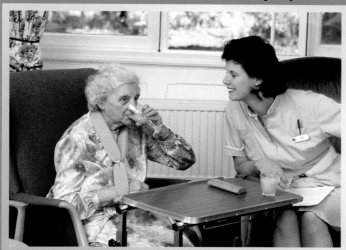

As a patient's dementia progresses, they will require more support in their daily lives from carers. Eventually, this care may need to be given on a 24-hour basis.

The clinical features of dementia relate to the progressive damage to the brain which occurs as the condition progresses. The symptoms do not differ from those of Alzheimer's disease, although the loss is often gradual with Alzheimer's disease and a step-by-step progression with vascular dementia. Deficits occur in:

■ Information processing
■ Memory
■ Expression of speech
■ Mobility and coordination
■ Continence.

Behavioural changes

There is disturbance in thinking, emotion and behaviour, and disinhibition means normal social constraints are lost. Skills required for activities of daily living disappear over time. A typical scenario would be:

■ Patient behaviour deteriorates and may become embarrassing, obstructive or annoying
■ Failure to dress or wash
■ Verbal abuse, screaming and physical aggression
■ Aimless wandering
■ Withdrawal from social contact.

Early symptoms of dementia may be noticeable as changes in personality and behaviour. Some patients may become socially withdrawn.

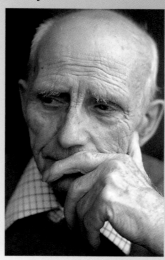

Diagnosing vascular dementia

The first signs of vascular dementia may be a change in a person's behaviour, loss of memory or decline in intellectual function. It is important that other causes of these symptoms are ruled out.

Vascular dementias may become apparent earlier than Alzheimer's disease, with an onset from age 55. There is often marked variation in the presentation of symptoms and fluctuation in the thinking process initially and over time. There may be a plateau when there is little change in symptoms and then a sudden worsening, followed by a period of stability before further deterioration.

COURSE OF THE DISEASE
The disease course relates to the occurrence of the brain infarcts. It can be abrupt, with an initial fall at the onset with intermittent confusion, speech difficulties and transient ischaemic attacks. Then there may be a step-by-step deterioration in brain function, skills and personality.

Ultimately there will be:
■ Deficits in cognition, the mental process by which knowledge is acquired, including perception, reasoning and intuition
■ Progressive memory loss
■ An inevitable decline in intellectual capacity.

Often there is high blood pressure and there may be evidence of vascular disease.

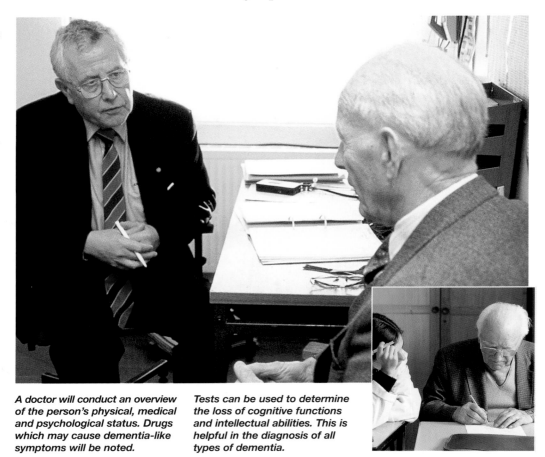

A doctor will conduct an overview of the person's physical, medical and psychological status. Drugs which may cause dementia-like symptoms will be noted.

Tests can be used to determine the loss of cognitive functions and intellectual abilities. This is helpful in the diagnosis of all types of dementia.

Investigations

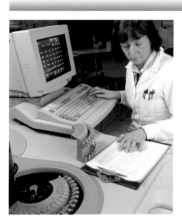

Blood testing can rule out many other causes of dementia-like symptoms. These may include thyroid disorders, anaemia and diabetes.

Initial investigation is directed towards exclusion of other causes of dementia and conditions which can mimic dementia. To this end, depression, vitamin deficiency, thyroid disorder, tumour, infection, repetitive head injury and confusional states have all to be considered and discarded or treated.

DIAGNOSTIC TESTS
Routine tests should include:
■ A memory test – the abbreviated mental test or the

mini mental status evaluation assessment tests are often used in primary care health checks
■ Blood tests for anaemia, thyroid function, glucose levels
■ Blood pressure monitoring
■ Liver function tests
■ Imaging techniques – X-rays

are required to exclude a tumour; if blockage of the carotid arteries is suspected, ultrasonography of the vessels will be indicated. CT and MRI brain scans are used to differentiate between Alzheimer's disease and vascular dementias.

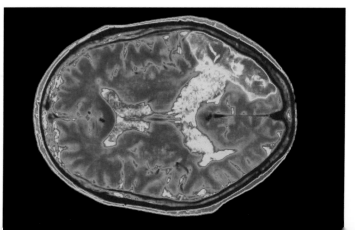

Imaging techniques such as MR imaging are useful in assessing areas of brain damage. This MR scan shows a region of the brain affected by a stroke (red).

Managing dementia

As yet, there are no drugs that can halt or cure dementia. Management aims to slow the progression of the disease and improve quality of life.

Good management of people with vascular dementia depends upon effective liaison between members of the primary care team. Continuing care is dependent upon the GP, community and practice nurses, health visitor, community psychiatric nurse, community social worker, occupational therapist, dietitian and the support of secondary health care facilities, such as respite care.

GOALS OF GERIATRIC CARE

All or a few specialists may be involved at any given time. Effort is directed at maintaining the patient in their own home for as long as possible and helping them to use their remaining skills and competence to best advantage.

As vascular dementia progresses, physical functions such as balance and movement may be affected. These patients will need help with mobility.

Community nursing and care in the home is necessary for patients who have lost the ability to carry out daily living tasks, such as preparing meals.

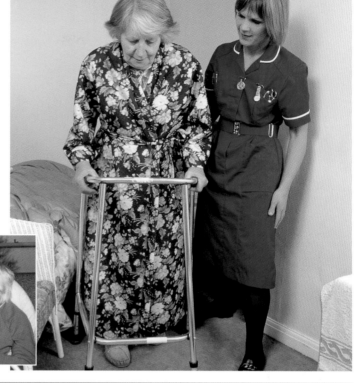

Drug therapies

Drugs can be taken to control or lower blood pressure; this may slow progression of the disease. Lipid-lowering agents – which reduce levels of lipids in the blood – may also be worthwhile in the early stages of decline. These are of particular value in people who have already had transient ischaemic attacks.

Antiplatelet drugs – for example, aspirin – which prevent blood clots may reduce the incidence of small strokes affecting the brain. Patients with narrowing of the carotid artery may benefit from surgery.

Some patients who are still able to live at home may still need community nurses to supervise them while taking drugs. This prevents accidental overdose.

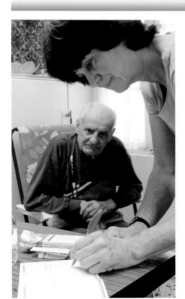

ASSOCIATED PROBLEMS

People with dementia often suffer from depression; antidepressant drugs may lift the depression and help some of the behavioural problems which occur with dementia.

Neuroleptic drugs, such as thioridazine and haloperidol, are often used to treat the behavioural disturbance associated with dementia, but their side effects can be serious and are a cause of agitation in people with dementia. When used, the dose should be small and under constant review. This type of drug should not be used in patients who have Lewy body dementia, as these people are very sensitive to them and can become seriously ill from side effects.

Aspirin is used in low doses in patients who have had, or are at risk of having, blood clots. Aspirin is an anticlotting agent and so inhibits coagulation.

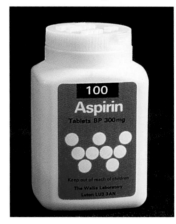

Non-drug treatments

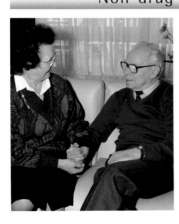

Non-drug treatments are often used in patients who react badly to drug therapy. Treatments include:
- Reminiscence work
- Reality orientation
- Music therapy.

Their value has been poorly researched but they, can be carried out by family carers and appear to improve quality of life.

Carers can help with a number of non-drug therapies in the home. These are believed to provide a higher quality of life.

Promoting healthy lifestyles

Vascular dementia is theoretically preventable. National health-promotion campaigns targeting hypertension, coronary thrombosis and cardiovascular disease should mean fewer people in future will suffer from this debilitating disease.

Changes in lifestyle may diminish its incidence. A low-fat diet, non-smoking habits and daily exercise decrease the possible occurrence of vascular dementia.

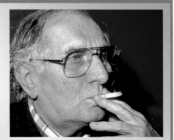

Preventative measures, such as giving up smoking, may reduce the incidence of vascular dementia in the future.

Temporal arteritis

Symptoms

Temporal arteritis is a condition that causes inflammation of the medium-sized blood vessels that supply the scalp, especially those in the temples. If the condition is widespread, it is known as giant-cell arteritis or cranial arteritis.

CLINICAL FEATURES
Symptoms of temporal arteritis include the following:
- Headache
- Intermittent impaired vision, such as double vision
- Sudden vision loss in one eye
- Jaw claudication (cramp) – affects 50 per cent of patients
- Tenderness on the scalp.

A quarter of patients also suffer from polymyalgia rheumatica (PMR), a condition that causes symmetrical pain and stiffness in the shoulders and hips.

Sometimes, patients with giant-cell arteritis have vague symptoms, such as tiredness, depression, prolonged fever, weight loss and reduced appetite

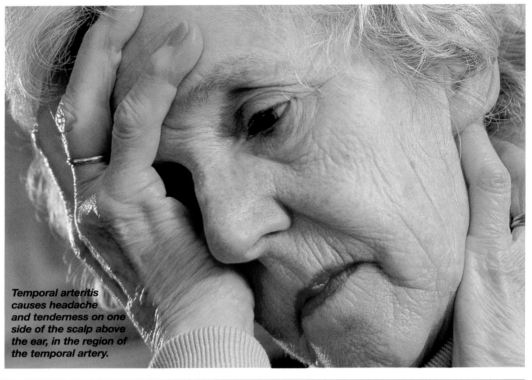

Temporal arteritis causes headache and tenderness on one side of the scalp above the ear, in the region of the temporal artery.

Diagnosis

It is essential to diagnose temporal arteritis as promptly as possible in order to reduce the risk of blindness. A medical history, an examination of the patient and a simple blood test are usually used to help diagnose temporal arteritis.

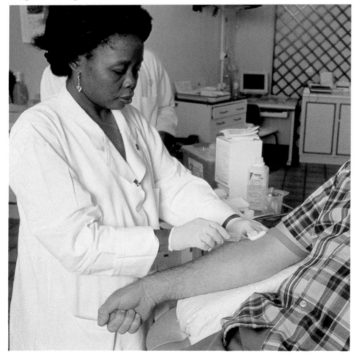

During the examination, the physician will check whether there is any tenderness over the superficial artery in the temple, and whether there is any loss of pulsation in the artery.

FURTHER TESTS
- An eye examination
- Blood tests – these will show mild anaemia and a raised platelet count if the disease is present. The most important indicator of temporal arteritis is a raised ESR (erythrocyte sedimentation rate). The ESR is markedly raised – above 50mm/hr – in temporal arteritis. However, in around 10 per cent of affected patients, the ESR may be normal; this complicates the diagnosis.

ARTERY BIOPSY
It is useful to perform a temporal artery biopsy to confirm the diagnosis. This procedure entails the removal of a segment of the artery, which lies just under the skin. It is performed under a local anaesthetic.

The biopsy will be analyzed to see whether there is an inflammatory arteritis along with the presence of multinucleated giant cells (hence the name giant-cell arteritis). The biopsies of the temporal

Blood tests may be used to confirm the diagnosis of temporal arteritis. Affected patients will have mild anaemia.

arteries of up to 20 per cent of patients with polymyalgia rheumatica are similar to those of patients with temporal arteritis.

Sometimes, biopsies are falsely negative in temporal arteritis due to 'skip lesions' with areas of normal artery, or because steroid treatment is already well established.

Swelling of the optic disc at the back of the eye may indicate temporal arteritis. This is detected by examination utilizing an ophthalmoscope.

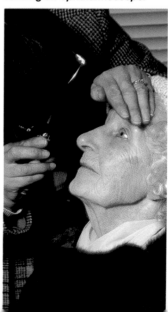

Causes

The cause of temporal arteritis is unknown, but the disease is thought to be due to an abnormal immune response within the wall of arteries. The same pathology is thought to cause polymyalgia rheumatica.

The loss of vision in temporal arteritis is caused by thrombosis (solidification) of the blood vessels that supply the retina at the back of the eye.

Intermittent symptoms of visual impairment or jaw pain are caused by partial blockage of blood vessels. There is no evidence to suggest that the condition is infectious.

Temporal arteritis is not a directly inherited condition, but variations in its incidence between different races suggests that genetic predisposition may play a part in the aetiology (origin) of the condition.

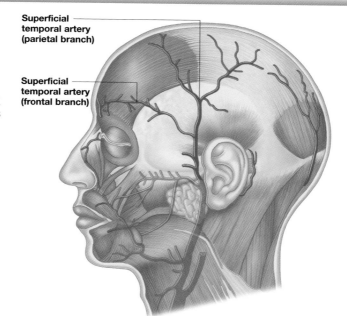

Superficial temporal artery (parietal branch)

Superficial temporal artery (frontal branch)

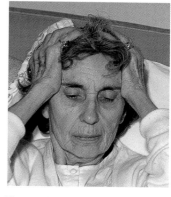

Temporal arteritis is rare in people under the age of 50. The headaches are a result of inflammation of the arterial walls.

The arteries most often affected are the two main branches of the superficial temporal artery, which supply the scalp.

Treatment

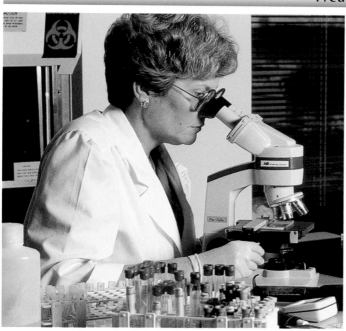

Giant-cell arteritis responds within two to three days to treatment with large doses of steroids. Some physicians advocate initially administrating it intravenously (directly into the vein) if they believe that vision may be threatened.

If there are visual symptoms, then oral doses of at least 60mg of prednisolone a day are recommended.

It is important that treatment is not delayed until a temporal artery biopsy has been carried out. The biopsy should be organized as soon as possible. It may still be positive for more than a week after starting steroids.

The progress of patients diagnosed with temporal arteritis is monitored by regular checks on their erythrocyte sedimentation rate (ESR).

LONG-TERM CONTROL
Once the disease has come under control, the physician will gradually reduce the intake of steroid tablets to a lower maintenance dose – 7.5mg to 10mg a day. The lowest possible dose is used to minimize the risk of the side effects of steroids, such as osteoporosis and infection.

Immunosuppressant drugs – such as azathioprine and methotrexate – are occasionally used as a substitute for steroids in patients who have difficulty coming off steroids.

Treatment needs to be continued for around two years in order to prevent relapse.

The progress of patients is monitored by:
■ Checking how much the patient's symptoms have come under control
■ Monitoring the patient's ESR.

Prognosis and incidence

The prognosis for temporal arteritis depends on the promptness of treatment. If sight is already severely affected, it is unlikely to completely return to normal. However, there may be partial improvement, and the disease is unlikely to get worse once the patient is on steroid treatment.

Lowering the dose of the steroid administered may trigger a relapse, but this is less likely after the first 18 months of treatment or over a year after stopping treatment. Typically, complete remission occurs after about two years.

INCIDENCE
Temporal arteritis almost always affects people over 50 years of age, with the average age of onset around 70 years. It is at least twice as common in women than in men. The incidence of temporal arteritis varies in different areas of the world. In northern Europe, the incidence of the condition is up to 20 cases per 100,000 in people aged over 50.

If temporal arteritis remains untreated, 50 per cent of patients may experience vision loss in one eye.

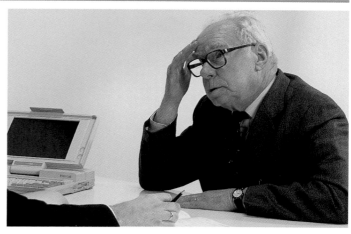

Parkinson's disease

Symptoms and signs

Parkinson's disease is a degenerative brain disorder associated with ageing. A distinction is often made between Parkinson's disease and parkinsonism, in which the same symptoms are produced by causes other than age.

A typical first sign is a slow tremor (shake) on resting, often initially on one side of the body. This is typically 'pill rolling' in form and diminishes on voluntary movement. It affects both sides involving the arms, legs and the jaw. Slowness of movement is often first noticed by the family rather than by the patient.

Rigidity ('cogwheel type') of the muscles occurs, which adds the general slowness and leads to a stooping posture and 'shuffling' gait. There is a noticeable loss of arm swing on walking. The patient develops monotonous speech, a masklike expressionless face and dribbles saliva because of difficulty in swallowing. Muscle aches and cramps occur, fatigue is often present and constipation is common. Writing becomes small, tremulous and untidy on account of the rigidity.

As the disease progresses, there may be major disability when the patient becomes immobile and chair-bound. The latter may lead to complications such as pneumonia, bedsores and urinary tract infections. Most patients have normal intellectual function but, with time, a proportion develop structural mental changes.

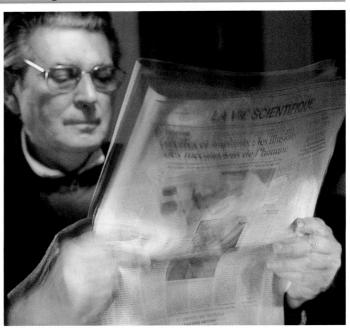

The most common initial sign of Parkinson's disease is a coarse, rhythmical slow tremor of the hands. It diminishes during conscious movement.

Diagnosis

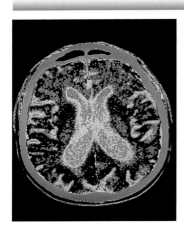

Diagnosis is made entirely on the clinical picture, which is usually characteristic. Careful history and examination are required to exclude causes of parkinsonism. These include:

■ Drugs – phenothiazines, reserpine, methyldopa
■ Infections – following brain swelling (encephalitis)

This coloured CT scan is from a Parkinson's patient. Loss of density in the brain tissue has caused the ventricles (blue) to increase in size.

■ Toxins – including carbon monoxide and manganese
■ Hypothyroidism
■ Vascular – cerebrovascular disease
■ Trauma to the head – particularly in boxers
■ In combination with other conditions, for example Alzheimer's disease or Huntington's chorea.

There are no diagnostic tests for Parkinson's disease, but CT and MR scans and biochemical tests may be necessary to exclude other causes.

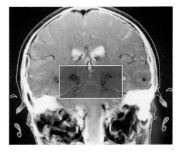

The boxed area in this MR scan is the basal ganglia of the brain. This area contains dopamine-producing cells, which are lacking in Parkinson's disease.

Causes and prognosis

Extensive microbiological studies have failed to find an infective cause. Degeneration of the brainstem, presence of large bodies within brain cells, and loss of neurones in important regions of the brain, causing severe loss of dopamine, are the main pathological changes. These important discoveries have led to treatment with L-dopa to replace the lost dopamine in the body.

The disease tends to be progressive and patients may become increasingly bedridden or chairbound on account of immobility. However, many patients remain reasonably active and the rate of progression varies greatly between individuals.

Since the introduction of L-dopa therapy, life expectancy in Parkinson's patients has increased. Studies have shown that with present day treatment, a person with Parkinson's disease is likely, on average, to live as long as an unaffected person of the same age. The average duration of the disease is 15 years, from diagnosis to death.

A Parkinson's patient undergoes a medical examination. The doctor is testing the rigidity of the wrist and the slow finger movement (bradykinesia); both are symptomatic of the disease.

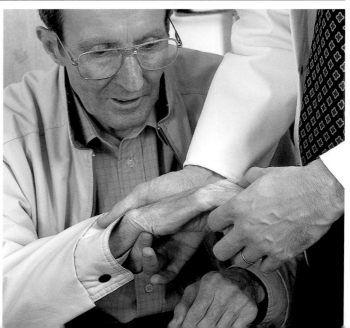

Treatment

DRUG TREATMENT

Specific treatment involves the use of anti-parkinsonian drugs. It is usual to start treatment when the symptoms become severe enough to interfere with the activities of daily living.

Treatment with L-dopa tablets begins with a small dose of L-dopa and a peripheral dopa decarboxylase inhibitor. Selegiline (MOA oxidase type B inhibitor) was thought to delay the progression of the disease, but this is now doubtful.

Dopamine agonists (stimulators such as pergolide, lysuride, bromocriptine and apomorphine) generally cause fewer side effects, but not all patients respond. Apomorphine is given by subcutaneous injection and is used for the troublesome 'on-off' phenomenon. This occurs when the effect of a drug wears off quickly, requiring increasingly frequent doses of medication.

Anticholinergic drugs, such as benzhexol and orphenadrine, are useful for treating prominent tremors. These drugs may cause increased confusion, blurred vision and a dry mouth, especially in the elderly.

Patients who respond well to L-dopa may find the duration of therapeutic effect from each tablet becomes shorter, leading to marked fluctuation of symptoms – this is the 'on-off' effect described above.

Other treatment

Supportive treatment
Occupational therapists and physiotherapists are important in helping to maintain independence in everyday activities for as long as possible.

In the later stages of the disease, when mobility is limited, family support and day care are very important.

Symptomatic treatment
Treatment may be required for constipation, depression or musculo-skeletal pain.

Surgery to the thalamus of the brain was popular in the 1950s and 1960s. Surgery is now considered only for patients resistant to drug therapy and whose tremor is severe.

Dopa
The chemical that begins the pathway (the substrate); L-dopa boosts the level of substrate

Dopamine
Dopa is converted into neurotransmitter dopamine; facilitates communication between cells

Dopamine re-uptake
Dopamine binds to dopamine receptors and is then recovered; amantadine blocks re-uptake

Dopamine receptor
Binding of dopamine to the receptor results in signal transmission along the adjoining cell; induced by dopamine agonists (pergolide, apomorphine)

Breakdown of signal
An enzyme called monoamine oxidase breaks down the nerve signal; inhibited by the drug selegiline

Nerve cell
The synaptic bulb at the end of the nerve cell releases neurotransmitter into the synapse

Synapse
Physical gap between two nerve cells

Nerve cell
Neurotransmitter binds to specific receptors

Parkinson's disease affects groups of nerve cells involved in movement, where the neurotransmitter dopamine facilitates signals across nerve junctions (synapses). Various drugs can partially restore this system.

Incidence and prevention

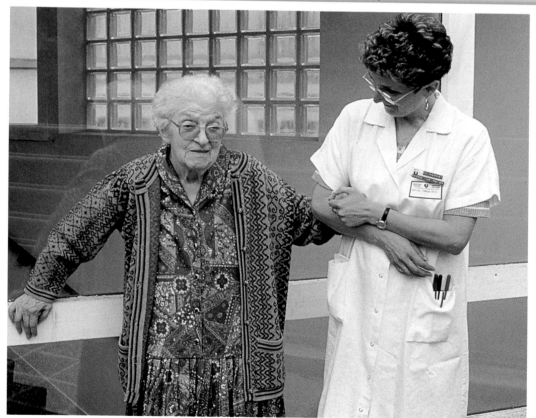

Parkinson's disease affects about 1 in 10,000 of the population. After the age of 50, the prevalence is about 1 in 200. It is slightly more common in men than in women and does not seem to run in families. Interestingly, patients with Parkinson's disease are less likely to die from lung cancer than the rest of the population.

As the cause of Parkinson's disease is currently unknown, prevention is not possible. The use of embryonic brain cell implants has been mentioned, but their use raises serious ethical issues, as their source would be aborted fetuses.

Parkinsonism occurring following the administration of antipsychotic drugs will usually resolve following cessation of the drug treatment.

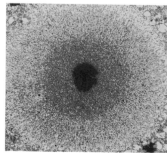

A sufferer of Parkinson's disease is helped to walk by a nurse. The shuffling, unbalanced walk and slow trembling are typical of the disease. This false-colour electron micrograph shows a structure found in brain cells called a Lewy body. This is a pathological feature of Parkinson's disease.

Huntington's disease

Symptoms

Huntington's disease (often known as Huntington's chorea) is a rare hereditary condition, affecting about one in 10,000 people worldwide. The disease causes progressive damage to the nervous system.

Nerve cell damage is greatest in two distinct masses of nerve cells located deep in the substance of the brain – the caudate nucleus and putamen. These areas are involved in the subconscious regulation of voluntary movements.

Symptoms of the disease usually start in early middle age and include:
■ Disturbances of movement
■ Progressive deterioration of mental function, leading to dementia
■ Other symptoms related to damage to the nervous system.

MOVEMENT
Involuntary jerky movements (chorea) affect about 90 per cent of patients and are often the first obvious symptom. Other movement disturbances include:
■ Loss of normal muscle tone or increased rigidity
■ Difficulties in posture and movement

■ Dysarthria (inability to pronounce words clearly, despite knowing their meaning)
■ Dysphagia (difficulty in swallowing)
■ Abnormal eye movements.

MENTAL DETERIORATION
Affected people invariably experience a gradual deterioration in mental ability and may develop psychiatric disorders. Symptoms include:
■ Impaired intellectual ability
■ Loss of concentration
■ Loss of short- and long-term memory
■ Loss of problem-solving ability
■ Dementia.

Some people may suffer psychiatric disorders, such as:
■ Personality changes, including irritability, apathy, aggression, changed sexual behaviour
■ Depression
■ Psychoses (illnesses in which the patient loses contact with reality, such as schizophrenia).

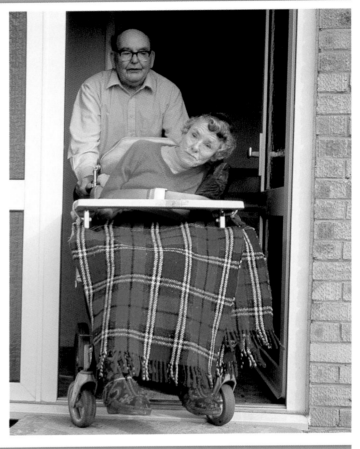

Huntington's disease is a rare genetic disorder that damages the nervous system. Symptoms include disturbed movement and impaired mental ability.

Causes

Huntington's disease occurs in individuals who inherit an abnormal gene on chromosome 4. This leads to the formation of abnormal proteins that invade and destroy nerve cell nuclei.

The defective gene is dominant (anyone who inherits the faulty gene will, at some stage, develop the disease). Children of an affected individual have a one in two risk of inheriting the gene.

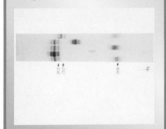

Huntington's disease is caused by an abnormal dominant gene. This gene can be detected using gel electrophoresis.

Diagnosis

A family history of Huntington's disease will suggest the diagnosis if an individual develops typical symptoms of the disease. However, an accurate family history may not always be available.

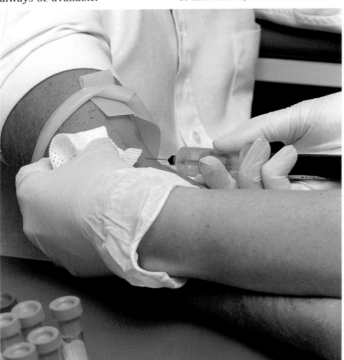

TESTS
In individuals carrying the Huntington gene, expert examination of the nervous system may identify subtle changes in speed and control of movement, and in reaction time long before chorea becomes very obvious.

GENETIC TESTING
Tests using blood DNA samples can now be used to identify the abnormal gene in the following groups:
■ Individuals who have symptoms
■ People who carry the abnormal gene but have, as yet, no symptoms
■ Unborn babies.

Genetic testing can, however, cause severe psychological distress and raises a number of issues, including ethical issues about abortion.

OTHER CAUSES
Other causes of chorea, such as a stroke, certain drugs or long-term alcohol abuse, must be excluded during diagnosis.

The diagnosis of Huntington's disease can be confirmed by taking a blood sample. The sample is then tested for the presence of the abnormal gene.

Treatment

Huntington's disease is, at present, incurable. Treatment therefore aims to reduce the effects of the disease as much as possible and to provide psychological support.

DRUG THERAPY

Some medications can minimize the unpleasant symptoms of the disease:
■ Treatments are available to relieve depression, anxiety, apathy, aggression and irritability
■ Phenothiazines, including pimozide and/or haloperidol, may be used to control the chorea if it is seriously incapacitating. Treatment should be carefully tailored to the patient's needs because side effects may be a problem
■ Dopamine agonists may be used to control rigidity. However, they are generally less effective in Huntington's disease than in Parkinson's disease.

SUPPORT

Patients and their families are likely to need skilled social and psychological support. Patients frequently become extremely depressed as they often retain a considerable amount of insight into their condition throughout a large part of their illness.

Speech therapy is sometimes helpful if a person has dysarthria and an occupational therapist can enable a person to lead as normal a life as possible. As the condition progresses, nursing care may be necessary.

FUTURE TREATMENT

Future therapies for the treatment of Huntington's disease which are currently being tested include:
■ Neuroprotective drugs, which may delay the onset of the disease
■ Neurotransplantation (the transplantation of fetal cells into the brain of a Huntington's disease patient)
■ Gene therapy.

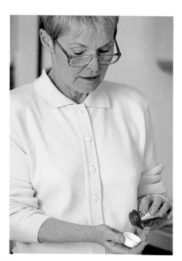

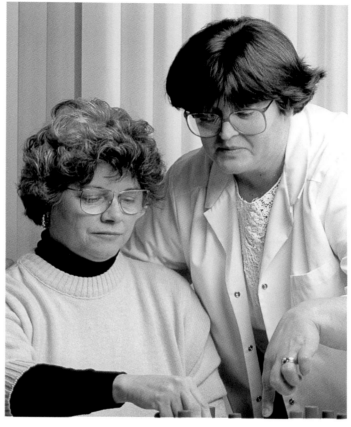

There is, at present, no treatment for Huntington's disease. However, medication can be used to control some of the unpleasant symptoms.

People with the condition may benefit from occupational therapy. This patient is receiving therapy to improve her coordination and muscle control.

Prognosis

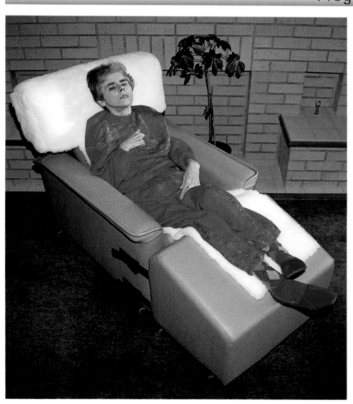

Once symptoms develop, Huntington's disease pursues a relentless course. Most patients eventually require full-time nursing and residential care.

People with Huntington's chorea often become less mobile as the disease progresses. Adapted furniture can help to maintain comfort.

The average time of survival from the time of diagnosis is about 16 years, but patients may live for much longer or shorter periods.

For many patients, the cause of death is pneumonia, which results from food and liquid entering their lungs after they lose their ability to swallow correctly.

Prevention

Prospective parents at risk of having a child with the disease may choose to have prenatal genetic testing to determine whether the fetus is carrying the abnormal gene. If tests prove positive, they may consider termination of the pregnancy.

GENETICS

As the symptoms of Huntington's disease usually do not appear until early middle age, an affected person will often have had children by the time the disease is diagnosed. This partly explains why the disease continues from generation to generation.

ETHICS

Ethical issues arise over the question of whether the offspring of affected individuals decide to remain in ignorance of their condition, or whether they choose to be tested for the presence of the abnormal gene before they decide to have children of their own.

Coping with depression

Depression is a mental illness that can take many different forms, and symptoms can range from mild to severe. Some forms of depression are connected with chemical changes in the brain.

Everyone experiences low moods from time to time, but this does not necessarily mean that they are suffering from depression. Their mood usually lifts after a few days and they return to their normal way of living. Depression, however, is a term used to describe a more severe illness that affects the body and the mind and lasts for a minimum period of a few weeks.

Sufferers experience persistent feelings of sadness, emptiness, loss and dread. They may also experience changes in appetite and weight, suffer from disrupted sleep patterns and have problems concentrating on daily tasks.

COMMON CONDITION

Depression is one of the most common psychiatric conditions, affecting one in five of the population at some time in their lives. Many people keep quiet about suffering from depression due to the stigma attached to the condition. Some sufferers tend to blame themselves and feel that depression is all their fault.

The effects of depression should never be underestimated – depression is a mental illness that can develop into an extremely serious problem, in some cases affecting all aspects of the sufferer's life. Each year there are 5000 suicides in England and Wales, and about 3000 of these are said to be the result of depression.

Depression can be a long-term recurring disorder, with the risk of a recurrence increasing with each new episode, and many different forms of this illness are now recognized. Reactive depression (exogenous depression) means coming from the outside. In this type of depression, a specific event triggers the lowering of the patient's mood. Such triggers range from bereavement to moving house or changing jobs. Some people appear to be more at risk of experiencing depression than others and different people react to life events in a variety of ways.

By contrast, endogenous depression, which comes from within, is more difficult to explain. Doctors ascribe it to a possible chemical or electrical imbalance in the brain.

SPECIFIC TYPES

There are other specific types of depression. Manic depressive illness is a very serious disorder. Sufferers experience mood disturbances consisting of depressive and manic phases. During the depressive phase, the sufferer slows down in mind and body and experiences feelings of worthlessness, despair and even suicidal tendencies. In the manic phase, judgement may be impaired, speech speeded up and the sufferer may have delusions of grandeur.

Some women suffer from postnatal depression after they have given birth. Levels of oestrogen and progesterone are

Postnatal depression may affect a woman after the birth of a baby. This is due to a drop in hormone levels; the feelings usually pass in a few weeks.

very high in pregnancy and drop dramatically after the baby is born and this sudden change can sometimes trigger a depression. About half of all women go through the 'maternity blues', but 15 per cent suffer from mild to moderate postnatal depression and one in 500 women experiences severe postnatal depression.

In some cases, people become depressed during the winter months because of the long, dark hours and the shorter days.

Twice as many women are thought to suffer from depression as men. Women are more willing to visit their GP and discuss the symptoms.

Coloured scans are shown of the brains of a depressed (above) and healthy (below) patient. Red/yellow areas show regions of low brain activity.

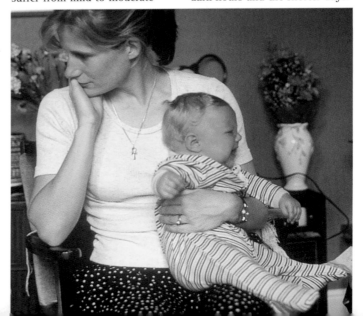

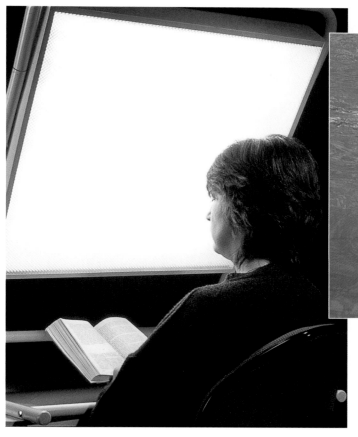

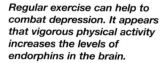

This type of depression is called seasonal affective disorder syndrome (SADS). SADS is thought to be related to levels of melatonin, a hormone that helps to control the body's daily rhythms. More melatonin is released by the pineal gland in the brain when it is dark, but production slows when the body is exposed to light.

Seasonal affective disorder syndrome causes depression in the winter months. Exposing sufferers to light is a successful treatment method.

MEDICATION

Antidepressants can help people to recover from depression, particularly if they are suffering from moderate to severe endogenous depression. In this condition, there are not enough neurotransmitters between interconnecting nerves in the brain. Antidepressants work by extending the life of chemicals in the brain that stimulate nerve activity. Most antidepressants need at least 10 days to work and they are effective only if they are taken over a long enough period of time.

There are three main classes of antidepressants: monoamine oxidase inhibitors (MAOIs), tricyclic antidepressants (TCAs) and selective serotonin re-uptake inhibitors (SSRIs). They are all effective, but side effects may occur. For instance, MAOIs can interact with food and other drugs. Tricyclics can make the patient drowsy, constipated and cause blurred vision and weight gain. They can also be

dangerous if taken in large doses, so they should not be prescribed to depressives with suicidal thoughts. Selective serotonin re-uptake inhibitors – the best known of which is Prozac – have fewer side effects than other antidepressants, but can still cause nausea, loss of appetite and allergic reactions.

Medication can help the symptoms of depression by lifting a patient's mood, but the underlying cause of the depression may need to be tackled in other ways.

THERAPY

Psychotherapy can be very helpful, especially when life events and the patient's attitudes are the root cause. Psychotherapists help to modify their patients' feelings, views and ideas about themselves through counselling. By talking things through, in the form of exploratory discussion, patients are able to find their own answers. And, by developing their own strategies, they will gain in maturity and strength and build the foundations for managing their future life.

Cognitive behavioural therapy is a more structured form of therapy. The therapist helps the patient to see the world from a different perspective, to try to

Regular exercise can help to combat depression. It appears that vigorous physical activity increases the levels of endorphins in the brain.

eliminate negative thoughts and to examine their own attitudes and beliefs in order to try to prevent feelings of depression arising in the future.

AVOIDING STRESS

People who have experienced depression need to take steps to avoid a recurrence of the problem. Stress should be avoided as far as is realistically possible, as this can trigger an episode. A well-balanced diet, plenty of sleep and regular exercise all help to counteract any stressful situations. Maintaining a good balance between work life, home life and 'personal time' is also essential in helping to beat depression.

FIGHTING DEPRESSION

Some people prone to recurrent depression find the company of a pet therapeutic. Looking after a pet can do wonders to help lift the sufferer's mood. Many kinds of pet are cuddly, reliable and responsive and can help to decrease levels of stress.

Depression can also be kept at bay through exercise. Prolonged exercise is thought to increase levels of the mood-raising endorphins in the brain. Endorphins are also natural pain-relieving substances in the body.

Less conventional approaches can help people suffering from depression in amazing ways. Pets can relieve stress and offer comfort to sufferers.

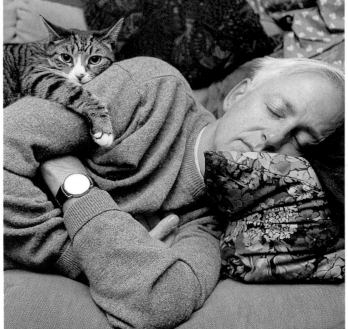

Stroke

A stroke is a disturbance in brain function due to either a blockage in a blood vessel supplying the brain or a haemorrhage. It is a major cause of disability and death among elderly people.

A stroke is a sudden, acute disturbance in brain function that can develop over a period of minutes or hours, and which lasts for more than 24 hours. It is a serious consequence of cerebrovascular disorders (disorders of the blood vessels of the brain and meninges), and is the third most common cause of death in the UK after heart disease and cancer.

WHO IS AFFECTED?

Stroke is the single greatest cause of physical disability, with an incidence of 5 per 1000 of the general population, and a higher incidence in elderly people. About half of those affected die, often within

24 hours of the event. A third are left with some functional disability and the remainder make a good recovery.

Doctors often refer to a stroke as a 'cerebrovascular accident' (CVA), the term indicating a problem affecting the blood vessels running from the heart to the brain.

Cerebrovascular events that last less than 24 hours are known as transient ischaemic attacks (TIAs); they are not usually associated with any obvious structural damage or lasting disability.

WHAT CAUSES A STROKE?

In older people, a stroke is the result of an interruption of the blood supply to the brain, or of a ruptured blood vessel bleeding deep within the brain.

An obstruction to the brain's blood supply (ischaemia) deprives nerve cells of vital oxygen and nutrition. Brain cell and nerve pathway damage occur, disturbing brain function and central control over the peripheral nerves and muscles.

In elderly people, stroke is often associated with high blood pressure and atherosclerosis. Blood from ruptured vessels (haemorrhage) within the cranium compresses brain tissue, with effects that can include paralysis and speech loss.

Risk factors

The likelihood of suffering from a stroke increases with advancing age. Other factors can also predispose to a stroke, such as:
- Previous TIA
- Previous stroke
- High blood pressure
- Heart failure
- Recent coronary thrombosis
- Atrial fibrillation (abnormal heart rhythm)
- Diabetes
- Family history of stroke
- High alcohol intake
- Smoking.

Blood supply to the brain

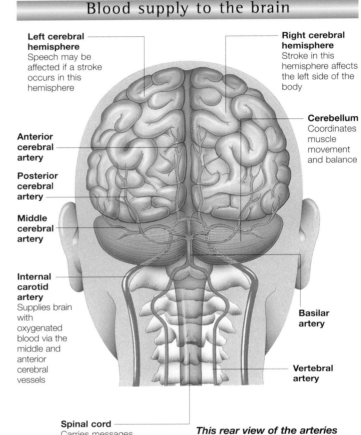

Left cerebral hemisphere
Speech may be affected if a stroke occurs in this hemisphere

Anterior cerebral artery

Posterior cerebral artery

Middle cerebral artery

Internal carotid artery
Supplies brain with oxygenated blood via the middle and anterior cerebral vessels

Spinal cord
Carries messages to and from the brain and body

Right cerebral hemisphere
Stroke in this hemisphere affects the left side of the body

Cerebellum
Coordinates muscle movement and balance

Basilar artery

Vertebral artery

This rear view of the arteries of the head shows the major arteries supplying the brain. A blockage of any of these major vessels can result in stroke.

Disruption of the brain's blood supply

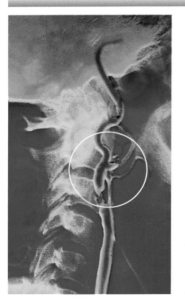

The left and right carotid arteries are the main arteries to the cerebral hemispheres. About 20 per cent of blood output from the heart goes to the brain.

The brainstem and cerebellum (the parts of the brain that govern movement) are supplied by the vertebral arteries, which fuse to become the basilar artery.

Eighty per cent of vascular events in the skull are due to cerebral infarction and 20 per cent are due to bleeding. Cerebral infarction occurs when the brain is damaged due to a lack of blood, such as when a

vessel becomes blocked. If the blood supply is not restored quickly, that part of the brain will die.

Blood vessel blockage may be due to thrombus or embolus. A thrombus (blood clot) may be formed by atherosclerosis (hardening and thickening of arteries with fatty deposits), which narrows and obstructs the vessel, starving the brain of blood, oxygen and nourishment. An embolus may be a tiny piece of clot that breaks away from an atherosclerotic neck artery, or even from the heart itself.

A false-colour angiogram reveals an obstruction (circled) in the carotid artery. This may be caused by atherosclerosis, a build-up of plaque in the vessels.

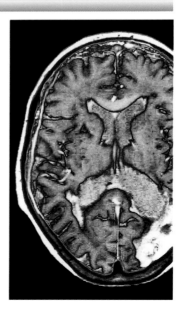

This false-colour MR scan shows a haemorrhage in the left hemisphere of the brain (the white area on the right of this image). The affected tissue often dies.

Symptoms and stroke diagnosis

The symptoms of a stroke directly reflect the area of the brain affected; a stroke in one cerebral hemisphere will show symptoms in the opposite side of the body. The clinical diagnosis of a stroke may be confirmed by examination and scanning.

The symptoms of a stroke are determined by the site of the brain infarct (tissue death) or the bleeding artery. Strokes that affect one of the two halves of the brain (the cerebral hemispheres) are five times more common than those affecting the brainstem.

SITE OF DAMAGE
Different parts of the body are affected, depending on the areas of damaged brain. If the front of the brain is affected, there may be personality changes and mood disturbance with poor emotional control, such as laughing or crying at inappropriate moments. The speech centre may be affected if there is damage in the left cerebral hemisphere.

PARALYSIS AND SENSATION
When the motor areas of the hemispheres (areas responsible for voluntary muscle movement) are damaged, the control of limb movements on the opposite side to the damage will be affected. This results in loss of power or paralysis of the arm, leg or both – this is known as hemiparesis or hemiplegia.

If the brain area responsible for governing sensation is disturbed, there may be interference with sensation of pain, touch and joint position. The latter causes imbalance, leading to falls.

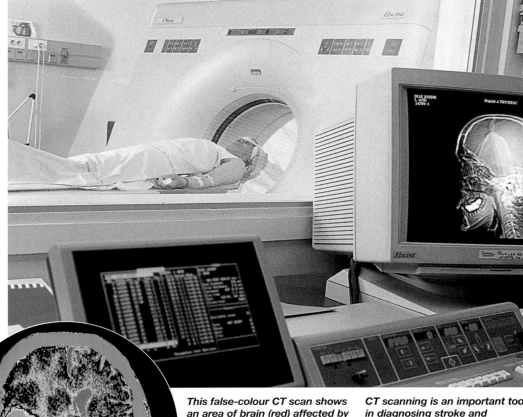

This false-colour CT scan shows an area of brain (red) affected by ischaemia or reduced blood flow. If left untreated, the brain tissue will eventually die.

CT scanning is an important tool in diagnosing stroke and determining the extent of brain damage. The images are seen as 'slices' through the head.

Diagnosis

A stroke is usually diagnosed from the signs and symptoms present, especially if the person has a pre-existing disease associated with risk of stroke. Such diseases include diabetes, hypertension (high blood pressure) and atherosclerosis. The condition can also be diagnosed if the person is known to have a source of emboli – in the heart, for example.

DIAGNOSTIC AIDS
To exclude the possibility of a rapidly growing tumour being the cause of symptoms, a skull X-ray may be required. To determine whether the cause is a haemorrhage or an infarct, CT scanning is a useful technique.

A further neurological examination of the motor and sensory systems and the eyes, and assessment of the mental state and physical function usually confirm the diagnosis.

Guidelines for good medical practice recommend that all stroke patients have blood investigations, blood pressure checks, an ECG (electrocardiogram to measure the electrical activity of the heart), or CT or MR scanning.

Echocardiography (ultrasound of the heart) may be undertaken when there is a suspected heart cause of emboli, such as after recent coronary thrombosis or where there is atrial fibrillation or known heart valve disease.

Onset of stroke

The onset of a stroke has several characteristics:
■ Cerebral infarction may take one or two hours to develop; embolic occurrences are often abrupt in onset. Intracerebral bleeding may occur suddenly, with headache, vomiting and impaired or lost consciousness.
■ There may be an associated paralysis with loss of muscle power on one side of the body. Disturbance in vision and impairment in speech, with slurring of words or even loss of speech can also occur. Urinary incontinence is common.
■ Reduced mental alertness and lost muscle power or limb paralysis can vary in the first few days after a stroke, or worsen due to swelling of brain tissue and, in some cases, the extension of the infarct.
■ If death does not occur, there is usually an improvement in function over days and weeks as the swelling in the brain subsides.

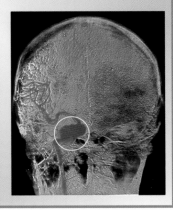

An aneurysm can be seen as a bulge (circled) in the carotid artery. If it ruptures, blood will haemorrhage into the surrounding brain tissue, causing a stroke.

Treating stroke patients

Treatment for stroke victims is based on rehabilitation to regain mobility and a level of independence in everyday tasks. For severely disabled patients, treatment aims to manage the symptoms.

The majority of patients are hospitalized after a stroke and need the services of a multidisciplinary team. Many patients also need help from a community rehabilitation team after discharge from hospital.

A person with previously good health suffering their first stroke has a good potential for survival and rehabilitation. However, no treatment can reverse or reduce local brain tissue damage.

DRUG TREATMENTS
Recurrence of an infarction is reduced by aspirin, which thins the blood. However, it should not be used if the stroke was caused by a cerebral haemorrhage, as it slows the action of clotting.

High blood pressure is treated with hypotensive drugs, although blood pressure is often raised in the two weeks after a stroke, so active blood pressure lowering should be delayed.

Physiotherapy to strengthen the muscles and improve coordination is a vital part of rehabilitation. Many ordinary tasks need to be relearned.

MANAGEMENT
The general management of stroke is aimed at maintaining the airway and breathing. Swallowing may be affected and a nasogastric tube may be passed into the stomach for feeding to avoid the inhalation of food and the development of pneumonia.

Urinary incontinence may need short-term catheterization. Good nursing care is required to avoid both the appearance of pressure sores and deep vein thrombosis.

A physiotherapist works with an elderly stroke patient. Paralyzed limbs must be exercised 'passively' from the onset of the stroke to avoid later spasticity.

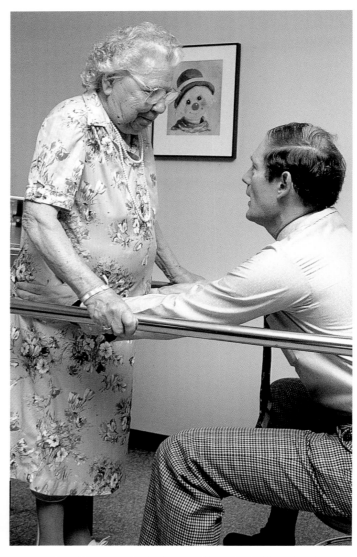

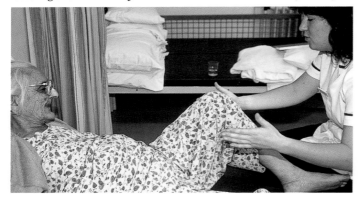

Rehabilitation

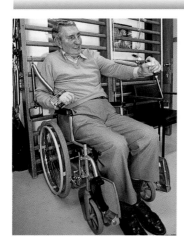

The objectives of rehabilitation are aimed at avoiding further physical and mental deterioration and achieving the best possible recovery of function for the activities of daily living. This involves a multi-professional team including physiotherapists, occupational therapists, speech therapists, prosthesis technicians and nurses.

Orthoses (surgical appliances, such as back splints and leg

Active exercises, where patients try to build strength and flexibility, are important in regaining independence.

braces) are often required to support unstable joints. Following a stroke, active interventions may be required over a period of six months. After this time, major improvement is unlikely.

Physiotherapy should begin soon after the stroke. The limbs are put through a full range of passive movements repeatedly each day. Of patients surviving the first two weeks after the stroke, two-thirds regain independence, despite some disability. The remainder will die in the next two months or become long-term disabled.

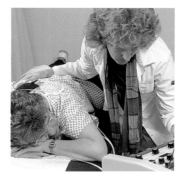

After a stroke, a patient may receive electrical stimulation of the affected muscles. This helps build up wasted muscles.

Prognosis

The prognosis immediately after a stroke is difficult to determine. Drugs can reduce the chance of another stroke, but functional recovery can be limited.

The presence of coma, complete hemiplegia (paralysis of one side of the body) and eye palsy suggest a poor prognosis for a stroke victim. Incontinence is also a poor prognostic feature and is associated with recurrent urinary tract infection. The onset of pneumonia can be a fatal complication.

PREDICTING RECOVERY
Neither the progression of symptoms nor the ultimate functional outcome of the stroke

An intracerebral haemorrhage caused by a major burst artery. Brain tissue has been pushed out of shape by the blood leaking from the vessel.

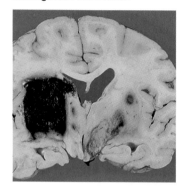

can be predicted in early post-stroke days. Recovery, and its extent, depends upon the site of the damage, the age of the person and the general state of their health.

Any functional disability existing after six months is likely to be permanent. About half of those affected with moderate or severe hemiplegia recover sufficiently to be able to walk and attend to basic activities of daily living. In general, the sooner an improvement in mobility occurs, the better the prognosis.

INCIDENCE
Mortality rates for stroke victims have been falling over the last 40 years, but the incidence remains the same, with more patients admitted to hospital as the number of elderly people in the population increases. In the absence of a cure for stroke and the damage that it causes, prevention is important.

Occupational therapy is another important treatment for patients recovering from a stroke. This patient is using an 'elevation board' to improve hand–eye coordination and grip.

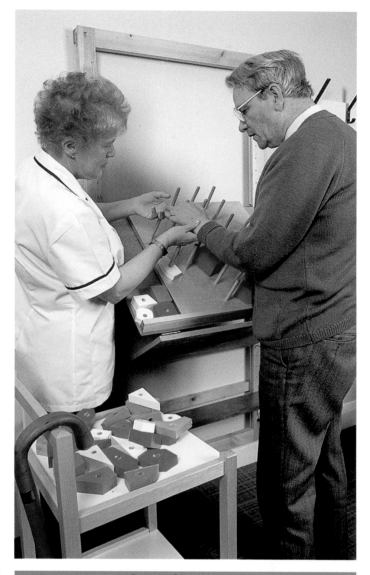

Preventing strokes

High blood pressure is the single most important risk factor for stroke in the elderly. Therefore, early treatment of high blood pressure, irrespective of age, is important, as is a reduction in smoking and alcohol habits. Reducing blood cholesterol and fats should also reduce the occurrence of stroke disease.

BLOOD PRESSURE
Comparative trials have shown a reduction of stroke by one third in people who have had high blood pressure significantly reduced. Blood pressure refers to the pressure of blood in a major artery and is read as two figures: systolic pressure is the first and highest figure, taken when the ventricles of the heart are contracting; diastolic is the lower figure, taken when the ventricles are relaxed. Blood pressure above normal (140mm Hg systolic and 90mm Hg diastolic) at whatever age should be treated to lower the risk of

stroke occurrence. Both fatal and non-fatal strokes are less likely to occur after blood pressure is lowered.

About a third of all people with transient ischaemic attacks (TIAs) suffer from a later stroke. TIAs should be investigated and any high blood pressure or carotid artery stenosis treated.

OTHER FACTORS
Heart irregularities increase the risk of stroke disease and irregular rhythms, such as atrial fibrillation (a type of heart arrhythmia with rapid, irregular beats), should be treated.

Environmental extremes can also affect the circulation, making the blood more viscous and the cells stickier. This means blood vessel blockage by means of a blood clot is more likely. For this reason, the elderly should avoid long exposure to direct summer sun and should use heating in living accommodation in the winter.

Complications

A stroke may have additional, longer-term effects, depending on the severity of the initial attack and the rate of recovery:

Neurological effects
■ Brain swelling, leading to confusion
■ Epilepsy
■ Depression
■ Mental impairment.

Deep vein thrombosis is caused by a blood clot in the leg. Symptoms include swelling and pain.

Other effects
■ Heart irregularity
■ Pneumonia
■ Contractures of the joints
■ Spasticity of the limbs
■ Deep vein thrombosis
■ Kidney failure
■ Urinary incontinence
■ Urinary infection
■ Pressure sores due to extended bed rest.

Pressure sores are a risk for any bedridden patient. Moving the patient regularly and good hygiene help to control sores.

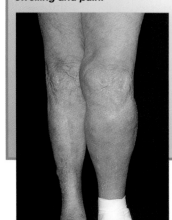

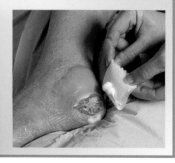

Prostate cancer

Prostate cancer appears to be on the increase among men. It is important to detect symptoms early before the cancer spreads and while treatment options can still offer a cure.

The prostate is the male gland that produces seminal fluid. It is about the size of a walnut and is situated below the bladder and in front of the rectum.

INCREASING PROBLEM

The incidence of prostate cancer is rising. Approximately 18,000 new cases of prostate cancer are diagnosed each year in the UK and about 10,000 men die each year from the disease. Prostate cancer accounts for 10 to 30 per cent of tumours in men and 13 per cent of all male cancer deaths, ranking third behind lung and large bowel cancer.

Lifetime risk of developing clinical disease is 10 per cent, while lifetime risk of dying from prostate cancer is three per cent. These figures may reflect an increasing ageing population, a greater diagnostic pick-up rate, and possibly a true increase in incidence in younger men.

The prostate gland secretes a fluid that forms part of semen. The prostate's position makes it accessible to examination through the rectal wall.

Location of the prostate

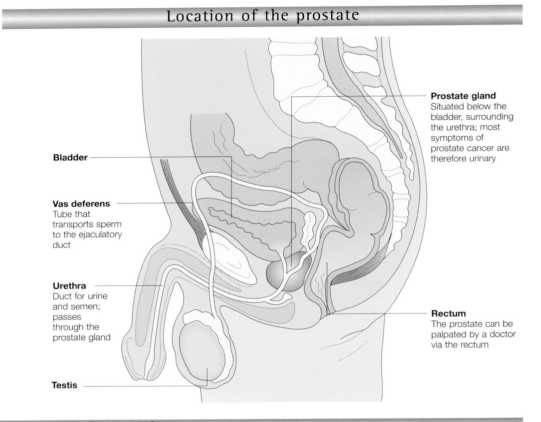

Prostate gland
Situated below the bladder, surrounding the urethra; most symptoms of prostate cancer are therefore urinary

Bladder

Vas deferens
Tube that transports sperm to the ejaculatory duct

Urethra
Duct for urine and semen; passes through the prostate gland

Rectum
The prostate can be palpated by a doctor via the rectum

Testis

Risk factors for prostate cancer

The established risk factors for prostate cancer are:

■ **Age**
Age is the single most important risk factor for the development of prostate cancer. Prostate cancer is rare under 45 years, but increases with age.

■ **Family history**
Nine per cent of cases have a genetic basis. Men with first-degree relatives suffering from prostate cancer, particularly if they were under 45 years, are at increased risk of developing the disease. This is related to carrying a specific inherited dominant prostate cancer gene.

In men with prostate cancer, there may be an association with breast cancer in female relatives.

■ **Diet**
Prostate cancer is associated with both total calorie intake and intake of saturated fat, specifically that of red meat. Vegetarians have a 25 to 50 per cent reduction in risk.

It has not been established whether anti-oxidant vitamins

(vitamins C and E) and carotenes (vitamin A), as well as plant oestrogens (contained in soya) and selenium (an essential mineral), are associated with decreased risk.

In a recent randomized trial, men who received vitamin E supplements had a 34 per cent reduced risk of developing prostate cancer.

■ **Ethnic origin**
There is an extraordinarily varied geographical incidence. The incidence of clinical cancer is low in Asia, intermediate in Latin America and Southern Europe, and high in Northern Europe and North America.

The highest incidence rates are in American Afro-Caribbeans; the lowest are in southeast Asia.

■ **Country of residence**
Observations in Japanese

A proportion of prostate cancer cases are hereditary. Men with relatives who have had prostate cancer are more likely to carry a certain cancer gene.

immigrants show that rates of prostate cancer rise when they move to the United States of America and also that rates increase with the number of generations living there.

LIFESTYLE FACTORS
These data demonstrate that the risk of prostate cancer is

partly dependent on lifestyle factors. Diet in particular is implicated.

The concept that low risk of prostate cancer can be achieved as a result of a diet containing potential anticarcinogenic agents, would suggest that a proportion of prostate cancer is potentially preventable.

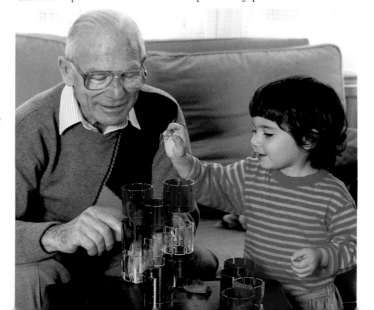

Detecting and diagnosing prostate cancer

Unfortunately, most of the symptoms of prostate cancer appear only when the disease is advanced. Investigation techniques are used to diagnose the stage which prostate cancer has reached and to determine the most suitable treatment.

The suspicion of prostate cancer may be raised by an abnormality on digital rectal examination (DRE) for the investigation of another condition, a raised prostate specific antigen (PSA) in the blood, or by development of urinary symptoms.

Unfortunately, however, many cases are asymptomatic and are only found at post-mortem.

SYMPTOMS OF CANCER
The presence of the following symptoms often indicates advanced disease:
■ Prostatic outflow symptoms – frequency, hesitancy, poor urinary stream, nocturia (urinating at night), haematuria (blood in the urine) and terminal dribbling (dripping urine after urination has finished).
■ Bone pain – (commonly in the back, pelvis, shoulders or ribs) is the most common complaint in patients with advanced cancer due to its spread to the bones (metastases)
■ The sudden onset of weakness in the legs, sensory loss and incontinence – due to compression of the nerves in the spinal cord caused by bone metastases
■ Hypercalcaemia (raised calcium level in the blood) – resulting in nausea, vomiting, abdominal pain and confusion
■ General symptoms of malignancy, which include malaise (a general feeling of being unwell), anorexia and weight loss.

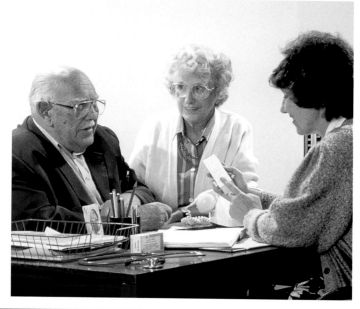

Men with early prostate cancer often have no symptoms, which makes it difficult to diagnose. When symptoms do occur, the disease is often advanced.

Investigations

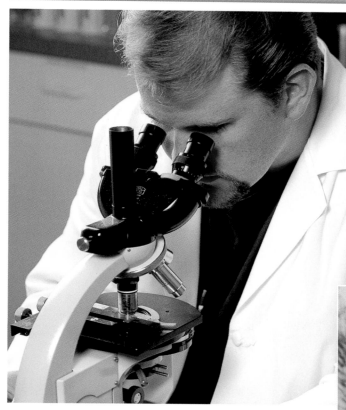

Prostate tissue removed during a biopsy procedure is examined under a microscope to diagnose cancer. This will indicate the aggressiveness of the tumour.

Cancer (circled) can be seen within the prostate on this ultrasound image. The transducer is the white circle at the top of the image.

Men with any of the above symptoms or who are suspected of having prostate cancer should undergo PSA testing and digital rectal examination.

If patients show signs of induration (abnormal hardening) of the gland or a PSA above the usual level of 4.0 ng/ml, they will usually be regarded as suitable for trans-rectal ultrasound and prostatic biopsy (known as TRUS).

BIOPSIES
The TRUS-guided and spring-loaded biopsy device allows a number of biopsies to be taken of the prostate without too much discomfort for the patient.

The diagnosis of prostate cancer has to be confirmed by histology (examining the prostate tissue taken by TRUS under the microscope).

The great majority of prostate cancers are adenocarcinomas, mostly arising from the periphery of the gland in the so-called peripheral zone.

DESCRIPTION OF CANCER
The histological appearance of the tumour is recognized as the best indications of prognosis. A grading system called the Gleason score (GL) is used to determine the aggressiveness of the tumour:
■ GL 2–4 – less aggressive
■ GL 5–7 – moderately aggressive
■ GL 8–10 – most aggressive.

SCANS
Once the prostate cancer diagnosis is confirmed after the biopsy, normally a bone scan and a CT scan or MRI of the pelvis and abdomen is undertaken. This will determine whether there is any local or distant spread of the prostate cancer in the body.

The MR scan gives more detail of the surrounding soft tissues around the prostate, and in particular can determine whether the seminal vesicles or lymph glands are affected.

Treating prostate cancer

A variety of treatments may be effective for patients with localized prostate cancer. Even when the cancer is advanced it may be possible to slow down its growth and control symptoms.

There are currently several treatment options for localized prostate cancer, these include:

■ Radical prostatectomy

This operation involves removal of the entire prostate and adjacent bladder neck, seminal vesicles and surrounding tissue. Provided the procedure is confined to younger men (aged under 70 years), death occurs in less than one per cent of patients.

Unfortunately, in 30 to 40 per cent of radical prostatectomy cases the cancer will have already spread to surrounding tissue. The obvious benefits are, however, that overall more than 70 per cent of men are cured by this form of surgery.

■ Radical radiotherapy

Radical radiotherapy can be delivered as external beam radiotherapy (EBRT), where radiation is targeted on the prostate from the outside.

External beam radiotherapy carries the advantage of being outpatient-based. It is also the only option for curing men who are not fit enough to have an operation, or do not want one. In addition, it has none of the risks of surgery, especially the risks of lung clots and infection.

However, there are other significant side effects. Another major disadvantage is its failure to achieve 100 per cent tumour cell kill in a significant proportion of cases, which leads to relapse.

In recent years, however, technical advances have been made which improve the outcome of EBRT.

■ Brachytherapy

Brachytherapy (transperineal prostate implantation) uses radioactive seeds, implanted in the prostate under general anaesthesia. This technique has a similar success rate to that of prostatectomy in patients whose cancer has been diagnosed early (with no metastasis or local spread only). The advantages are the decreased incidence of impotence compared to EBRT and prostatectomy, and the fact that it can be given as a single day outpatient treatment.

CONSIDERING OPTIONS

Individual treatments are very different in terms of side effects and the effects on quality of life. It is thus important for each patient to discuss the treatment options with specialists.

Radical prostatectomy is a surgical procedure used to treat localized cancer. The operation involves removing the whole prostate gland.

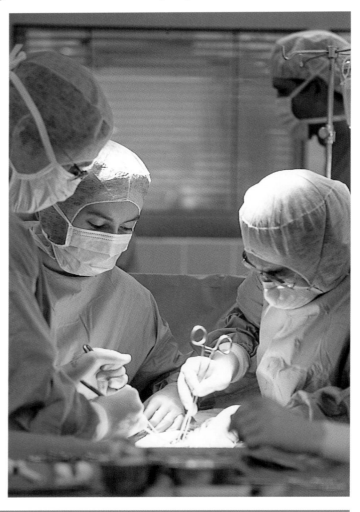

Palliative treatment

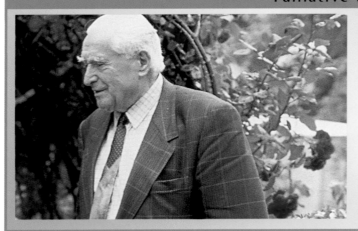

A 'wait and watch' policy, or palliative care, may be justified for men with a life expectancy of less than 10 years, due to other medical conditions, or old age.

This is appropriate for men not likely to live long enough for the cancer to grow and cause harm. In other words, they may die with prostate cancer rather than from it, and 'watch and wait' saves

For some older patients with prostate cancer, palliative care may be most suitable. This involves treating symptoms rather than curing the disease.

them the toxic effects that radical treatment entails.

Regular checks

With this policy, men are checked at regular intervals, and only when there is a change in their condition, with a rise in the PSA or evidence of progressive disease, is medical treatment in the form of androgen ablation (lowering testosterone levels) initiated. This policy is, however, not acceptable generally for younger men, as by deferring treatment the opportunity for curative treatment might be lost.

Treating advanced prostate cancer

Advanced prostate cancer is the extension of disease beyond the capsule surrounding the prostate. The term encompasses the spectrum between direct spread into local tissue to widespread metastases (distant spread via the blood or lymphatic systems).

HORMONAL THERAPY
For patients with metastatic disease, the standard treatment is hormonal manipulation. This is because prostate cancer cells are stimulated by the male hormone testosterone (an androgen). By decreasing testosterone levels in the body (androgen ablation), prostate cancer can be effectively treated, as it has no stimulus to grow.

This can be achieved either by the use of injections of drugs called LH-RH antagonists (these are hormones produced by the brain, which stimulate testosterone production) or by surgical removal of the testicles (orchidectomy). Both of these are equally effective and the choice will be based on suitability for each individual patient.

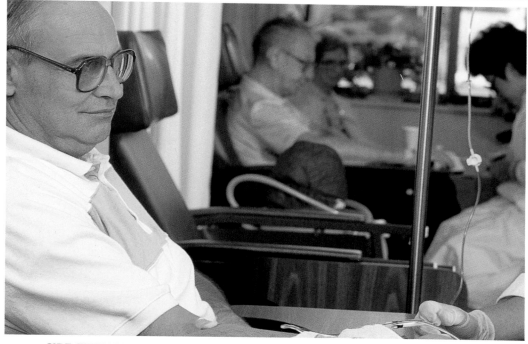

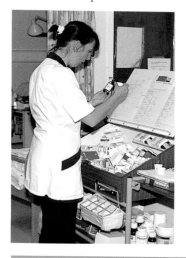

In hospital, analgesics (painkillers) are given to patients with advanced prostate cancer. Nurses will adjust the dose according to the level of pain.

SIDE EFFECTS
The side effects of hormonal manipulation include impotence, loss of libido, hot flushes, weight gain and gynaecomastia (growth of breasts).

SUCCESS OF TREATMENT
Hormone treatment benefits 70 to 80 per cent of patients with metastatic disease. The average time for a patient to be in remission is 18 months and inevitably many will relapse.

Further hormonal manipulation, with the addition or withdrawal of an anti-androgen and the use of steroids or female hormones, is normally tried, but unfortunately it is often disappointing.

CONTROLLING SYMPTOMS
Further treatment, at this stage, is aimed at controlling symptoms. Bone pain and tiredness are the most crippling effects of terminal prostate cancer. In addition to the appropriate use of painkillers, radiotherapy to the painful areas can be very effective.

Chemotherapy may also be tried, resulting in improvement of symptoms for some patients and a reduction in the PSA levels. However, no benefit in overall survival has been proven as yet, and therefore doctors should consider the toxicity of the treatment as well as its effect on quality of life.

Chemotherapy involves the used of drugs to control the symptoms of advanced prostate cancer. This treatment also reduces PSA levels in patients.

MEDICAL PRIORITIES
In cases of advanced prostate cancer, which are usually incurable, high priority is given to improving quality of life.

In addition to the necessary supportive treatments (painkillers, steroids and radiotherapy), medical staff should pay particular attention to the nutritional and psychological state of patients.

The involvement of a specialist palliative care team including doctors, nurses and dietitians, is crucial in facilitating delivery of this care during the terminal illness.

Screening for prostate cancer

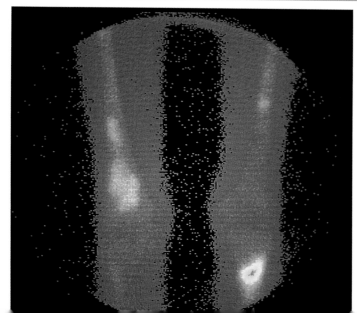

A hot spot (shown here in yellow) on a bone scan indicates spread of the cancer to bone. The disease is usually already incurable at this stage.

Prostate cancer is a slow and insidious disease. Symptoms normally develop only when the disease is either locally advanced within the pelvis, or after metastases in the bone have occurred. By this stage, the disease is incurable.

LACK OF EVIDENCE
Screening, which is aimed at finding cancer in the early and curable stages of the disease, would seem to be the obvious solution. However, there is lack of evidence from randomized trials that PSA screening reduces prostate cancer mortality. There is also the concern that screening would result in the diagnosis of tumours that do not, in fact, need treatment.

FUTURE ADVANCES
It remains to be seen, from the ongoing clinical trials, whether screening will have an impact in reducing deaths due to prostate cancer. In the USA, where PSA testing is widespread, prostate cancer is being detected at an earlier stage, with a reduction in mortality from the disease recently having been reported.

Lung cancer

Lung cancer causes non-specific symptoms and presents at a very advanced stage. Reducing smoking, use of technology for earlier diagnosis and more effective drugs all help to combat the disease.

Lung cancer causes non-specific symptoms, and for this reason it is generally not diagnosed until a very advanced stage. Only 10 per cent of patients in the UK are operable at the time of diagnosis; most of the remainder will succumb to the illness within six to nine months.

DEFINING LUNG CANCER
There are many different types of growth or tumour that can occur in the lungs. It is conventional to divide growths into benign and malignant, and into primary and secondary. A benign tumour is one that is

Certain occupations increase the risk of contracting a respiratory disease. Miners exposed to radon may develop lung cancer. Coal miners are at risk of other respiratory diseases.

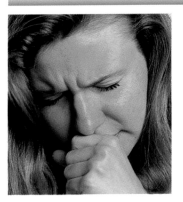

unlikely to spread to become life-threatening, whereas a malignant tumour grows rapidly, and spreads (metastasizes), thereby threatening life. This happens by direct invasion of surrounding structures or by spreading through the blood or lymphatic system.

A primary tumour of the lungs is one that has arisen first within the lung tissue; a secondary tumour is one that has arisen elsewhere in the body, but has then spread to the lungs.

Lung cancer is the term given to a primary malignant tumour arising from the lungs. It is responsible for more deaths than any other form of cancer, and accounts for 900,000 deaths per year worldwide.

INCIDENCE
In 1992, lung cancer was estimated to account for 37,000 deaths in the UK, with the highest rates occurring in the Merseyside region of northwest England. Here, it is estimated that nearly 12 per cent of the male population and seven per cent of the female population will develop lung cancer before the age of 75.

The incidence rates for lung cancer in men is declining slowly; however, in women the rates continue to rise.

RISK FACTORS
The most common cause of lung cancer is tobacco smoke. It is estimated that about 80 per

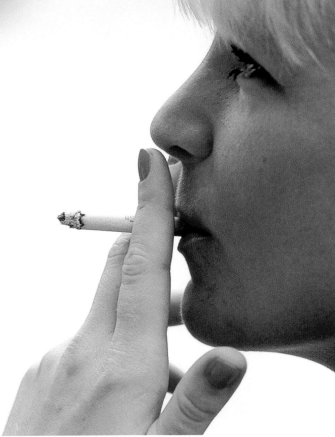

cent of all lung cancers are attributable to tobacco smoking. There are, however, other known factors associated with an increased risk of lung cancer:
- Dietary factors (deficient in vitamins, high in cholesterol)
- Radon (radioactive gas, found in increased amounts in mines)
- Ionizing radiation

The number of women that are diagnosed with lung cancer is rising. This is due to increasing numbers of women smoking.

- Occupational carcinogens, such as industrial chemicals
- Genetic factors (that is, an inherited predisposition to developing lung cancer).

Symptoms of lung cancer

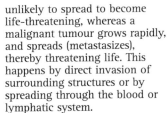

The symptoms of lung cancer are very non-specific. This is the reason that many patients with lung cancer present at an advanced stage of the disease.

The symptoms include: breathlessness, cough, chest pain, lethargy and weight loss. All these symptoms are very common and are present in

One factor hindering the early diagnosis of lung cancer is that the symptoms, such as a cough, are common to other conditions.

numerous other conditions. Even coughing up blood (haemoptysis), which is assumed by many people to be a defining symptom of the condition, is not present in the majority of patients who are diagnosed with lung cancer.

Any one of these symptoms may be caused by many other conditions, the most common being chest infections. The percentage of patients with each of these common symptoms is shown in the table (right).

Presentation

Symptom	Percentage of patients
Cough	40–75
Shortness of breath	30–40
Coughing blood	15–35
Weight loss	40–50
Loss of appetite	35
Lethargy	35
Chest pain	25–40

Primary investigations

The majority of lung cancers are discovered after a patient goes to see their GP or hospital accident and emergency department with one or more of the symptoms discussed. In the presence of such symptoms (particularly in a smoker), a chest X-ray is mandatory.

X-RAY CONFIRMATION

The majority of lung cancers will be visible on a chest X-ray, either as an obvious mass or as abnormal shadowing that is regarded as non-specific (but needing further investigation). Following an X-ray, the patient is usually referred to a specialist for further investigations.

A small number of lung cancers are picked up when a chest X-ray is performed for another reason – for example, prior to a routine operation or during health screening programmes. Diagnosis may then be confirmed by microscopic examination of a sputum sample. The further investigation of these tumours

is identical to the investigation of those that are found to be causing recognized symptoms. Guidelines suggest that a patient with suspected lung cancer should be referred to a specialist urgently, preferably within a week of initial diagnosis.

PATIENT HISTORY

Initially, the specialist will take a full history from the patient during the first consultation to ascertain which symptoms are present and what risk factors for lung cancer may be present, such as cigarette smoking.

A full physical examination is performed to look for clinical evidence of tumour spread. Further investigations will be performed to assess the tumour type and the extent of the spread.

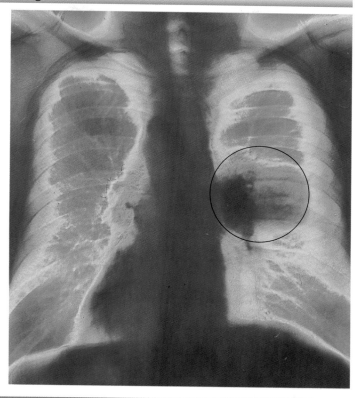

Lung cancer is evident on this false-colour X-ray, appearing as an isolated, solid mass on the patient's left lung (circled). Confirmation may be by tissue biopsy and sputum analysis.

Origins and types of lung cancer

All lung cancers arise from an abnormal division of one of the cells within the lung. From that point, they divide at a constant rate, thus doubling in size over a fixed period of time. This means that it takes the same for the tumour to increase in size from 6cm (2⅜in) in diameter to 12cm (4¾in) in diameter as it did to develop from four cells to eight cells.

Lung cancers may grow for many months (or even years) before being diagnosed. From the patient's point of view, once the tumour is diagnosed, it seems to worsen very quickly, as its growth in size terms is exponential.

Classifying tumours

Although the term lung cancer is used to describe all primary malignant tumours of the lungs, there are a number of different types of tumour contained within this definition. The main division is between tumours that have small cells when examined under a microscope (termed small-cell lung cancer) and those which do not (termed non-small-cell

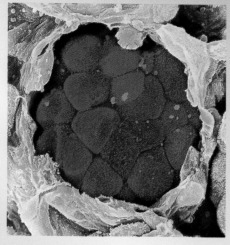

lung cancer). This division of lung cancer is necessary because the two types of tumour probably arise from different cells within the lung, and they certainly respond differently to various treatments.

■ Small-cell lung cancers are thought to arise from the nerve and glandular cells within the lungs and account for about 15 per cent of all lung cancers

■ Non-small-cell lung cancers arise in the main from cells lining the air passages in the lung and account for approximately 85 per cent of all lung cancers.

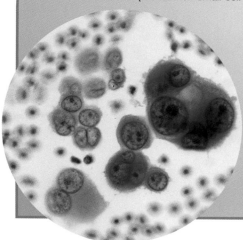

This is a light micrograph of clusters of cells from a mesothelioma, a lung cancer caused by asbestos. The malignant cells, of varying sizes, are stained blue.

The nuclei (dark blue) of these squamous cells of a non-small-cell lung cancer are enlarged. This, and the abnormal cell shapes, are characteristic of cancer.

This coloured scanning electron micrograph shows a lung tumour (red) filling an air sac in the lungs. Each cancer cell is covered by hairlike microvilli.

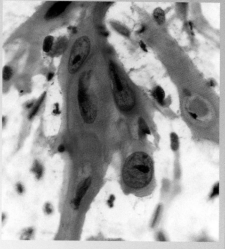

There are also a number of sub-divisions of the group of non-small-cell lung cancers. This is because the tumours arise from different types of cell within the air passages of the lungs, and they are classified according to cell type. However, the response to treatment is very similar for all of them. Tumours of this group include adenocarcinoma, squamous cell carcinoma, large-cell carcinoma and undifferentiated non-small-cell carcinoma.

Treating lung cancer

If lung cancer is suspected, a patient will be referred to a respiratory specialist. Investigations confirm the diagnosis, but treatment depends on the stage the disease has reached.

A variety of investigative tools are used by the respiratory specialist to confirm a diagnosis of lung cancer. These include:

■ Fibre-optic bronchoscopy
The larger air passages within the lungs are inspected using a flexible fibre-optic camera. This is usually performed under a local anaesthetic. The flexible bronchoscope is passed through either the nose or the mouth, then through the vocal cords, into the windpipe (trachea) and finally into the larger airways of either lung. The majority of lung cancers are visible in the larger airways.

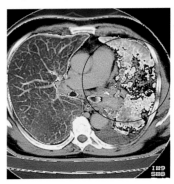

A respiratory specialist may need to use a bronchoscope to examine the larger bronchial branches of a patient's lungs.

■ CT scanning
The patient lies flat and is passed slowly through a circular scanner. The scanner takes X-rays in slices 1cm (³⁄₈in) in thickness and usually 1cm (³⁄₈in) apart. With the aid of specialized computer software, the lungs can then be viewed in three dimensions.

■ MR scan
Occasionally, this type of scan is used to assess invasion of the tumour into adjacent structures. This is not necessary in the majority of cases.

■ Bone scan
A radioactive isotope is injected into the bloodstream and is taken up by the bones. Areas of tumour spread show up as areas of increased uptake ('hot-spots').

This CT scan reveals cancerous tissue in the patient's left lung (circled), in contrast to the healthy right lung.

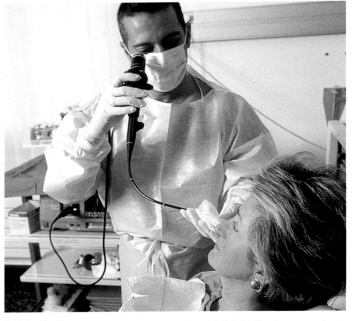

■ Needle biopsy
If the tumour is not visible at bronchoscopy but is visible on the CT scan, a needle biopsy may be performed through the chest wall. Local anaesthetic is applied to the skin and muscle of the chest wall and the needle is guided into the tumour using either conventional X-ray or CT scanning.

■ Abdominal ultrasound
Used to look for tumour spread to the liver; it is the same type of scan used during pregnancy.

Progression of lung cancer

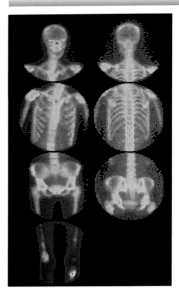

This coloured gamma camera scan reveals areas of secondary bone cancer. The spread of the cancer throughout the body is shown as the bright patches.

The outlook for patients with lung cancer depends on how far the tumour has spread before diagnosis. This is assessed using the tests outlined above.

The tumour may spread into adjacent structures, or it may spread into local lymph nodes within the chest. Both scenarios are assessed with CT scanning, and occasionally MR imaging. Any spread to the liver or adrenal glands (situated above the kidneys) is also assessed using the CT scan or ultrasound.

Spread to the bones is assessed with a bone scan. The stage of cancer will then be classified as either:
- Small cell
- Limited: confined to one side of the chest
- Extensive: spread beyond one side of the chest.

Stages of the disease

Non-small-cell lung cancers

Stage I	Tumour confined to the chest No evidence of distant spread
Stage II	Larger tumour than in stage I, or local lymph node enlargement No evidence of distant spread
Stage IIIA	More extensive lymph node enlargement No spread outside the chest
Stage IIIB	Lymph node spread into other side of the chest No spread outside the chest
Stage IV	Spread outside the chest, for example to the brain, liver, adrenal glands or skin

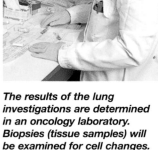

The results of the lung investigations are determined in an oncology laboratory. Biopsies (tissue samples) will be examined for cell changes.

Treatment and prognosis

The treatment of lung cancer depends upon the type of tumour, the stage of disease at diagnosis and the general fitness of the patient.

If the tumour is small and there is no evidence of spread to local lymph nodes, surgical removal of the tumour is usually performed. Chemotherapy is used in all other cases, as small-cell tumours respond reasonably well to this type of treatment. Roughly 75 per cent of tumours will respond to chemotherapy, but relapse is very common and the period of remission may last for only a few weeks. The prognosis is generally poor, the average survival from the time of diagnosis being nine months.

Non-small-cell lung cancer makes up about 85 per cent of all lung cancers. Treatment of the non-small-cell tumours can be divided into radical treatment

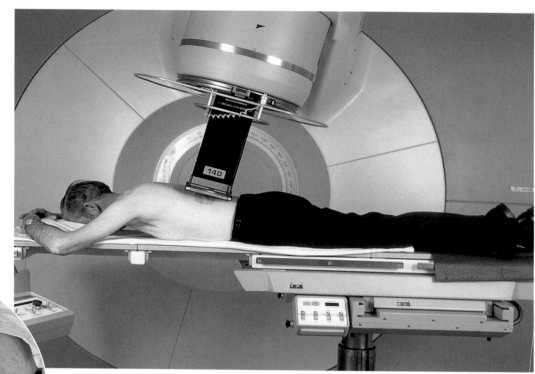

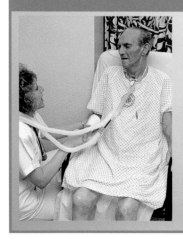

Chemotherapy is used in many countries to treat inoperable lung cancer. Recent studies suggest this treatment can prolong the lives of patients by six weeks.

with the intent to cure, or palliative treatment to alleviate the effects of the symptoms only.

SURGERY

When there is no evidence of cancer spread, or this is limited at the time of diagnosis, the treatment of choice is surgery to remove the tumour. This requires a general anaesthetic and usually a thoracotomy operation, in which a part of the lung is removed. This ranges from a lobe (of which there are three in the

right lung and two in the left) to a whole lung, depending on the site of the tumour.

Only 10 per cent of patients presenting to hospitals in the UK are both fit enough and at an early enough stage of the disease for an operation. Survival to five years after surgery varies from 80 per cent of those patients who present with stage I disease to 45 per cent in those presenting with stage IIIA disease. Therefore surgery, despite being the best option available, cannot cure all patients.

Radiotherapy involves bombarding the lung tumour with high-dose radiation. The aim is to kill all the cancer cells.

RADIOTHERAPY

In patients who decline, or who are not fit for surgery but have stage I, II or IIIA disease, high-dose (radical) radiotherapy is the treatment of choice. This consists of giving multiple high doses of radiation (X-rays) on consecutive days. However, the results, in terms of overall cure rates, are not as good as those achieved by surgery.

Palliative treatment

Non-radical treatment of lung cancer aims to improve the symptoms caused as the tumour progresses. Unfortunately, this type of treatment is the only option for the vast majority of non-small-cell lung cancer patients (in excess of 80 per cent). Without radical treatment, the average survival from the time of diagnosis is between three and six months.

This patient with advanced lung cancer is connected to a ventilator. Symptomatic relief is the aim of palliative care.

There are a variety of drugs available for the treatment of pain (including morphine and its derivatives), lethargy and anorexia (steroid tablets), cough (morphine derivatives) and breathlessness (morphine derivatives, asthma medications and oxygen). Radiotherapy, in doses much smaller than those used for radical treatment, is also used to improve cough, coughing blood, pain and, to a lesser extent, breathlessness. Chemotherapy for inoperable lung cancer is currently under evaluation in the UK.

Non-medical intervention is extremely important in this context. Access to community nursing support(either through district nurses or the Macmillan service), along with advice regarding social services and benefits, may improve the health status of lung cancer patients immensely.

It is important to recognize that the vast majority of symptoms associated with advanced lung cancer are manageable with the medications available and the strategies currently in use.

Bladder cancer

Symptoms and causes

By far the most common symptom that brings people with bladder cancer to their GP is blood in the urine. There are usually no other symptoms, although if small clots are being passed there may be some pain and difficulty in passing urine. Large tumours can block the urethral orifice, causing urine to stagnate; some people develop a urinary infection (cystitis).

CAUSES
The causes of bladder cancer are not fully understood. Certain risk factors render people more likely to develop the disease, but not all people with these factors develop bladder cancer.

Risk factors include:
■ Smoking – there is a consistent, but relatively low, risk among smokers, who are two to five times more likely to develop bladder cancer than non-smokers
■ Occupation – may be relevant in up to 20 per cent of cases.

There is an increased risk to workers in the chemical dye, solvents or rubber industries
■ Chronic inflammation – an infection such as the tropical parasitic infection schistosomiasis can cause long-term inflammation and a resulting risk of malignancy.

CARCINOGENS
The risks to industrial workers arise because they handle potentially cancer-causing substances called carcinogens. These substances are absorbed during a working lifetime and then excreted in the urine, which means that they have contact with the bladder lining. In developed countries, workers will be offered regular urine screening tests.

The presence of blood in the urine is often the first sign of bladder cancer. GPs will then refer patients for further specialist investigation.

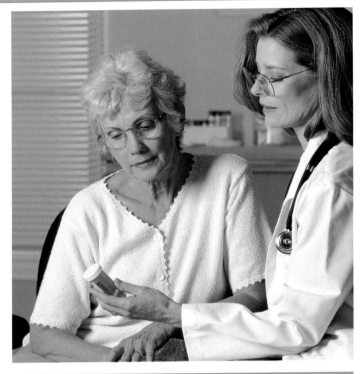

Diagnosis

GPs will not be able to make a diagnosis of bladder cancer themselves – they can only suspect that the disease is present, so referral is usually made to a urologist.

CYSTOSCOPY
The diagnosis is made by a urological surgeon, who will

arrange to look inside the bladder with an instrument called a cystoscope. This is a hollow viewing tube, which is inserted into the bladder under local or general anaesthesia.

A small sample (biopsy) of any suspicious tissue is sent to the pathologist for examination under a microscope.

On this X-ray of the bladder, the cancer is evident as the large, dark mass on the right-hand side. A cancer of this size is likely to be quite advanced.

DIAGNOSTIC IMAGING
Special X-rays called cystograms and excretion urograms may be employed, as well as CT scans, MRI scans, bone scans and chest X-rays to look for the spread of the cancer.

STAGING THE CANCER
Once bladder cancer has been confirmed, it is important to establish the grade of the disease and the stage or extent that it has reached. Low-grade cancers (where the tissue removed at biopsy is nearly normal) will spread more slowly than high-grade cancers.

The staging is important as a guide to how far the cancer has spread to nearby tissues or to other parts of the body. Treatment therefore depends on the size and stage of the tumour.

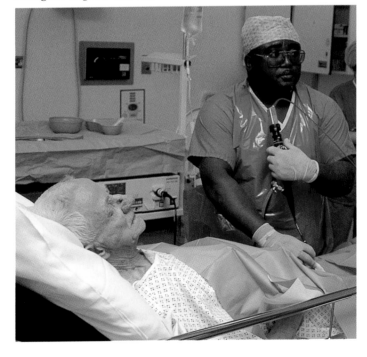

If doctors suspect a bladder tumour, cystoscopy is usually carried out. In this procedure, a flexible fibre-optic tube is passed up the urethra into the bladder to allow direct viewing.

Incidence
Incidence data includes:
■ Bladder tumours are second only to prostate tumours as sites for cancers within the urinary tract
■ Three-quarters of all cases occur in men, usually after the age of 50
■ In England and Wales, bladder tumours account for about seven per cent of all cancer in men and 2.5 per cent in women
■ Bladder tumours are 50 times more common than those of the ureter or renal pelvis.

Bladder cancers have a tendency to recur, and regular follow-up checks on all patients are therefore important.

Treatment

The treatment of bladder cancer depends on whether the tumour has infiltrated the muscle of the bladder wall and the type of cell of which the tumour consists.

TREATMENT OPTIONS
In the case of an early superficial tumour, the following treatments may be used:
■ Diathermy (or burning away of the tissue) – there are few post-operative problems. Patients may have some blood in their urine and there may be slight discomfort for a few days
■ Insertion of radioactive material – into the bladder to destroy the tumour.

For more extensive tumours, surgery is the most common form of treatment:
■ Partial cystectomy – the part of the bladder containing the tumour is removed and the remainder left in place
■ Total cystectomy – complete removal of the bladder may be carried out when tumours recur after megavoltage irradiation or when multiple tumours are too extensive for diathermy.

AFTER SURGERY
After total cystectomy, patients need an alternative storage reservoir for urine. One such alternative is to bring the ends of both ureters out through an opening in the abdominal wall, (an ileal conduit) so that urine can be drained into a bag.

RADIATION
Radiation therapy is the use of high-energy X-rays to kill cancer cells. External megavoltage irradiation is reserved for tumours that invade bladder muscle and those that are more malignant. Patients often become very tired after

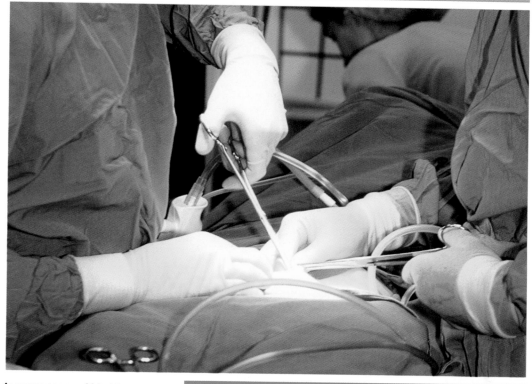

In some cases of bladder cancer, the removal of the whole bladder may be appropriate. This operation is called a total cystectomy.

radiotherapy and there may be permanent darkening of the skin in the treated area. It is also common to lose hair and the skin may become dry, tender and itchy. There may also be nausea, vomiting and some urinary discomfort.

CHEMOTHERAPY
Chemotherapy is the use of drugs to destroy cancer cells. The drugs are usually given orally or intravenously and absorbed through the body.

Prevention

Stopping smoking reduces the risk of bladder cancer, lung cancer and several other types of cancer as well as other problems such as heart disease. People who work in industries that are associated with an excess risk of developing the disease should avail themselves of all the screening tests on offer through their employers.

People whose work involves regular contact with potentially carcinogenic substances should take suitable precautions.

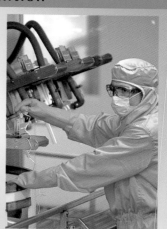

Prognosis

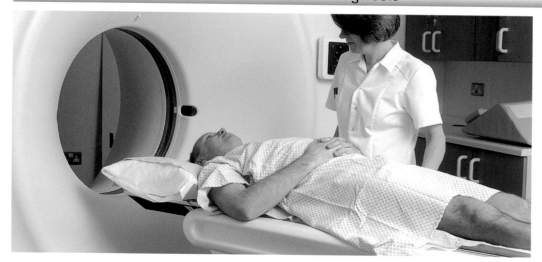

Once bladder cancer has been diagnosed, cystoscopic follow-up, usually at six-month intervals, must continue for life. Tumours may recur 13 years or so after first diagnosis.

Approximately 80 per cent of patients with superficial tumours and 60 per cent of those having had interstitial irradiation are still alive after five years, and around 30 per cent of those who have had a total cystectomy are still alive after three years.

Patients who have been treated for bladder cancer may need regular follow-up scans. These will reveal whether the cancer has spread.

Breast cancer

Breast cancer is the most common female cancer in the UK, affecting about 1 in 14 women at some stage in their lives. However, there are a variety of treatments and over two-thirds of patients are cured.

Breast cancer is the most common female cancer by far, with more than 30,000 new diagnoses every year in the UK. It is also the leading cause of cancer deaths in British women.

However, unlike many other types of cancer such as lung or pancreatic cancer, which kill the vast majority of the patients who develop them, breast cancer is cured in around two-thirds of cases.

AT-RISK WOMEN
Despite concern among many young women about developing breast cancer, predominantly it is a disease of older women who have passed the menopause.

The risk of developing breast cancer before the age of 35 is only about 1 in 2500. It rises to 1 in 50 by the age of 50, and is 1 in 10 for women who reach the age of 80.

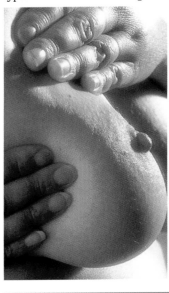

◀ *Regular self-examination can help to detect breast cancer early. The earlier a malignant abnormality is detected, the more effective the treatment.*

▶ *Mammography is an X-ray technique that reveals the presence of breast abnormalities. Many countries have breast screening programmes for at-risk women.*

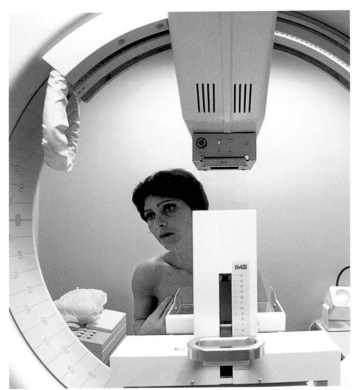

Risk factors for breast cancer

Although in the majority of patients the development of breast cancer is a chance event, there are a number of clearly documented risk factors for its development. These include:
■ Family or personal history of breast cancer

■ Increasing age
■ Previous non-cancerous breast lumps
■ Excessive exposure to the female sex hormone oestrogen – this means that women who start their periods early, go through the menopause late, or who take hormone replacement therapy (HRT) after the menopause have a slightly increased risk of developing breast cancer
■ Diet and alcohol intake – these have also been implicated.

CANCER GENES
Women from families with several members who develop breast cancer, particularly young first-degree relatives (mothers, sisters or daughters), have an especially high risk of developing the disease themselves. This is related to carrying an inherited breast cancer gene.

Two breast cancer genes have been identified, and these are known as BRCA1 and BRCA2. The chance of breast cancer developing during the lifetime of a patient carrying either BRCA1 or BRCA2 is 87 per cent.

The BRCA1 gene has been linked to the development of breast cancer. The gene is the red band (circled) on this fluorescent micrograph of chromosome 17.

Thus it is important to identify affected families and offer genetic counselling and, if appropriate, testing.

If a breast cancer gene is found in a patient with breast cancer, their offspring have a 50 per cent chance of inheriting that gene. Those family members inheriting the gene have a high risk of developing cancer.

OTHER FACTORS
Although the breast cancer genes are a very important cause of breast cancer, it should also be remembered that less than 10 per cent of all cases of breast cancer occur in individuals from families in which a specific breast cancer gene can be found.

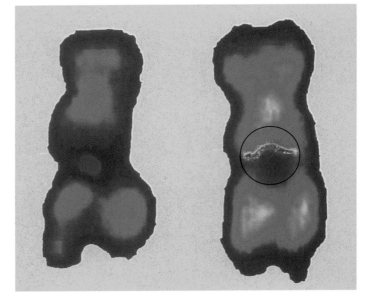

Risk of breast cancer by age	
AGE	RISK
30	1 in 2525
40	1 in 217
50	1 in 50
60	1 in 24
70	1 in 14

Breast cancer prevention

There are several strategies that may be employed to reduce the chance of developing breast cancer. Their use is generally confined to women in high-risk groups, particularly those individuals who have been shown to have inherited one of the breast cancer genes.

TAMOXIFEN

The anti-oestrogen drug tamoxifen has been used in breast cancer prevention trials. A recent US trial in women at a moderately increased risk of breast cancer showed that those who took tamoxifen for five years were less likely to develop breast cancer than those who did not. However, there was an increased risk of endometrial cancer (cancer of the inner lining of the uterus) and thromboembolic disease (blood

Removal of breast tissue is an effective method of preventing recurrence of breast cancer. The reduction of risk is linked to the amount of tissue removed.

clots in the leg veins or lung) in women taking tamoxifen. Women who took tamoxifen have not been shown to be less likely to die of breast cancer than those who did not.

Preliminary results from an ongoing UK study in women with a family history of breast cancer have shown no advantage from the use of tamoxifen. This collection of conflicting trial results makes it hard to formulate clear treatment guidelines.

Women contemplating tamoxifen chemoprevention for breast cancer should discuss this with an appropriate specialist and should, ideally, be treated in a relevant clinical trial.

PREVENTIVE SURGERY
■ Mastectomy
The most effective preventive strategy, supported by the best evidence, is bilateral mastectomy (or second mastectomy for patients who have already been treated for a first breast cancer). The removal of normal breasts cannot be undertaken lightly, however, so it is vital that

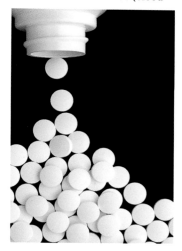

Tamoxifen is an anti-oestrogen drug that may prevent breast cancer in some women. However, the results of clinical trials have not been conclusive.

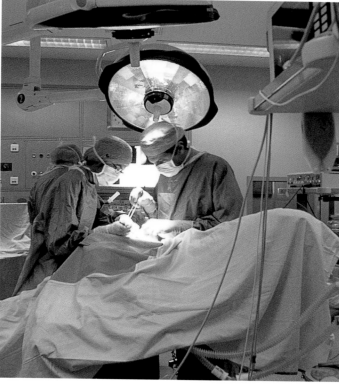

women considering this procedure receive adequate pre-surgical counselling.

The reduction of cancer risk is directly related to the amount of glandular breast tissue removed. Thus subcutaneous mastectomy, which leaves the nipple intact, is not generally recommended as it leaves about 10 per cent of this tissue behind. A traditional mastectomy leaves about one per cent of the glandular tissue.

■ Oophorectomy
For BRCA gene carriers, there is also an increased risk of ovarian cancer and consideration should also be given to prophylactic oophorectomy (preventive removal of the ovaries).

Oophorectomy reduces the risk of breast cancer by reducing the main source of oestrogen production and has been shown to reduce the risk of breast cancer in BRCA gene carriers.

Detecting and diagnosing breast cancer

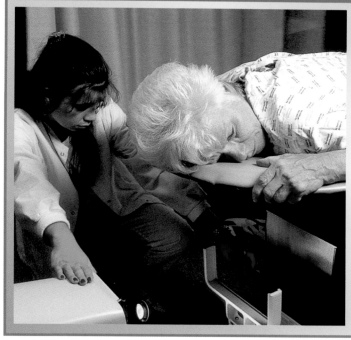

Patients can be alerted to the suspicion of breast cancer in one of two ways:
■ An abnormality can be detected on a screening mammogram, usually in the NHS Breast Screening Programme
■ A breast abnormality is noticed by the patient herself.

The commonest symptoms and signs of breast cancer are the presence of a lump, a change in shape of the breast, abnormalities in the skin of the breast, changes in the nipple or nipple discharge.

The diagnosis of breast abnormalities is usually made by a 'triple assessment', which includes clinical examination, mammogram and a needle

A breast biopsy may be taken under X-ray guidance. The biopsy needle takes a small tissue sample from the breast to be analyzed for cancer cells.

biopsy. Mammography may not, however, be useful in some women – particularly before the menopause when normal breast tissue is more dense – and ultrasound or magnetic resonance imaging offer an alternative means of diagnosis.

After these investigations, the majority of women, particularly those who notice a breast lump, are found not to have cancer. For those with a positive diagnosis, the emphasis moves on to treatment.

Patients need a multi-disciplinary approach to treatment, with input from surgeons, oncologists (cancer specialists), physiotherapists and other allied healthcare professionals. Specialist breast care nurses have an important role in counselling and helping patients to select appropriate treatment options.

Renal tumours

Symptoms

Renal (kidney) tumours may be non-cancerous (benign) or cancerous (malignant).

Benign tumours seldom cause any symptoms and they are usually discovered only incidentally, when the kidneys are being investigated for some other reason.

Malignant tumours that arise in the kidney include renal cell cancers (previously known as hypernephromas or Grawitz tumours) and nephroblastomas (Wilms' tumours).

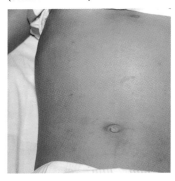

Nephroblastomas mostly occur in young children. Swelling of the abdomen, due to malignant growth, is often the first clear indication of a tumour.

RENAL CELL CANCERS

Renal cell cancers mainly affect older adults and cause:
- Blood in the urine (haematuria) – a common symptom
- Pain and swelling in the loins
- Fever – in about 20 per cent of patients
- Anaemia
- Weight loss
- Polycythaemia – raised haemoglobin and red blood cell levels due to the overproduction of erythropoietin, a hormone produced by the kidney
- Swollen veins in the testicle – due to tumours on the kidney obstructing the neighbouring renal vein.

In addition, about 25 per cent of patients with renal cell cancer first consult their doctors about symptoms such as swollen glands, cough or bone pain. This is a result of secondary cancers (metastases) in the lungs, bones or liver due to spread via the lymphatic system (to the lymph nodes) or the blood.

NEPHROBLASTOMAS

Nephroblastomas, also known as Wilms' tumours, usually occur in children up to the age of three; they are rare over the age of eight. In a few cases, tumours develop in both kidneys. Children with nephroblastomas develop:
- A large mass in the abdomen – this is usually the first and principal symptom. The mass is usually painless but may bleed internally, causing some pain
- Blood in the urine – this is rare in the early stages

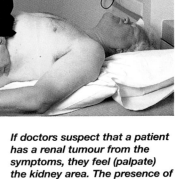

If doctors suspect that a patient has a renal tumour from the symptoms, they feel (palpate) the kidney area. The presence of a lump can indicate cancer.

- Loss of appetite
- Nausea and vomiting
- A feverish illness
- Raised blood pressure – due to kidney damage.

Causes

The cause of renal tumours varies according to the nature of the disorder.

SMOKING

Little is known about the cause of renal cell cancer, except that current cigarette smokers are at approximately double the risk of developing the disease compared to those who have never smoked.

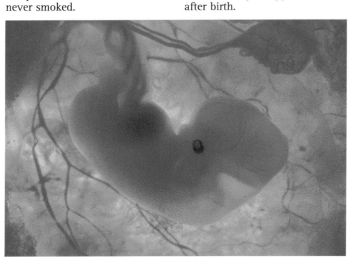

GENETIC ABNORMALITIES

The underlying cause of nephroblastomas is unknown. However, genetic abnormalities, particularly of chromosome 11, have been found in children with nephroblastomas. The tumours develop from cells involved in the development of the kidneys before birth, which usually disappear after birth.

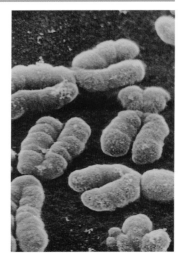

Genetic disorders, usually of chromosome 11, have been linked to nephroblastomas. About two per cent of cases have a relative with the disease.

Nephroblastomas are tumours arising from the embryonic tissue that develops into the kidneys during gestation (seven-week-old embryo shown).

Incidence

Renal cell cancer is about twice as common in men as in women. This type of cancer is rare under the age of 40, and usually occurs over the age of 50 years. The average age for first seeking medical advice is 55 years.

The number of cases occurring each year has increased in recent years, particularly among people of Afro-Caribbean origin in the United States.

Childhood malignancy
Nephroblastomas are the most common abdominal tumours in childhood, affecting about 75 children in Britain each year. About 10 per cent of cases occur in children born with other abnormalities, such as absence of the iris (the coloured part of the eye), abnormalities of the genito-urinary tract or learning disabilities. Around 1–2 per cent of patients have a family history of nephroblastoma.

Diagnosis

Renal cell cancer may be diagnosed by an X-ray of the urinary tract using a radiopaque medium (excretion urography). This is effective at visualizing large masses, although small tumours may not show clearly. An ultrasound or CT scan may confirm the diagnosis. Secondary deposits in the lungs from a renal cell cancer have a characteristic 'cannon-ball'-like appearance on a chest X-ray.

NEPHROBLASTOMA TESTS
Nephroblastomas are often first diagnosed clinically when a child develops a large smooth abdominal tumour or, in a few cases, large tumours on each side. Investigations include blood and urine tests, chest X-rays to see if the disease has spread to the lungs, ultrasound and CT scans.

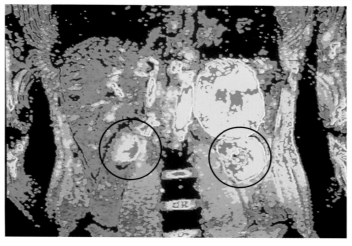

This MR image shows the kidneys (circled) on either side of the spine. A large malignant tumour can be seen above the right kidney.

MR imaging produces cross-sectional images through a person's body. These images can reveal diseased internal organs, such as the kidneys.

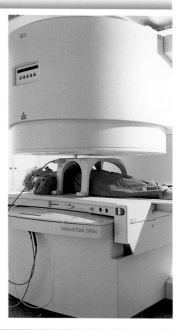

Treatment

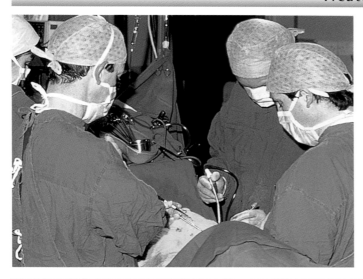

Surgery to remove a renal cell tumour gives the only chance of a complete cure. Unfortunately, by the time of diagnosis, many tumours are too advanced to be totally removed or have already metastasized. However, surgery may still be indicated as the metastases sometimes shrink if the primary tumour in the kidney is removed.

Chemotherapy and radiotherapy have little effect in renal cell cancer. Some tumours respond to hormones, such as

Surgical removal of a renal cell tumour is often the only option. A cure may not be possible, however, if the cancer has spread beyond the kidney.

progesterone. Treatment with interferon-alpha (a substance produced by the body which is able to inhibit viral growth) sometimes produces a short-term response.

NEPHROBLASTOMA
Treatment involves surgery, chemotherapy, which may be given before surgery to shrink the tumour or after to help prevent recurrences, and sometimes radiotherapy.

Prevention

Since renal cell cancer is more common in people who smoke, it is likely to be prevented by not taking up smoking or by ceasing to smoke.

There is at present no known method of preventing a nephroblastoma.

Prognosis

The outlook for those with renal cell cancer depends on how closely the cancer cells resemble normal kidney cells and whether the disease has already spread from the kidney. If the cancer cells are very dissimilar to normal cells (poorly differentiated), the outlook is worse than if they are similar (well differentiated).

If the tumour is confined to the kidney at the time of diagnosis, about 60–70 per cent of patients survive for at least five years and 50 per cent are alive 10 years later. The outlook is less optimistic for people whose lymph nodes contain cancer cells or who have metastases in distant organs, such as the lungs, when the disease is first diagnosed.

HIGH CURE RATE
The outlook for most children with a nephroblastoma is good. A combination of surgery, chemotherapy and radiotherapy cures about 90 per cent of children, including those who have metastases at the time of diagnosis. A few children do, however, develop recurrences or a second tumour so careful follow-up treatment is needed.

The presence of a particular genetic abnormality, loss of heterozygosity of 16q, appears to be more common in children with a poor outlook than in children who do well. The abnormality is more common in children who develop a nephroblastoma when over the age of two.

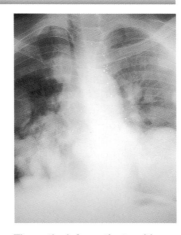

The outlook for patients with renal tumours worsens if the cancer spreads. In this case, secondary tumours have developed in the patient's lungs.

Cataracts

Symptoms

A cataract is an opacity of the lens of the eye that causes blurred vision. The normally transparent lens lies immediately behind the pupil and focuses light on the retina. It has a transparent capsule that is attached to the ciliary muscle, which contracts to make the lens more convex, and thus focus the eye on near objects.

SIGNS OF CATARACTS
Cataracts interfere with the passage of light through the eye. Small cataracts may not cause any noticeable problem to sufferers, but larger cataracts can be the cause of:
■ Reduced visual acuity (blunted vision) – interferes with everyday activities such as reading or driving; eyesight is often worse-affected in a bright light, and distant and central vision are affected first
■ Spots – these may appear in a fixed place in front of the eyes
■ Diplopia (double vision) – this may affect only one eye and remains when the other eye is covered

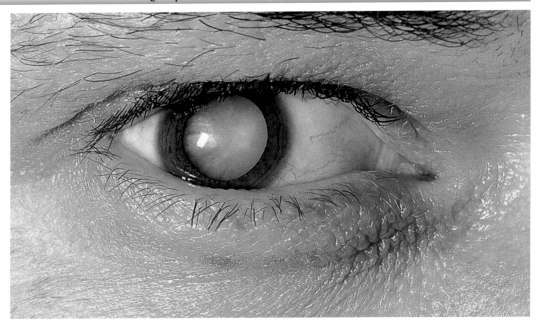

■ Halos – orange halos may seem to appear around lights or any bright areas, and everything in the patient's general environment may look as if it has a slightly orange glow

■ Easier reading – people who previously needed reading glasses sometimes no longer need them; a cataract-related change in the shape of the lens makes them more short-sighted.

A close-up of the eye shows a cataract with its distinctive milky glaze. The term 'cataract' derives from the original idea that the condition was like a little waterfall that fell inside the eye.

Causes

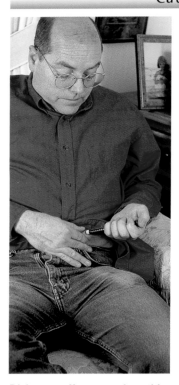

Diabetes sufferers, such as this man self-injecting insulin, can be affected by cataracts due to under-nourishment of the lens of the eye.

Opacities of the lens may be:
■ Age-related – the lens degenerates with age
■ Congenital – these may result from intrauterine viral infections, such as rubella (German measles), or from metabolic disorders such as galactosaemia, in which the sugar galactose accumulates in the blood
■ Inherited – a genetic tendency to develop cataracts at an early age occurs in some families
■ Traumatic – secondary to bruising of the eye, penetrating injuries from windscreen glass or metal fragments, or previous eye surgery
■ Inflammatory – patients with persistent inflammation of the iris (iritis) have an increased risk
■ Diabetic – high blood sugar levels may adversely affect the nourishment of the lens
■ Radiational – from prolonged exposure to sunlight or other ionizing radiation
■ Corticosteroid-induced – prolonged courses of corticosteroids can cause cataracts
■ Associated with skin disorders, such as atopic dermatitis.

Diagnosis

Cataracts are diagnosed by a full eye examination – this will also check for other problems, such as glaucoma or retinal disease.
　Patients with cataracts should be able to point to the position of a light and their pupils should react normally. In advanced cases, the lens may appear brown or white.

USING AN OPHTHALMOSCOPE
The use of an ophthalmoscope, (a specialized instrument for examining the interior of the eye) will confirm the presence of a cataract. When the light beam is shone through the pupil from about 60cm (2ft) away, the back of the eye normally appears red

(the 'red eye' that appears in some photographs); cataracts will show as dark patches.

CONGENITAL CATARACTS
All babies should be examined at birth and at six to eight weeks for cataract and other eye conditions. Congenital cataracts must be treated within the first three months of a baby's life. If treatment is delayed, normal vision may not develop, even if the cataracts are removed at a later stage.

Opticians use specialized ophthalmoscopes to examine the interior of the eye. This can be used to confirm a diagnosis of cataracts.

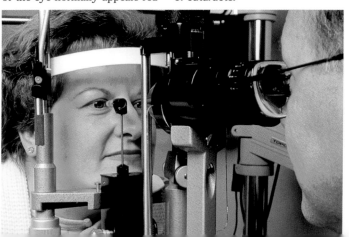

Treatment

There is no medical cure for cataracts. In the early stages, tinted glasses may prevent the dazzle from bright light. Good illumination from above and behind will help reading.

SURGERY
Surgery to remove the cataracts (cataract extraction) is safe and very effective. It is the most common non-emergency operation performed on older people: 105,000 cataract extractions are performed in the UK each year on the NHS.

Patients used to be told that surgery was inadvisable until the cataract had become very advanced and sight was very poor. With modern operating techniques, this delay is no longer necessary. The operation is usually performed as a day case under a local anaesthetic.

SURGICAL TECHNIQUES
■ Extracapsular extraction is the most commonly used procedure – using microsurgery techniques, the surgeon removes the lens through a small incision in its capsule

In an extracapsular cataract extraction, the central, more solid part of the lens (the nucleus) may be liquefied before removal by ultrasonic probe.

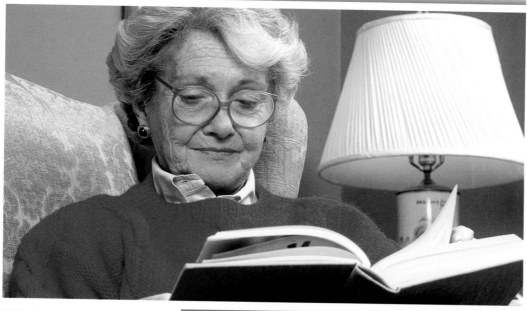

Following a cataract operation, most patients will notice a substantial improvement in their vision. Glasses may still be needed for reading, however.

■ Intracapsular extraction involves the removal of the entire lens within its capsule, usually with a cryoprobe; this technique is not now commonly used.

Patients recover rapidly, but may need to use anti-inflammatory and antibiotic eye drops for several weeks.

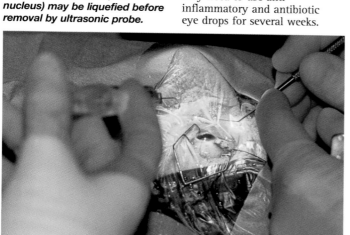

Optical correction after surgery

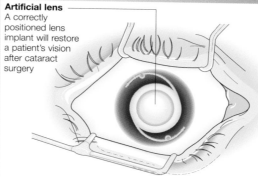

Artificial lens
A correctly positioned lens implant will restore a patient's vision after cataract surgery

Without a lens, the eye has distant vision but cannot focus on near objects. Spectacles or lens implants will correct vision:
■ Spectacles – the spectacles needed after cataract surgery are cumbersome and restrict the field of vision while magnifying near objects; intraocular lens implants means that they are now rarely needed
■ Intraocular implants – the development of intraocular lens implants followed on from the

There are various types of lens implant, including rigid polymethylmethacrylate (pMMA) lenses and foldable silicone lenses, inserted through a minute incision.

Second World War discovery that fragments of Perspex from aircraft windscreens remained safely in the eye, unlike many other foreign bodies; most lens implants are now placed in the empty lens capsule.

Prognosis and incidence

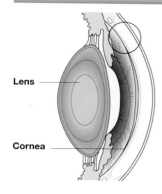

Lens

Cornea

Cataracts tend to grow in size over time and may eventually cause blindness. By blocking the view of the inside of the eye to medical examination, they may also prevent the diagnosis of other treatable eye conditions. Fortunately, surgery restores

During corrective surgery for cataract, an incision is made near the edge of the cornea (area circled). This allows the wound to heal without sutures.

good vision if the eye is otherwise healthy.

After a lens implant, the capsule may thicken, causing a progressive deterioration in vision. This may respond to laser treatment. Cataracts are a very common cause of impaired sight among the elderly. Between the ages of 50 and 59, 65 per cent of people have lens opacities, not necessarily causing any trouble. Over the age of 80, 100 per cent of people are affected.

Age-related visual disorders

A number of conditions affect the eyes with increasing age.
Regular check-ups in the early years will ensure that visual disorders
are detected before vision is significantly impaired.

People gradually become aware of their advancing years with the slow realization that their sight is no longer as sharp as it once was. Age-related visual loss is often so subtle as to be almost unnoticed in its advance, but progressive decline is inevitable.

Age-related visual loss ultimately brings the need for visual aids such as spectacles and contact lenses. Many elderly people often fail to appreciate how even marginally impaired vision can add to other infirmities associated with ageing. Falls and fractures can both result from poor sight.

ANATOMY OF THE EYE
A number of visual disorders can result from the natural degenerative changes that occur in the structure of the eye as a result of ageing. The eye is a complex organ, consisting of the transparent cornea at the front of the eye, behind which are the anterior and posterior chambers, separated by the lens and iris (which lies in front of the lens).

The iris regulates the amount of light entering the eye by adjusting the size of the pupil (central opening of the iris). The image seen through the lens is focused onto the retina, which is made up of many rod and cone cells that respond to dark and light. Tiny muscles change the shape of the lens to alter its focus on the retina.

MESSAGES
The retinal cells, activated by the light, pass messages along the optic nerve to the brain, where they are interpreted to provide a view of the world. At the centre of the retina is the macula, which is responsible for central visual tasks such as reading.

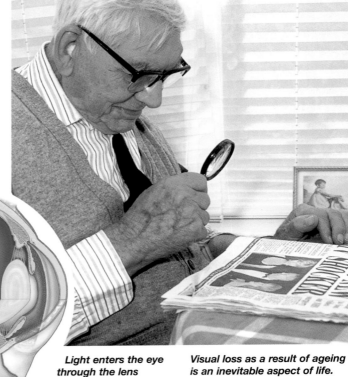

Light enters the eye through the lens (white). The lens focuses this light onto the retina, the structure at the back of the eye.

Visual loss as a result of ageing is an inevitable aspect of life. Reading aids, such as a magnifying glass, become increasingly necessary.

Causes of visual degeneration

Normal ageing of the eye is caused by genetic and environmental factors.

GENETICS
The eyes may be predisposed to degenerative disease due to small abnormalities present in an individual's genes.

ENVIRONMENT
One environmental factor is the effect of intense and prolonged sunlight on visual acuity. The thinning of the ozone layer allows more of the sun's harmful radiation to reach the earth. In addition, many older people now spend long vacations in, or retire to, countries with near-constant high-intensity daytime sunlight.

Many ophthalmologists suspect that these two factors bring about a rise in cataract formation and macular degeneration. This is backed up by reports of increased cataract incidence in parts of the world where inhabitants are exposed to strong sunlight for long periods.

Light radiation reaching the eye passes to the retina and the macula in particular. Here, it is absorbed by photoreceptors, usually protected from the harmful effects of ultraviolet radiation. With age, the efficacy of this protection declines.

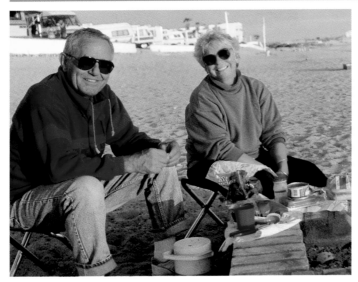

Ageing of the eye can be caused by exposure to sunlight. This is particularly relevant today, when many older people retire to or holiday in sunny climates.

Investigating visual disorders

Regular eye check-ups should mean that any visual disorders are detected in the early stages.

A number of diagnostic techniques are helpful in the investigation of visual disorders. These include:

■ Ophthalmoscopy – used to view the blood vessels of the retina as well as to observe the optic nerve.

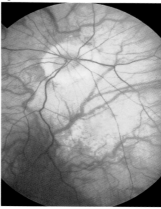

■ Slit lamp biomicroscopy – can be used to examine structures at the front of the eye such as the cornea, iris and lens.

■ Fluorescein angiography – fluorescent dye is injected into a vein and passes through the blood vessels in the eye. When a light is shone into the eye, the dye fluoresces, revealing any abnormal blood vessels.

■ Applanation tonometry – measures the pressure in the eye. Elevated intraocular pressure is characteristic of glaucoma.

Ophthalmoscopes are used by doctors to examine the interior of the eye. The instrument directs a fine beam of light into the patient's eye.

Using an ophthalmoscope, the doctor is able to obtain a view of the back of the eye. This image shows the network of blood vessels supplying the retina.

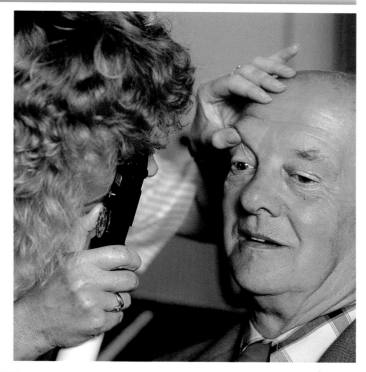

Focal disorders

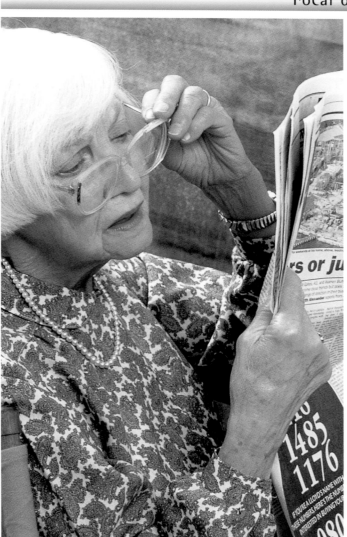

Long-sightedness in elderly people causes a blurring of near vision. Corrective spectacles with convex lenses restore normal vision.

There are three main types of focusing disorders that may occur in elderly people. These are:
■ Hypermetropia
■ Myopia
■ Presbyopia.

HYPERMETROPIA

Hypermetropia (long-sightedness) is the most common refractive (focal) defect among the elderly.

Parallel rays of light are focused behind the retina, and in elderly people near vision becomes more blurred than distance vision.

This condition is treated by placing convex corrective lenses in front of the cornea.

MYOPIA

Myopia (short-sightedness) occurs when parallel light rays are focused in front of the retina. Consequently, distant objects become blurred and, to enable a clear image to be obtained, concave corrective lenses should be placed in front of the cornea.

PRESBYOPIA

Presbyopia occurs with advancing age and is caused by the fact that the lens of the

eye becomes increasingly less flexible.

The result is that the eye is less able to alter its focus, with the consequence that reading and close work, such as sewing, becomes difficult.

This condition can be treated by the placement of a convex lens in front of the eye. Regular eye check-ups will help to ensure that prescribed lenses are of the correct strength.

Floaters

Another common, but usually minor, problem of older age is the appearance of spots or 'floaters' before the eyes.

Seeing floaters in the field of vision is more frequent in the very myopic and the old.

Cell debris
Floaters tend to be worse in bright light and are usually of little significance. They are caused by cell debris floating in the vitreous body and usually disappear over time.

If they are large enough, floaters can impair vision by clouding it temporarily; they will, however, eventually float out of the visual field.

This condition can prove a nuisance when reading, although head movement can move floaters out of the immediate visual field. There is no curative treatment.

Treating progressive blindness

If left untreated, certain visual disorders affecting the elderly can lead to blindness. Cataracts and macular degeneration are two such conditions, which can be treated effectively if detected early.

There are a number of degenerative conditions affecting the eyes in old age. If these conditions are left untreated, they can lead to blindness and have a huge impact on quality of life. Examples of conditions that cause progressive blindness are glaucoma (elevated pressure in the eye, which can damage the optic nerve), cataracts and retinal degeneration.

CATARACTS
A cataract is an opacity in the lens of the eye, which leads to a gradual, painless loss of vision. Cataracts may be caused by senile degeneration, although the condition is treatable with surgery. Cataract surgery is the most frequently performed operation in Western society and few operations bring such an improvement in quality of life.

SURGERY
Doctors and opticians should refer people for surgery if:
■ The cataract is causing a visual problem, even if accompanied by macular degeneration, for this may improve with cataract removal
■ The eye is red and painful

■ The person is fit enough for surgery.

TREATMENT OPTIONS
Two surgical techniques are currently available:
■ Extracapsular cataract extraction involves removing the cataract, leaving the lens capsule behind with surrounding tissue
■ Intracapsular cataract extraction involves removing the lens and surrounding capsule.

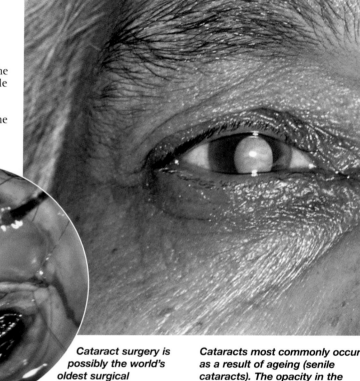

Cataract surgery is possibly the world's oldest surgical procedure. This cataract is being extracted from the eye.

Cataracts most commonly occur as a result of ageing (senile cataracts). The opacity in the lens of the eye, shown here, results in blurred vision.

Secondary diseases affecting the eye

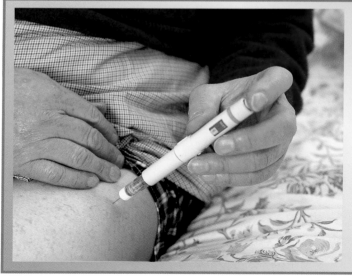

A number of diseases indirectly affect the retina:

■ High blood pressure and generalized arteriosclerosis (thickening of the arteries) can cause the blood vessels supplying the retina to become thickened and tortuous.

With severe high blood pressure, the area around the optic nerve becomes swollen. Vision is not initially affected, but a blind spot develops, which gradually increases in size.

The retina can become damaged as a result of diabetes. Careful control of blood sugar levels with insulin will prevent this damage.

Controlling high blood pressure
Treatment is directed at controlling arteriosclerosis and high blood pressure with the cessation of smoking, weight reduction, a low-cholesterol diet and the use of blood pressure-lowering drugs.

■ Diabetes mellitus is a major cause of blindness and is often associated with chronic adult onset diabetes. The degree of retinopathy (damage to the retina) seems dependent upon the duration of the disease, and is worsened by accompanying high blood pressure. Treatment involves effective control of blood pressure and good management of blood sugar levels.

Macular degeneration

Macular degeneration is the commonest cause of loss of central vision in people over 50 years of age in the Western world. The disorder results in a painless, slow or sudden loss in central visual acuity. There is no known predisposing factor for the disorder, which affects both men and women and is more common in fair- than dark-skinned people.

NEW BLOOD VESSELS

In older people, the degeneration is usually due to the proliferation of new blood

This view of the eye shows macular degeneration (dis-coloured area, centre right). The image has been obtained by means of an ophthalmoscope.

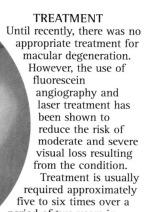

vessels at the back of the eye. The visual loss results from a deterioration in function of the macula, that part of the eye which is primarily concerned with vision involving the ordinary activities of everyday life, such as reading.

EARLY SIGNS

In about 10 per cent of people over 65 years of age, macular degeneration begins as small yellow deposits (drusen) which appear in the centre of the retina. These can be identified using an ophthalmoscope.

Abnormal new blood vessels grow into the drusen (choroidal neovascularization). Bleeding then collects beneath and within the retina. The photoreceptor cells are damaged and an acute loss of central vision occurs.

TREATMENT

Until recently, there was no appropriate treatment for macular degeneration. However, the use of fluorescein angiography and laser treatment has been shown to reduce the risk of moderate and severe visual loss resulting from the condition.

Treatment is usually required approximately five to six times over a period of two years in order to prevent recurrence of the disorder. However, in people who already have

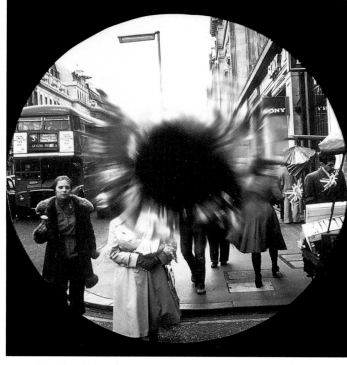

extensive visual loss, this treatment is not effective.

CHECKING FOR PROBLEMS

Early warning signs of macular generation may be detected by identifying abnormalities when looking at straight lines (such as those on a piece of graph paper or between tiles in a bathroom). Any sudden development of blank spots or distortion of the lines may be a sign of the growth of new blood vessels at the back of the eye.

Macular degeneration causes a breakdown of the central part of the retina. The result is a central blind spot, as illustrated by this simulated effect on vision.

Developing new blood vessels in one eye is associated with a 50 per cent chance of the same happening in the other eye.

Regular eye tests in people with a high risk of developing macular degeneration may mean that it can be halted before vision becomes too impaired.

Maintaining visual health

Good vision is important for driving, using tools, reading and carrying out daily activities.

When added to other age-related problems such as arthritis, visual problems can result in falls and fractures, and impact on the quality of life.

Elderly people should therefore:
■ If over 75, have the annual medical health check available from the doctor and also have their blood pressure checked

■ Undergo the free annual eye test available to elderly people
■ Wear wraparound sunglasses when in strong sunlight, especially when abroad.
■ Wear appropriate visual aids for focal disorders.

Ophthalmology test frames have been fitted to this elderly man to help assess his vision. Annual eye tests are an important part of maintaining visual health.

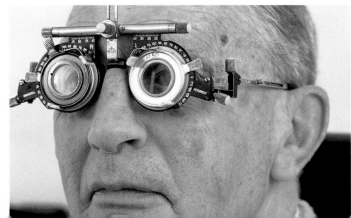

Laser surgery

The advent of laser surgery has revolutionized the way in which visual disorders are treated, and a number of conditions can now be effectively corrected using this procedure.

In a disorder such as macular degeneration, the effects of the condition can be halted thus preventing further damage.

Light beams

Lasers produce high-energy beams of light which, when directed through an optical fibre, become a precise surgical tool.

The laser is focused onto a specific part of the eye using a contact lens placed on the cornea. Using this technique, the laser can be used to treat tiny areas of the eye without damaging other areas.

Conditions commonly treated by laser treatment range from leaking blood vessels in the eye

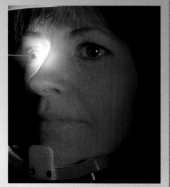

A number of visual disorders can now be treated quickly and effectively using laser surgery. High-energy beams of light are directed at the eye.

(often caused by diabetes mellitus), to correcting focal disorders such as short-sightedness and astigmatism (spoon-shaped cornea).

Glaucoma

Symptoms

Parts of the eye affected by glaucoma

Glaucoma is a condition in which the pressure inside the eye (intra-ocular pressure) becomes abnormally high, leading to visual impairment and sometimes blindness.

PRIMARY GLAUCOMA
In most cases, there is no other associated eye disorder, and the condition is termed primary glaucoma. There are two main classifications:

■ **Angle-closure glaucoma** (acute or congestive glaucoma). In this medical emergency, the angle where the aqueous humour (fluid in the front chamber of the eye) drains closes, leading to a rapid increase in intra-ocular pressure. This results in pain and blurring of vision. Nausea and vomiting may occur if the pain is severe.

■ **Open-angle glaucoma** (chronic simple glaucoma). This is a common cause of blindness and affects both eyes. The drainage of aqueous humour

Angle between cornea and iris
Contains drainage channel for aqueous humour; in glaucoma, the fluid cannot drain away, leading to a build-up of pressure within the eye

Anterior (front) chamber
Filled with aqueous humour; this fluid normally drains at the angle, but cannot in glaucoma

Iris
Coloured part of the eye

Cornea
Transparent cover of eye; often has an abnormal appearance in glaucoma and may be hazy or swollen

Optic disc
Where blood vessels and the optic nerve pass into and out of the eye; becomes 'cupped' in congenital glaucoma and open-angle glaucoma due to atrophy of the nerve fibres

Vitreous body
Largest chamber of the eye; pressure here rises in glaucoma – raised intra-ocular pressure

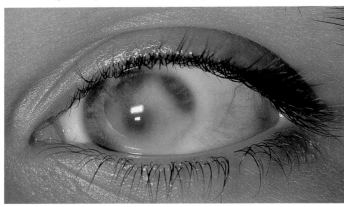

is blocked, although the angle remains open. Raised intra-ocular pressure leads to 'cupping' of the optic disc (dipping of the centre of the optic disc) due to thinning of the nerve fibre layer. This causes abnormalities in the visual field and often blindness.

SECONDARY GLAUCOMA
Glaucoma may arise as a result of other conditions and diseases affecting the eye. Like primary glaucoma, secondary glaucoma occurs when the drainage of aqueous humour is impaired, resulting in raised intra-ocular pressure. Examples include:
■ Pigmentary glaucoma, when pigment is present in the

In certain cases, glaucoma is congenital, as in this teenage girl. The clouding of the iris is a result of the abnormally high pressure within the eye.

anterior chamber of the eye, deposited on the corneal surface
■ Exfoliation syndrome, in which white flakes are deposited on the surface of the lens and in the drainage angle.
Glaucoma may also be secondary to changes in the lens of the eye or the uveal tract, or following trauma or eye surgery; it may also be induced by steroid drops or ointment used around the eye for more than a week.

CONGENITAL GLAUCOMA
Otherwise known as buphthalmos, this condition is present at birth. The baby's eyes are watery, red and painful, with an enlarged cornea and cupping of the optic disc.

Incidence

Glaucoma is the leading cause of preventable blindness, and the third commonest form of blindness after cataract and age-related macular degeneration.

Primary open-angle glaucoma is the commonest form, affecting approximately two per cent of people over the age of 40. Angle-closure glaucoma is very rare, especially below the age of 60.

People with a family history and/or hypermetropia (long-sightedness) have a tendency to develop primary open-angle glaucoma.

Causes

In all forms of glaucoma, the outflow of aqueous humour from the eye is impaired as a result of abnormalities within the drainage system of the front chamber of the eye or impaired access of the aqueous humour to the drainage system. The reason for the defect depends on the type of glaucoma, but the pain and deterioration in vision arise from the abnormally high pressure within the eye.

Characteristic of glaucoma is 'cupping' of the optic disc (the central yellow circular area). Surrounding blood vessels are hooked over the disc's edge.

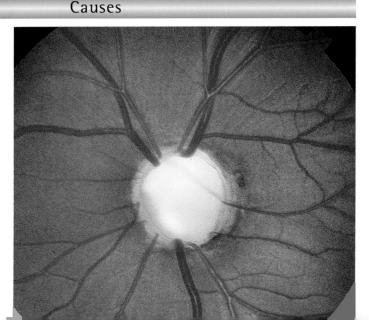

Diagnosis

Diagnosis is made when there is a typical history in the acute types of glaucoma; otherwise, routine examination of vision and visual fields determine a particular pattern of visual field loss. Tests include:
■ Measurement of the intra-ocular tension (tonometry) and examination of the back of the eye (fundus) using an ophthalmoscope are essential
■ Gonioscopy – an examining technique of the front chamber of the eye, utilizing a corneal contact lens magnifying device, allows direct visualization of the angle structures and the tissue at the junction of the cornea and sclera, where aqueous humour drains
■ Optic disc assessment is essential with the visual fields, as visual field defects cause tunnel vision and may progress to blindness; in the absence of symptoms until relatively late in the disease, screening is necessary for the detection of primary open-angle glaucoma.

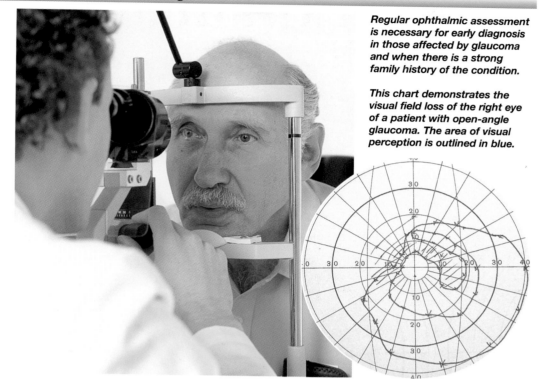

Regular ophthalmic assessment is necessary for early diagnosis in those affected by glaucoma and when there is a strong family history of the condition.

This chart demonstrates the visual field loss of the right eye of a patient with open-angle glaucoma. The area of visual perception is outlined in blue.

Treatment

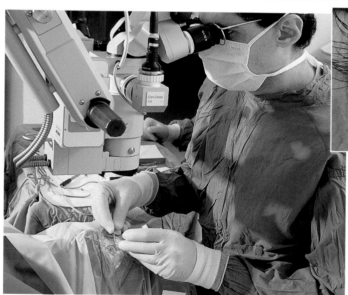

Acute glaucoma is a medical emergency, requiring immediate treatment to reduce the intra-ocular pressure. Laser surgery may be offered subsequently.

Chronic, open-angle glaucoma may be treated by an operation known as a trabeculectomy. This is designed to improve the drainage of fluid within the eye.

Treatment of chronic, open-angle glaucoma is aimed at reducing the intra-ocular pressure:
■ By suppressing production of aqueous humour; for example, with drugs such as beta-blockers applied topically
■ By increasing the outflow of aqueous humour with parasympathomimetic agents such as pilocarpine
■ By reducing aqueous volume with hyperosmotic agents.
Pupil constriction is important in angle-closure glaucoma; for instance, by using a mydriatic drug for pupil dilation.
Surgical treatments include laser iridotomy and surgical peripheral iridectomy for chronic glaucoma; laser trabeculoplasty removes a small segment of the eye to facilitate aqueous outflow.

Prevention

Regular eye tests, especially in those with a family history of chronic open-angle glaucoma, are essential to ensure the early recognition of the onset of the disease. This also ensures regular supervision and should help to avoid what is a very common form of blindness.
Early diagnosis offers the best chance of successful treatment. The identification of other risk factors for chronic glaucoma, such as ischaemic heart disease, may also aid prevention.

Prognosis

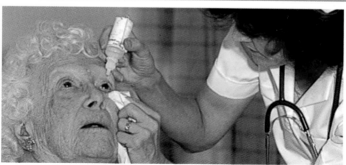

In at-risk patients, preventative medication (eye-drops) may help delay the progression of open-angle glaucoma.

Without treatment, open-angle glaucoma may progress to complete blindness. If anti-glaucoma eye-drops are used, and the eye has not suffered extensive damage, the prognosis is good. When the condition is detected early, medical management is most successful. It is imperative that patients receiving topical or systemic steroid therapy undergo periodic tonometry and ophthalmoscopy, particularly if there is a family history of glaucoma.

127

Hearing loss in older people

As the body ages, there is a gradual decline in the senses, with marked functional loss occurring in hearing. This hearing impairment can greatly affect the quality of older people's lives.

Hearing loss is a common consequence of ageing, and may be due to two types of disorders:
■ Conductive – affecting the external and middle ear
■ Sensorineural – affecting the inner ear. This is also known as presbyacusis and is the most frequent cause of hearing loss in older people.

WHO IS AFFECTED?
After about age 50, the proportion of deaf people rises

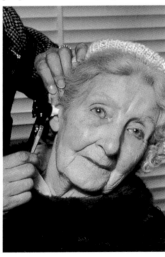

sharply. One in five adults and half those over 60 have some degree of hearing loss for high frequency sound.

In those aged over 65 years, 294 people per 1000 will suffer auditory impairment, and this rises to 437 over age 75. There are estimated to be about 8.5 million deaf and hard of hearing residents in UK, few of whom are of young age.

PARTS OF THE EAR
Anatomically the ear is divided into three parts:
■ External ear – the auditory canal running to the eardrum
■ Middle ear – containing three tiny bones (ossicles), the malleus, incus and stapes – these transmit sound vibrations from the eardrum to the inner ear
■ Inner ear – contains the organs of hearing and balance. Inside the cochlea, the sound vibrations are converted into sound impulses, which travel via the auditory nerves to the brain.

Hearing loss is a common symptom of old age. In most cases it is caused by presbyacusis, a gradual loss of hair cells from the cochlea.

Anatomy of the ear

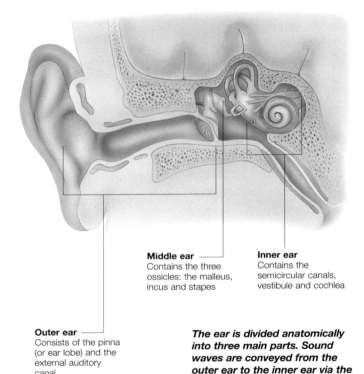

Middle ear
Contains the three ossicles: the malleus, incus and stapes

Inner ear
Contains the semicircular canals, vestibule and cochlea

Outer ear
Consists of the pinna (or ear lobe) and the external auditory canal

The ear is divided anatomically into three main parts. Sound waves are conveyed from the outer ear to the inner ear via the eardrum and ossicles.

Natural hearing loss

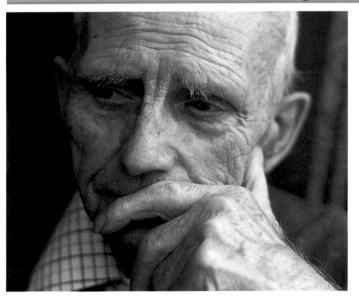

Presbyacusis results from the loss of hair cells in the cochlea, the part of the ear where sounds are processed for the brain to interpret. With ageing, the hair cells begin to die and sounds, particularly high frequency ones, are heard less clearly.

UNDERSTANDING SPEECH
As speech contains many high frequency sounds in consonants, such as 't', 'p', 'k', 'f' and 's', the first sign of hearing loss is some difficulty in understanding what people are saying. This is more likely to happen in men.

An uncorrected hearing deficit can have a major impact on an older person's life. Hearing loss is often associated with social isolation and depression.

Symptoms

Elderly people with hearing loss often find that:
■ Other people's speech seems less clear
■ Hearing conversation in noisy places becomes difficult
■ There is a need to ask people to repeat words before they are comprehended
■ Listening to conversations requires concentration and becomes tiring
■ The television or radio has to be be played at a level too high for other listeners
■ Hearing a telephone ringing becomes difficult
■ Conversation with several people all talking together becomes hard to follow
■ Failure to hear others' speech leads to frustration.

Treating hearing loss

Hearing tests are used as a means of determining the exact cause of a hearing disorder. Once the extent of hearing loss has been determined, a hearing aid may be prescribed to improve symptoms. Modern, efficient digital aids are now available.

Five million people in Britain have hearing loss sufficient to merit the use of a hearing aid. However, only two million people have a hearing aid and only about two in three use them regularly.

HEARING TESTS
Hearing by air conduction is assessed by presenting an acoustic stimulus – a sound – in the air, to the ear.

Hearing by bone conduction is measured by placing a sounding source – a tuning fork, for example – in contact with the head. This causes vibration throughout the skull and stimulates the inner ear, bypassing the middle and external ear to test the integrity of nerve paths.

ASSESSING HEARING LOSS
An audiometer is used to find out how loud a sound has to be for the patient to hear it. Sounds of specific frequencies are transmitted through headphones at specific intensities to determine the person's hearing threshold for each frequency. This is a painless procedure requiring the person being tested to record when they have heard the sounds emitted.

Test results are plotted on a graph called an audiogram and the degree of hearing loss is measured in decibels. The test can be done in GP surgeries.

CONDUCTIVE LOSS
In older people, hearing loss may be due to conductive loss – for example, an obstruction, usually wax, in the outer ear. The most likely location for this is the ear canal. The obstruction can be visualized by a nurse or a doctor with an audioscope (also known as an otoscope), and removed with hot water and wax solvent syringing.

Wax drop solvents are available from pharmacist stores but if wax has been lodged in the ear for years, syringing of the canal is usually necessary to move the obstruction.

Tinnitus

Tinnitus is the perception of sound in the absence of an acoustic stimulus. The sound may be a buzzing, roaring, whistling, ringing, or intermittent or continuous noise in one or both ears experienced in the absence of external sounds. The incidence of tinnitus increases with age.

Causes of tinnitus
The cause of tinnitus remains obscure, but it can be very annoying or distressing for the sufferer. It can occur as a symptom of most ear disorders and may last for months or even years.

Relief may be obtained by wearing a tinnitus-masking device, which is worn like a hearing aid and produces a noise that masks the tinnitus.

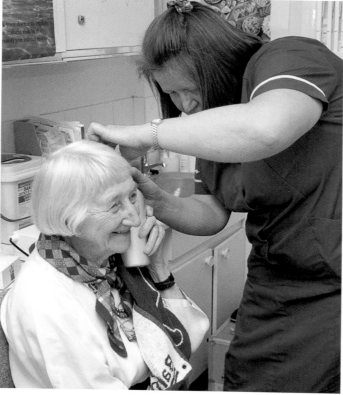

SENSORINEURAL LOSS
Sensorineural hearing loss occurs in presbyacusis. It initially affects higher frequencies (18–20 kHz) and then the lower range (4–8 kHz) by age 55 to 65, although there is variation in individuals.

OTHER CAUSES
Long-term use of a few drugs, such as aspirin and quinine

In some cases, hearing loss may be due to an obstruction in the outer ear canal, such as impacted wax. This can be treated by syringing the ears.

(used to treat leg cramps), can cause reversible and irreversible hearing loss. Exposure to very noisy environments for prolonged periods may also lead to the onset of deafness.

Hearing aids

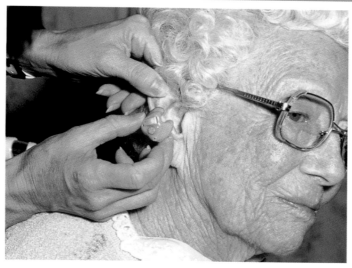

Hearing aids do not restore hearing to former acuity levels, but they can improve hearing. These devices contain a tiny microphone, amplifier and speaker and run on battery power. They can be placed in the ear canal or behind the ear.

NEW TECHNOLOGY
More people who are hard-of-hearing may use a hearing aid in the future as technology improves and digital hearing aids are introduced.

Hearing aids can be an effective means of improving hearing. Sound vibrations entering the ear are amplified, allowing them to be detected by the brain.

Modern hearing aids use digital technology and have microphones with a better directional focus.

OTHER AIDS
Even using a good hearing aid, people with impaired hearing may still have difficulty with communication and will also use lip reading skills. Telecoils are present in most hearing aids and can be used with induction loop systems. These cut out background noise and pick up particular sounds – for example, the television and radio.

Telephone amplifiers also provide enhanced bell sounds and some telephones are hearing-aid compatible.

Age-related foot disorders

Elderly people are particularly vulnerable to problems involving the feet. In old age, the effects of foot disorders can be far more debilitating than for younger people, so rapid treatment is important.

The ageing process affects the foot just as it does every other part of the body. The effect may be minor, or severe enough to disturb walking and may even result in immobility due to inflammation and pain.

Loss of muscle mass and tendon tone causes dropping of the arches of the foot in elderly people such that it becomes flatter and loses some flexibility. Also, as skin ages it is less able to cope with trauma and infection in the feet.

DISEASE

Diseases associated with old age, such as diabetes and osteoarthritis, can have a debilitating effect on the circulation to the feet and on the joints within them, which can seriously disturb mobility. There can be knock-on effects on foot shape, skin quality and joint movement.

Minor disorders of toes, nails and feet which, in younger people, normally heal quickly, can lead to major loss of function in older people. This is due to poor blood circulation and to difficulties many elderly people have in reaching their feet to wash and treat them and even to cut their toenails.

FOOT CARE

A lifetime's use of the feet may have caused deformity, calluses, corns and chronic infection of

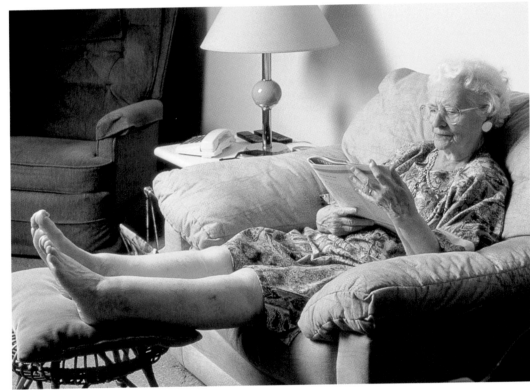

Poor blood circulation in elderly people can cause swelling in the feet and lower legs. Lack of exercise and sitting for too long can aggravate the problem.

the toes and toe spaces. All require personal attention and hygiene, which older people are often unable to provide.

The feet may no longer be accessible or visible to the individual, who will be dependent on a nurse or podiatrist (foot specialist) for appropriate attention.

Regular nail-cutting and good foot hygiene are vital to avoid the overgrowth of nails, skin injury and infection. Deformed

ingrowing nails digging into the skin, distorted toes, infected web spaces and inflamed toe and foot joints can cripple an otherwise healthy elderly person.

Fortunately most of these conditions may be prevented or alleviated with prompt and appropriate treatment, thus maintaining mobility.

Structure of the foot

The foot is made up of many bones, including: the 14 phalanges of the toes; the five metatarsals of the forefoot, which create an arch across the foot (transverse arch) and along it (longitudinal arch), with the intervening joints providing the 'spring' in the step; and the seven tarsal bones.

Tendons from the leg with some fatty padding, a blood nerve supply and overlying skin complete the anatomy of the foot.

TOENAILS

The toenails are specialized, thickened skin. Their lifetime growth demands regular trimming. Toenails should be cut in such a way to prevent overgrowth, which can result in skin damage and infection.

Bones in the foot create arches that provide the 'spring' in a step. In old age, the loss of muscle mass and tendon tone causes the arches to flatten.

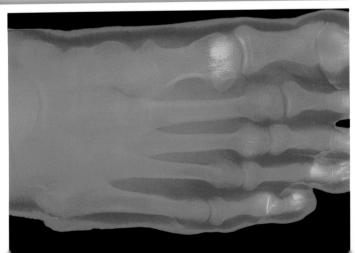

Causes of foot disorders

During the ageing process, a number of conditions may occur which affect the feet. Other factors, such as hygiene considerations, may exacerbate the problem.

Foot disorders in the elderly can be caused by many factors:
■ Ageing of the heart and the onset of arteriosclerotic disease – this can lead to poor blood circulation, which can result in swelling of the feet and lower legs
■ Lack of mobility in elderly people – this means that the circulation to the feet is further reduced, exacerbating foot problems
■ Diabetes mellitus, a disease often associated with old age – this is another cause of bad circulation to the feet
■ Smoking for many years – this makes vascular disease of the feet more likely in old age.

Without blood circulating properly, it takes longer for cuts and sores to heal and this can lead to serious infection.

In addition to this, elderly people may not be able to reach their feet to wash them and thus prevent fungal infections.

In some cases, elderly people who are not always able to take care of themselves may be neglected and so foot problems which should have been treated go unnoticed.

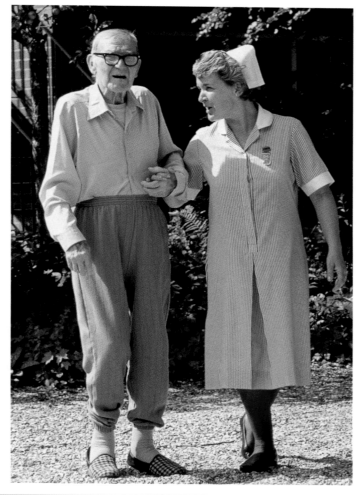

Lack of mobility with ageing aggravates circulatory disorders that underlie many foot problems. These problems can further reduce mobility.

Effects of systemic disease

Gout, osteoarthritis and rheumatoid arthritis can all affect the feet, with gout causing very painful swelling of the great (big) toe. Anti-arthritic drugs are helpful in treating these conditions and simple painkillers may alleviate pain that impairs normal walking.

Psoriasis sometimes affects the nails, causing pitting.

The poor blood supply to the lower limbs and delayed healing in diabetes brings a constant threat to the well-being of the feet, so good foot care is very important in those with this disease. Diabetic foot ulcer healing can be improved by treatment with platelet-derived growth factor; this is now licensed for use in Britain.

Soft-tissue disorders

The most common avoidable afflictions of the foot are corns, callosities, fungal infections and ingrowing toenails. All of these can be treated by a podiatrist or a doctor.

These disorders are the end result of constant or repetitive pressure from ill-fitting shoes or friction from toes rubbing together.

CORNS

Corns are of two varieties – hard and soft. Both can result in pain, which may interfere with walking. Treatment, once they are present, requires paring off the accumulated hard skin using a scalpel; this is best left to skilled podiatrists.

Soft corns develop an infected centre and the hard skin has to be removed, the pus cleaned out and a dressing applied. This is a simple procedure in the young, but in older people there is an increased risk of infection if sterile instruments and antiseptic procedures are not used.

Diabetic patients are exposed to serious health risk if cuts and sores of the feet are not treated correctly and hygienically, as their poor healing ability may allow the spread of infection with gangrene developing in the foot.

CALLOSITIES

Callosities (or calluses) develop over points on the foot where shoes pinch or toes override each other. A thickening of the skin from constant pressure brings more thickening and roughening of the skin, which creates more pressure and pain.

Podiatrists treat corns by removing the hardened skin with a sharp scalpel. The pus at the centre will then be removed and a dressing applied.

Removal of the affected skin with a surgical scalpel by a podiatrist will do much to alleviate the problem. Steps should also be taken to remove the source of the unwanted pressure, preventing recurrence.

Neglect of the feet by elderly people may result in the formation of corns and callosities. Regular visits to a doctor or podiatrist are advised.

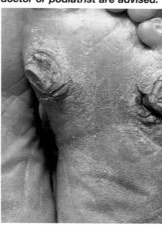

Common foot conditions in elderly people

Foot disorders can be classified into several types, including nail problems, fungal infections and joint disorders. The treatment for each of these is aimed at reducing pain and discomfort.

Nail problems

Damage to the nail bed can lead to the overgrowth and thickening of the nail. In time, it may grow down under the toe or sideways into other toes. A nail rasp can be used to thin down the nail and chiropody nail cutters can be used to shorten it.

NAIL DAMAGE
Damage to the nails and the surrounding skin often arises when people inadequately groom their nails, and this is particularly true with older people struggling to reach their toes. Nails should be cut transversely across, just behind the border of the toe. The angles should be rounded to ensure that the sharp edges do not embed in

Overgrowth and the thickening of the toenail must be treated to avoid infection occurring. Problems can be reduced with proper toenail grooming.

the surrounding skin, as this can cause painful infection. Treatment sometimes requires removal of the nail before the infection can be eradicated.

If an elderly person has difficulty cutting their toenails correctly, a doctor or nurse can do it for them. This will help to avoid ingrowing toenails.

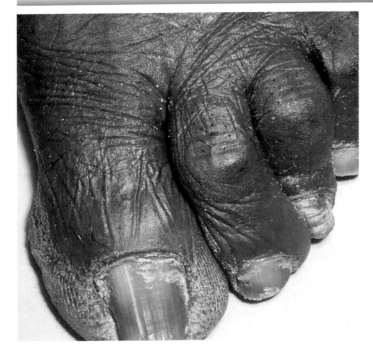

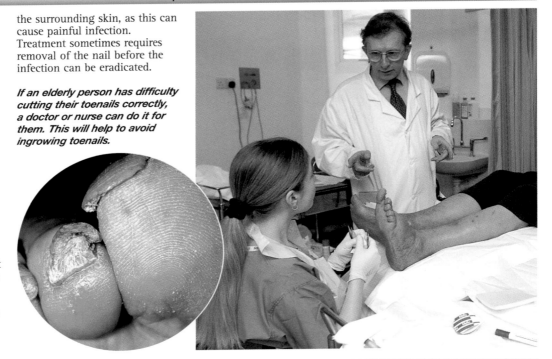

Fungal infections

The hot humid area between the toes – the web – is very attractive to micro-organisms (bacteria and fungi), which thrive there. Fungi, in particular, can cause chronic infection.

Poor foot hygiene encourages the growth of fungi, and failure to dry the webs of the toes after washing helps to maintain and spread the infection.

Tinea pedis (also known as ringworm) is the main culprit. Persistent treatment with antifungal ointments can eradicate it, although treatment is often prolonged. The fungus will spread to the nails; affected nails often become brown and crumbly and erode away – a process called onycholysis. It is

Fungal infections occur most frequently in the webs between the toes. It is common for elderly people to have such infections due to poor hygiene or diabetes.

not uncommon to find very elderly people with all their toenails infected.

Oral medicines are available to treat fungal nail infections, but side effects contra-indicate their use in elderly people.

DIABETES SUFFERERS
People with diabetes mellitus are particularly likely to have monilial (yeast) infections affecting the feet. Scratching and skin breakdown can lead to affected areas becoming sore. Ulcers, if formed, heal slowly and are a serious problem.

Poorly controlled diabetics may cause the development neuropathic ulcers of the toes – usually painless but dangerous and requiring prompt medical attention. The risk of gangrene developing in the foot means that all diabetics should have regular podiatry care from a skilled and qualified podiatrist.

Joint disorders

Bunions are often associated with hallux valgus, which usually results from wearing high-heeled shoes earlier in life, causing the big toe (hallux) to be displaced inwards. This may result in callosities, corns, skin abrasions and ulcers. Foam padding that takes pressure off the deformity and wide-fronted shoes may alleviate this problem.

HALLUX VALGUS

Hallux valgus is a swelling of the joint between the big toe and the first long foot bone (metatarsal) caused by ill-fitting shoes. Appropriate footwear and foam padding may help to diminish pain and make walking easier but sometimes only surgery can improve symptoms.

HALLUX RIGIDUS

Hallux rigidus is a painful condition in which there is a stiffness of the metatarso-phalangeal joint of the big toe.

This often causes a disability in which sufferers are unable to bend the big toe properly. The condition is related to osteoarthritis, and patients may therefore benefit from anti-arthritic medication.

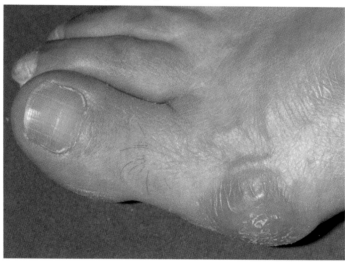

A bunion is a swelling of the joint between the big toe and the metatarsal bone. Bunions are frequently caused or exacerbated by ill-fitting shoes.

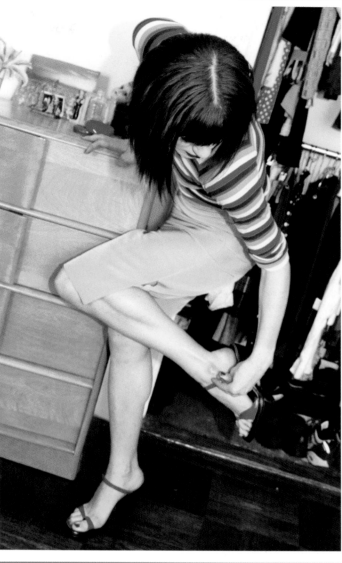

Women who regularly wear high-heeled shoes are particularly vulnerable to hallux rigidus in old age. This condition may impair walking severely.

Preventing foot disorders

To prevent foot disorders, there are a number of measures which can be taken. These include:
■ Wearing sensible, well-fitting foot wear in youth and middle age – this will minimize foot problems in later life
■ Observing meticulous foot hygiene – this is important in older people
■ Drying feet, and especially toe webs, properly after washing
■ Taking great care when cutting toenails or paring corns
■ Cutting toenails properly – not leaving unseen and/or sharp edges, which may grow into surrounding skin
■ Protecting friction points of bunions and displaced toes from trauma with padding
■ Removing debris regularly from nail borders, together with regular grooming of nails
■ Ensuring that any soreness or infection of the toes or skin of the feet is taken seriously and seen by a professional.

Patients with diabetes must take particular care of their feet. They should:
■ Be especially careful to avoid injury and infection of the feet
■ Receive regular foot care from a health professional with expertise in diabetic care
■ Seek professional help for any infection or injury affecting the feet
■ Check their feet regularly or, if unable to do so, have someone else inspect them daily
■ Avoid using a hot water bottle to warm the feet.

Good foot hygiene will help to reduce the occurrence of foot disorders. Regular checks mean that any problems can be identified and treated early.

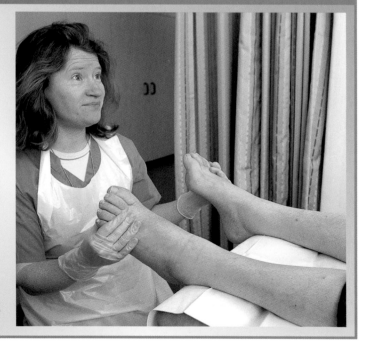

Age-related mobility problems

As we grow older, our ability to get around tends to diminish. This may be due simply to the effects of ageing, or to health problems, such as strokes. The aim of treatment is to maximize quality of life.

With advances in medicine, the population of elderly people in Britain is predicted to increase greatly over the coming decades.

INCREASED LONGEVITY
While the period of healthy living and independence is lengthening, an extension in living time will inevitably mean an increase in the number of elderly people who suffer from age-related disability and therefore become dependent on others.

DEFINING DISABILITY
It is extremely difficult, however, to define disability. This is because it is not an attribute that is clearly present or absent. It is, rather, more a matter of degree of infirmity, with a range of disability extending from minor to severe.

A moderate disability may hardly affect the lives of some individuals, while for others the same disability can lead to immobility and complete dependence on others.

QUALITY OF LIFE
Though ultimately the aim of increasing lifespan is a desirable one, it is the quality of that life which really matters.

Quality of life can be defined as an individual's ability to lead an independent life, enjoying mental and physical fulfilment. The quality of an individual's life will be enhanced if a period of disability and dependence with increasing age is delayed or avoided.

ADDRESSING THE CAUSES
It is important, then, that the underlying causes of age-related mobility problems are identified and addressed, enabling elderly individuals to carry out the ordinary activities of daily living, such as personal care, shopping, housework and walking without aids.

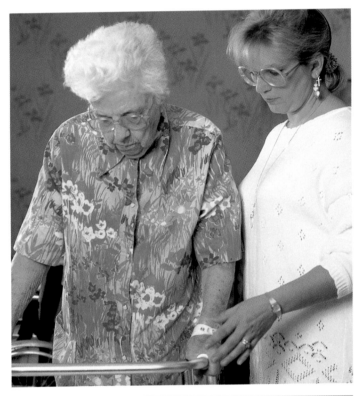

The effects of ageing can have a considerable impact on the quality of an individual's life. Age-related disability can lead to immobility and dependence.

Causes of age-related disability

Disability can be a result of many of the changes that occur in elderly people, including:

■ The ageing process
■ Frailty
■ Medical conditions affecting the feet, legs, lower joints and co-ordination
■ Localized ailments, such as bunions, hammer toes, tendinitis
■ Generalized disease, such as malnutrition and diabetes mellitus
■ Strokes – where there is weakness and paralysis of muscles and loss of proprioception.

People can compensate for many of these changes; in the case of diseases, however, some of these will be not only debilitating but disabling.

Many of the changes of advanced age make falls more likely. Such accidents are a major source of disability, immobility or impaired mobility, and the consequent loss of independence.

STATISTICS
In a recent study of those aged 65 and over in England and Wales, 11 per cent of men and 19 per cent of women (1.3 million people in total) were recorded as disabled physically, with 38 per cent of these over 85 years old.

Of these, 80 per cent needed external help to maintain the activities of daily life, with a third requiring personal care. The majority of them were living in their own homes, however.

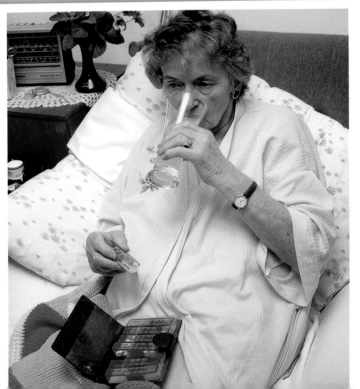

As people age, they become susceptible to various conditions that are associated with impaired mobility. These include strokes and foot problems.

Effects of ageing on the musculoskeletal system

Between 20 and 25 per cent of visits from elderly people to the family doctor relate to problems associated with the musculoskeletal system, which comprises bones, cartilages, muscles, tendons and ligaments.

Any disturbance to the system which can occur as a result of the ageing process may interfere with physical function and result in disability, impaired mobility and loss of independence. The main areas affected are:

■ **Bones** – there is shortening of the vertebrae in the spine and thinning and flattening of the intervertebral discs. This leads to a loss of height and a more stooping posture. Bone mass is reduced, and, in many women, hormonal changes lead to osteoporosis (thinning of the

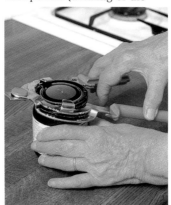

bones), which is the result of a gradual loss of calcium from the bones.

■ **Joints** – the ageing process leads to increased wear and tear on the joints, which causes destruction of the cartilage layer covering the ends of the bones where they articulate with each other. This leads to stiff and often painful joints.

■ **Muscles** – muscle fibres degenerate and fat and fibre are deposited, with a resultant loss in strength. The spring is lost from the step and there is a decrease in suppleness. Posture can be altered and the gait can become more shuffling.

Added to these changes are losses in visual acuity and proprioception – the feedback to the brain about joint, foot and body position. As a result, uneven footways and minor obstacles become more difficult to negotiate successfully.

Conditions such as arthritis can lead to the inability to carry out everyday tasks. Treatment will help the individual achieve a better quality of life.

The affects of ageing upon the skeleton can lead to conditions such as osteoporosis. Sufferers from this condition are more prone to fractures.

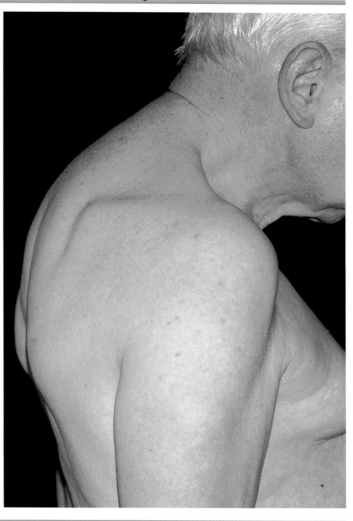

Dangers associated with falls

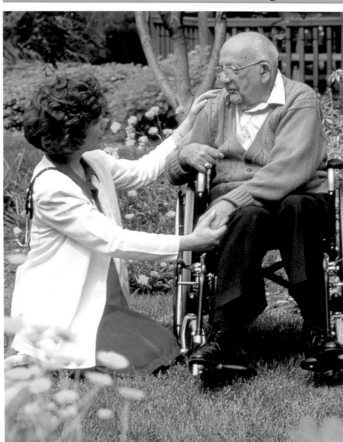

Elderly people are more likely to suffer falls – poor coordination may follow a stroke, for example. The recovery time may sometimes be prolonged if there are underlying conditions present, such as osteoporosis or rheumatoid arthritis.

EFFECTS OF FALLS
Falls are a dominant cause of disability and even death. When an older person falls to the ground, a bone fracture is very likely. This will result in hospitalization, operation, prolonged rehabilitation (with perhaps a change in gait), increased frailty and possible further falls and fractures.

PRECAUTIONS
As falls can often be traced back to fairly simple causes around the home, such as tripping over

When an elderly person suffers a fall, the consequences are often serious. Bone fractures easily occur, frequently resulting in increased immobility.

a carpet or doorstep, a number of simple precautions can be taken to minimize risk:

■ Remove loose carpets from the home
■ Ensure prescription of spectacles is appropriate to the extent of visual impairment
■ The home and its immediate surroundings should be well lit at night
■ Consider installing ramps to negotiate rather than stairs
■ Remember the adverse effect on balance of certain medications, such as sedatives and hypnotics
■ Avoid trailing electric leads in the home
■ Install grab rails on stairs, corridors and round the bath
■ Use appropriate supporting shoes
■ Keep the feet healthy with regular chiropody care
■ Use balance and walking aids when necessary
■ Seek early treatment for rheumatoid arthritis, osteoarthritis and osteoporosis.

135

Treating the causes of impaired mobility

Age-related disability is often associated with specific medical problems. Addressing these conditions directly – with drugs or physiotherapy, for example – will often enhance individuals' mobility.

There are a number of medical conditions that can lead to disability. These conditions can be divided into three categories:
■ Chiropody problems
■ Stroke disease
■ Joint problems and degenerative conditions.

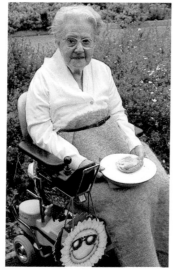

Elderly people who have suffered a stroke may have mobility problems as a result. Physiotherapy can often help to rehabilitate stroke patients.

CHIROPODY PROBLEMS

Certain foot conditions are common in the elderly, such as bunions, ingrowing toenails and hammer toes. These simple but painful conditions often deter individuals from walking. All are amenable to chiropody treatment, however, freeing the affected area from pain.

STROKE DISEASE

Strokes cause weakness, paralysis and spasticity of muscles and fixed flexures of the joints. They can result in a change in gait and can cause major problems in the discernment of joint positioning.

This brings a high possibility of falls and therefore further disability in those who can walk, leading to impaired mobility and even immobility in the worst afflicted.

Prompt, appropriate physiotherapy and active rehabilitation can minimize disability and thus reduce dependence on other people.

Disability in the elderly may be caused by several conditions relating to foot and joint problems. Rehabilitation may reduce dependence.

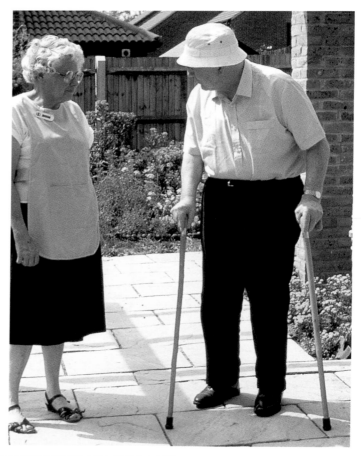

Preventing disability

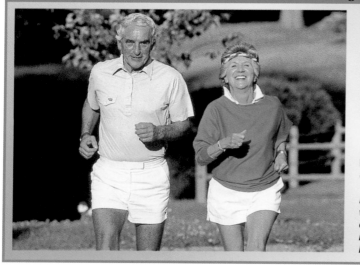

Disability and loss of mobility result both from simple factors and more complex medical conditions. All are treatable although not perhaps curable.

There are measures the individual can take to prevent or delay both the loss of function and independence associated with these conditions.

In particular, older people are advised to:
■ Keep fit with active, daily exercise for as long as possible,

Leading a healthy and active life will help to reduce the likelihood of developing mobility problems in old age. Exercise serves to keep the body supple.

especially walking and swimming to maintain the musculature and the joints
■ Be aware of the symptoms of osteoporosis, rheumatoid arthritis and osteoarthritis and be ready to seek medical help promptly when these appear
■ Seek referral to a rheumatologist for current drug therapy, which often delays or stops progression of the disease
■ Keep the feet healthy with chiropody care
■ Ensure that dietary intake contains adequate vitamin D and calcium
■ Check out the home environment and ensure that the risk of a fall is minimized.

Treating joint problems and degenerative conditions

There are several musculoskeletal conditions that may cause a loss of mobility in later life, including osteoporosis, rheumatoid arthritis and osteoarthritis. These can usually be controlled with medication to reduce their effects and minimize disability.

Joint problems can be caused by rheumatoid arthritis (RA), osteoarthritis (OA) and gout. These diseases cause swelling and disruption of the small joints of the toes and ankle, accompanied by pain and severe stiffness. These changes can bring permanent change to the shape of the foot and cause painful walking. Gout can be treated with medication with good results. OA and RA are treatable, especially in the early stages of the disease.

Hip, knee and ankle joints can be affected by degenerative joint disease – mainly OA and RA – and destruction of the joints can lead to major disability. Joint replacement of hips and knees is very successful in restoring function: a total hip replacement may last for over 15 years.

The treatment of osteoarthritis with anti-inflammatory drugs can help to relieve symptoms. This will enable sufferers to achieve a better quality of life.

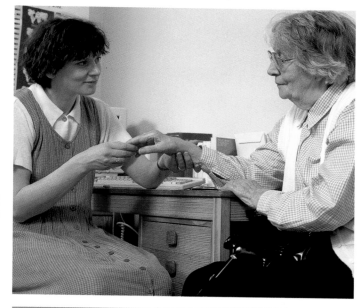

Osteoporosis

Osteoporosis (OP) is a common medical disorder in which there is bone loss, with the resultant bone weakness often causing many falls and associated loss of function and impaired mobility. The prevalence rate is 31-40 per cent in women, but is much less in men because they have a higher peak bone mass and do not experience the menopause, which is associated with rapid bone loss.

Most fractures occur at the wrist, spine and hip, with the latter leading to a high incidence of illness and even death. OP can progress rapidly

Osteoporosis is common in elderly women, causing bones to weaken. Early diagnosis using bone densitometry will enable more effective treatment.

and there is a high risk that a patient who has had one osteoporotic fracture will have another in the following year.

RISK
The risk is best determined by the measurement of bone mineral density (BMD). Risk factors include:
- Family history of osteoporosis
- Low dietary intake of calcium
- Obesity
- Taking glucocorticoid drugs.

TREATMENT
Currently, the main therapies available are vitamin D and calcium supplements and oestrogens (hormone replacement therapy) for post-menopausal women. New antiresorptive drugs have also been shown to be effective.

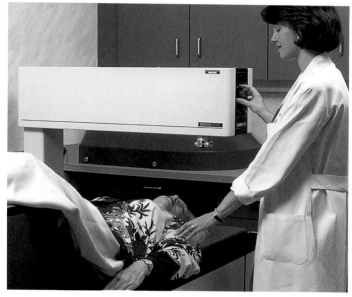

Rheumatoid arthritis and osteoarthritis

Rheumatoid arthritis (RA) is the most common inflammatory joint disease, having a prevalence of 5600 cases per 100,000, with a peak onset in the sixth decade of life. Women are affected three times more frequently than men, but in the elderly the incidence in men and women is more equal. It is a chronic disabling disease, but many people have only mild symptoms. In others, there can be serious joint destruction and loss of function.

In severe cases, 90 per cent of sufferers may become very disabled within 20 years of onset, life expectancy in these cases being reduced by four years in men and 10 years in women.

X-rays may be taken and blood testing for the presence of rheumatoid factor is often performed, but may be negative.

TREATING RA
Non-steroidal anti-inflammatory drugs can give symptomatic relief to RA but do not change the long-term outcome. Increasing evidence suggests that treatment with new disease-modifying antirheumatic drugs (DMARDs) leads to less joint destruction and a better treatment outlook. Early treatment is important if the disease process is to be slowed or halted.

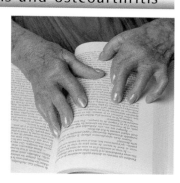

Rheumatoid arthritis causes joints to swell, commonly affecting the hands. This can be disabling, and prevent sufferers from carrying out simple tasks.

OSTEOARTHRITIS
Osteoarthritis involves the gradual degeneration of the cartilage covering the bone ends within the joints, resulting in pain, deformity and swelling of the involved joint. It is more common than any other rheumatological problem and typically affects the hip, knee and base of the thumb.

Most OA joint problems can be managed medically and few people have a relentless progression of the disease. OA cannot be cured, but most patients are helped with drug injections into the joint, medication and exercise.

Urinary incontinence problems in old age

Urinary incontinence is the complete or partial loss of voluntary control over bladder function. The problem occurs more frequently in the elderly, and can cause distress and embarrassment.

In medical terms, urinary incontinence is defined as the involuntary loss of urine, with disturbing social consequences for the individual. Urinary incontinence is not uncommon, but it can present minor or major difficulties.

An occasional leak may perhaps be tolerable, whereas recurrent loss of control has a great personal impact. If severe, incontinence can determine whether an elderly, ill person is cared for at home or requires nursing care.

PREVALENCE

Incontinence occurs more frequently in women than in men, and in the elderly of both sexes. At least six per cent of elderly people are affected by incontinence, and the incidence is rising as the population ages.

The ageing process alone does not bring inevitable urinary incontinence, but illness and health disorders associated with old age can precipitate symptoms. For example, medications used to treat some illnesses can create incontinence problems. The causes should therefore always be identified, as

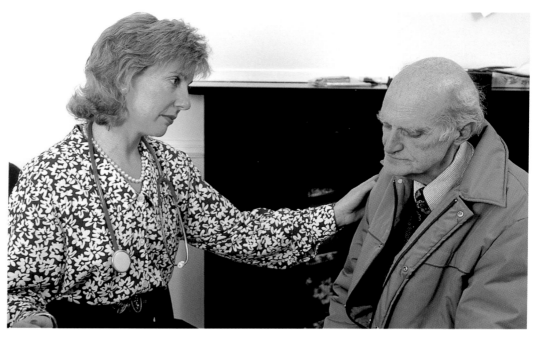

many can be treated successfully with medicine or surgery.

EMBARRASSMENT

Many people find it difficult to discuss incontinence. Over half of those afflicted are too embarrassed to consult a doctor,

with many patients believing that nothing can be done. As a result, some people fail to seek medical aid.

In most cases, however, incontinence responds well to treatment. Continence clinics report that half of their patients

A large number of people find it embarrassing to seek medical advice for incontinence. However, the problem usually responds well to treatment.

are completely cured and almost two-thirds show an improvement.

Types of incontinence

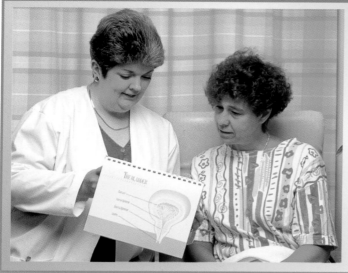

Incontinence can be divided into four main types:

Stress incontinence
Stress incontinence is the involuntary leaking of small amounts of urine. Stress incontinence is the most common type of incontinence and generally affects women.

Urge incontinence
Urge incontinence is the sudden desire to urinate, closely followed by the involuntary loss of urine.

Often, urinary incontinence has a treatable cause. It is therefore vital to identify the problem with the patient and take steps to improve the incontinence.

This type of incontinence is more common in the elderly and women are usually affected more frequently than men.

Overflow incontinence
Overflow incontinence is the inability of the bladder to empty due to a blockage or weak bladder muscle. Overflow incontinence is more commonly found in those aged over 50 years and affects men more than women.

Total incontinence
Total incontinence is a complete lack of control of bladder function. There may be a number of causes, such as dementia or cancer.

Causes of incontinence

The causes of urinary incontinence in the elderly vary according to the type of incontinence suffered.

STRESS INCONTINENCE
Stress incontinence is caused by weakened pelvic floor muscles. Generally, old age brings replacement of muscle tissue with fat and, in women particularly, the muscles in the pelvis become weak.

The pelvic floor muscles assist in the closure of the bladder sphincters. If these muscles are lax, a cough, sneeze or sudden movement can cause small amounts of urine to be squeezed out of the bladder.

URGE INCONTINENCE
Urge incontinence may have a number of causes. Usually, the muscle of the bladder wall becomes irritated, which leads to involuntary contraction of the muscle and a resulting loss of urine. This type of incontinence is often due to inflammation or infection, such as cystitis. It may also be caused by bladder stones, stroke or spinal injury.

OVERFLOW INCONTINENCE
Overflow incontinence occurs when the bladder is unable to empty due to the presence of a blockage in the neck of the bladder or urethra. The result is a build-up of pressure in the bladder as it fills, leading to a constant leak of urine.

The flow of urine may be restricted by bladder stones. Men may also be affected by an enlarged prostate gland. A weakened bladder muscle may be the result of an obstruction, pelvic surgery or diabetes mellitus.

The severity of overflow incontinence varies between individuals. Some people retain a certain amount of control over their bladder function, while others are unable to prevent

Overflow incontinence can be caused by bladder stones. This urogram X-ray shows a number of bladder stones nestling in the bladder cavity.

A stroke occurs when the blood supply to the brain is interrupted, leading to damaged tissue. People who have suffered a stroke may develop incontinence.

the loss of urine while the bladder empties.

TOTAL INCONTINENCE
Total incontinence usually arises as a result of nerve damage following a stroke, neurological trauma, such as spinal injury, or pelvic surgery, such as that performed to treat cancer. A person with dementia may also suffer from total incontinence.

Bladder function

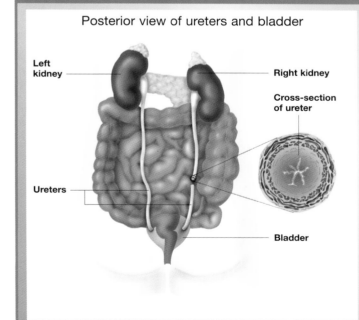

Posterior view of ureters and bladder

Left kidney

Right kidney

Cross-section of ureter

Ureters

Bladder

Urine is created by the kidneys and flows down the ureteric tubes to the bladder, a distensible muscular 'bag' in the pelvis.

Emptying the bladder
Strong muscular contractions of the bladder walls squeeze the collected urine into a tube called the urethra and expel it from the body. This act of emptying the bladder is known as micturition.

Bladder control is exercised voluntarily via nerves that run from the brain to the detrusor muscles in the bladder and a muscular ring at its base – the sphincter. This voluntary control can be lost if the nerve supply is damaged. For example, a spinal

Urine is stored in the bladder – a strong muscular sac. When full, the bladder is emptied under voluntary control by relaxing its sphincter.

cord injury may damage the nerves or a stroke may disturb the nerve centre and pathways in the brain.

Function in women
In women, the urine is voided through a short urethra. The female bladder and urethra are closely associated with the reproductive organs and damage to them, particularly during childbirth, may weaken muscle structures, which can create future continence problems.

Function in men
In men, the urethra traverses the penis on a longer course than in women. The prostate gland in men surrounds the urethra below the bladder. If the gland is diseased or enlarged, the passage of urine will be obstructed, with resultant micturition problems.

Management of incontinence

Most people with incontinence respond well to treatment.
Individuals can be taught how to manage the problem themselves,
by performing pelvic floor and bladder retraining exercises.

An individual seeking medical attention for urinary incontinence should be given a full medical examination.

EXAMINATION

A medical examination includes:
- General medical appraisal
- Review of current medication
- Psychological assessment
- Social assessment
- Rectal/vaginal examination
- Urine testing.

Further investigations might include prostatic ultrasound examination and urodynamic assessment, to determine the type of incontinence. However, in older people, it should be possible to diagnose the cause without the aid of urodynamic assessment, which should be reserved for those in whom treatment is unsuccessful.

TREATMENT

Many women with stress incontinence can be treated with pelvic floor exercises (Kegel exercises). Almost all women should receive instruction in these exercises before they are considered for gynaecological surgery.

Any disorder causing urge incontinence should be treated as a priority. Various measures

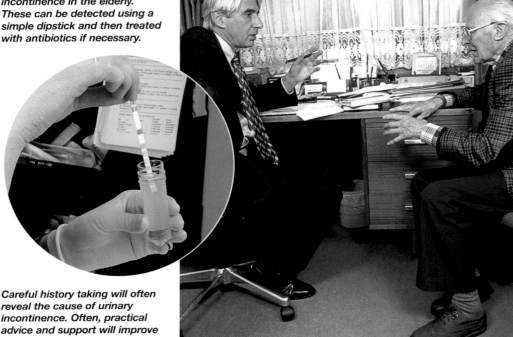

Urine infections are a cause of incontinence in the elderly. These can be detected using a simple dipstick and then treated with antibiotics if necessary.

Careful history taking will often reveal the cause of urinary incontinence. Often, practical advice and support will improve distressing symptoms.

can be taken by the patient to improve the problem, such as performing Kegel exercises to strengthen bladder muscles.

For overflow incontinence that is caused by prostate

obstruction, the treatment is surgical intervention. If the incontinence is caused by bladder stones, these should either be treated by lithotripsy or surgically removed.

Total incontinence may respond to surgery to improve bladder muscle tone. Bladder catheterization to continuously drain the bladder may also be necessary.

Bladder retraining

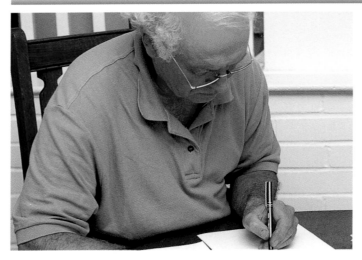

Bladder retraining (bladder drill) can be helpful in the management of both urge and stress incontinence.

REGULAR TOILETING

In urge incontinence, which affects older age groups particularly, there is the sudden, immediate need to urinate. This problem can be eased if a sufferer is taught to go to the toilet only at specified times. These times become less rigid as

People with incontinence may be asked to keep a personal flow chart. This helps the doctor to ascertain the pattern and frequency of micturition.

dry days become progressively more frequent.

At least one-third of patients are cured and others helped considerably by this process, although retraining requires significant cooperation and determination on the part of the patient.

INTERRUPTED URINATION

Individuals affected by stress incontinence should be instructed to practise interrupted micturition every time they go to the toilet. This technique involves voluntarily stopping urination mid-flow. Patients are often also asked to keep a personal frequency/flow chart.

Treating resistant incontinence

Urinary incontinence is occasionally resistant to intervention. In these cases, the patient has to resort to continence devices.

AIDS

Non-invasive treatment of incontinence is preferable to catheterization. Such treatment involves the use of a great variety of incontinence aids.

Aids range from incontinence pads that can be placed inside regular underwear, to briefs that have a special pouch into which a pad can be positioned. Re-usable incontinence shields provide 24-hour protection, and all-in-one absorbing pants are obtainable for those with heavy or total loss of urine.

In men, a penile urosheath can be rolled onto the penis like a condom, draining into a bag attached to the leg. The drainage bag is emptied when necessary.

URINARY CATHETERS

An permanent in-dwelling catheter is usually the last resort in the management of urinary incontinence; a catheter is a 'foreign intrusion' into the urinary tract and can become a source of infection. Catheters are therefore used in the community only under the supervision of the community nurse.

A catheter can allow free drainage into a bag attached to a leg or it can be closed off with a spigot and released at intervals to drain into a suitable container or the toilet.

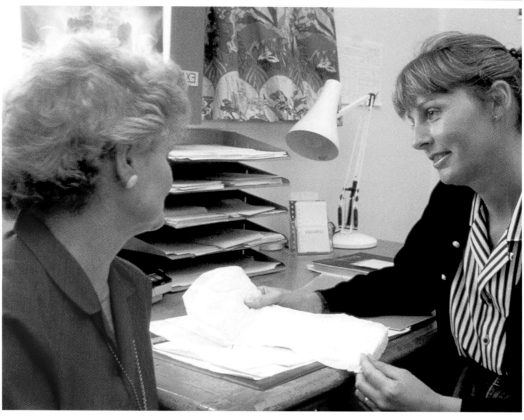

SKINCARE

Incontinence can cause odour and infection in the genital area. Ammonia in urine can also cause the skin to break down. It is important, therefore, to pay special attention to skincare in this sensitive area.

Medicated barrier creams protect the skin from infection and bed sores, eliminate bacteria and prevent rashes, urine burn and rectal itching. Special body washes remove infectious micro-organisms and eliminate odour.

PROTECTIVE DEVICES

A range of specially designed protective devices can be used by people with incontinence to enhance day-to-day comfort and cleanliness.

Nurse advisors can help people with resistant incontinence to lead a normal life. Continence devices range from pads to indwelling catheters.

Waterproof sheet protectors protect bedding and mattresses from bedwetting. Special waterproof chair pads can also be used to protect furniture.

Pelvic floor exercises

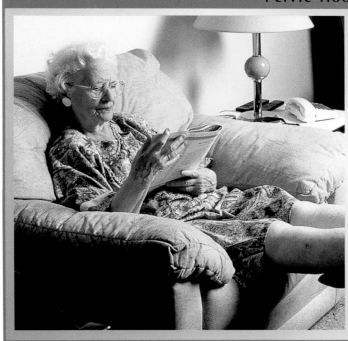

Strengthening the pelvic floor muscles by regularly practising pelvic floor (Kegel) exercises can be very effective in the treatment and prevention of urinary incontinence. Stress incontinence, in particular, responds well to Kegel exercises.

Kegel exercises can be performed while sitting, standing or lying down. It is usually recommended that the exercises are performed as often as possible, and at least eight to 10 times a day.

Identifying the muscles

The pelvic floor muscles are those muscles that are used should it be necessary to

Pelvic floor exercises can be performed at any time, even while relaxing at home. To be effective, they should be carried out several times a day.

suddenly stop urinating during the urination process. When these are tensed, a tightening sensation will be felt around the vagina, urethra and rectum.

About one third of women begin by squeezing the wrong muscles. It is therefore helpful to seek medical guidance initially, to be taught the correct technique.

Strengthening the muscles

The pelvic floor muscles can be strengthened by performing the following exercises:
- The pelvic floor muscles should be contracted and held for at least 10 seconds
- The muscles should then be relaxed slowly
- This procedure should be repeated 5–10 times, as often as is practicably possible.

It usually takes from six to 12 weeks for most women to notice an improvement in urine loss.

Diabetes mellitus in the elderly

Non insulin-dependent diabetes usually occurs after the age of 40 and affects one tenth of those over 70. Treatment focuses on stabilizing glucose levels within the bloodstream.

Diabetes mellitus is the inability of the body to utilize glucose (a sugar) for energy, due to a lack of the pancreatic hormone, insulin. This occurs for two reasons; the pancreas produces inadequate amounts of insulin or the body's cells lose their sensitivity to the hormone.

GLUCOSE BUILD-UP
In healthy individuals, insulin is produced by the pancreas and allows the cells of the body to absorb glucose from the blood. In people with diabetes, glucose accumulates in the blood (a condition known as hyperglycaemia) and urine, leading to excessive thirst and urine production.

INCIDENCE
There are two main types of diabetes: type I (insulin-dependent) diabetes and type II (non-insulin-dependent) diabetes. Type I diabetes usually develops in childhood or adolescence, and often starts suddenly. Type II diabetes, which accounts for 70 per cent of all cases, occurs when the pancreas is still able to produce insulin, but the body's cells have become resistant to its effects.

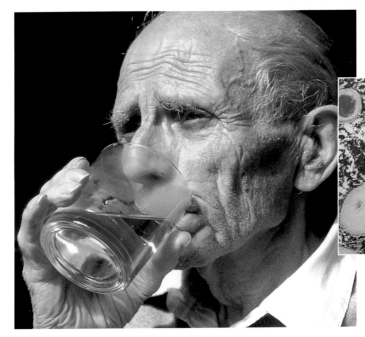

◄ One symptom of diabetes is excessive thirst, due to a build-up of glucose in the blood. People with diabetes are unable to utilize glucose for energy.

▲ The islets of Langerhans (shown here magnified) are cells in the pancreas that secrete insulin. Insulin is vital in controlling body glucose levels.

Type II diabetes mainly affects people over the age of 40 – it is found in 10 per cent of individuals over the age of 70.

CAUSES
Genetics, obesity and ageing are all important factors in understanding the causes of type II diabetes:
■ Approximately one-third of affected individuals have a relative with the same form of diabetes
■ The condition is on the increase in Western societies due to the combination of high food intake and a high-fat, low-fibre diet, both of which predispose individuals to obesity. A lack of physical exercise also increases the risk of developing the condition
■ The prevalence of increased glucose intolerance rises with advancing age; hence the high incidence in the elderly.

Effects of diabetes

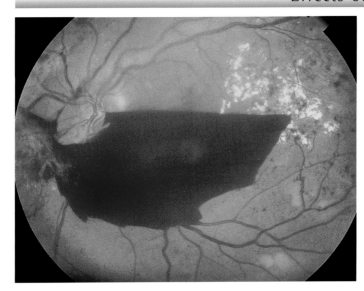

Diabetic retinopathy, in which haemorrhaging (shown in red) around the retina may result, is a complication of diabetes. It is a common cause of blindness.

The symptoms of both types of diabetes mellitus are similar. Whereas type I diabetes tends to develop rapidly, the symptoms of type II diabetes commence slowly and the condition may not be diagnosed for a number of years.

SIGNS
The main symptoms of diabetes mellitus include:
■ Thirst
■ Excessive urination
■ Loss of weight
■ Tingling in hands and feet
■ Lack of energy
■ Blurred vision
■ Frequent infections, which are slow to clear.

COMPLICATIONS
Type II diabetes is often wrongly regarded as a mild form of diabetes, but people with the condition are susceptible to chronic diabetic complications.

Short-term complications include hypoglycaemia (a low level of glucose in the blood) which, if left untreated, can lead to seizures and coma.

Long-term complications include cardiovascular disorders, hypercholesterolaemia (high cholesterol), hypertension, diabetic retinopathy, neuropathy (nerve damage) and kidney failure.

Diagnosing the condition

Early diagnosis and treatment of diabetes mellitus is important as timely intervention may delay the progress of the disease and minimize complications.

URINE SAMPLE
Those who suspect that they may have diabetes should go to their doctor. They will be asked to provide a urine sample, which will be tested to determine the level of glucose.

BLOOD TESTS
The diagnosis will then be confirmed by a blood test, which measures the glucose level. The blood is also tested for glycosylated haemoglobin. This is a changed form of the pigment in red blood cells, which becomes more concentrated when the level of glucose in the blood has been high for a period of weeks or months.

Those over the age of 75 should have a routine health check, in which a test for diabetes is automatically undertaken.

MONITORING
Once the condition has been diagnosed, affected people should be monitored for life by their doctor, diabetic clinic or hospital diabetic department. Individuals are taught to check their glucose levels on a daily basis by means of finger-prick and/or urine tests.

The British Diabetic Association (BDA) recommends reviews at least twice a year for patients who are well controlled and without cardiovascular problems, and three or more times annually for others. The tight control of blood glucose and blood pressure considerably reduces microvascular complications.

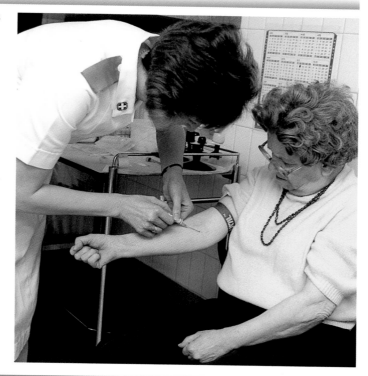

A blood test confirms the diagnosis of diabetes, once a urine sample has been carried out. It is important that the condition is diagnosed early.

Treatment

The treatment of diabetes mellitus centres around maintaining a satisfactory level of glucose in the blood. This may be achieved by the use of insulin injections in those with type I diabetes, while for individuals with type II diabetes, glucose levels can usually be controlled by regular exercise and a healthy diet.

Exercise
Regular exercise is important, as it lowers the risk of stroke, heart disease and high blood pressure. It also helps people to lose weight, which is very beneficial in the treatment of diabetes.

Diet
Three out of four newly diagnosed patients are obese and a diet considered healthy for the general population is thought to be best for the diabetic. Calorie requirements for each individual have to be assessed and designed to achieve weight loss.

Those with type II diabetes should try to eat a low-fat diet, and derive their energy from complex carbohydrates, such as bread or rice.

Alcohol should be consumed in moderation since it may cause a reduction in blood glucose levels in excess. It is also likely to lead to weight gain as it is high in calories.

People with diabetes should stop smoking as it increases the risk of long-term complications, such as stroke and heart disease.

Medication
If exercise and diet are not helpful in controlling glucose levels, various drug treatments may be prescribed to augment, rather than replace, these treatment methods.

Oral medications are usually tried initially. These include sulphonylureas, which act directly on the pancreas to enhance insulin secretion. They can sometimes cause hypoglycaemia, resulting in dizziness and black-outs, which can be easily reversed by the ingestion of sugar or sweets.

Another oral drug is metformin, which helps body tissues to absorb insulin and is a more suitable drug for obese patients.

Regular exercise can be beneficial in the treatment of diabetes. It reduces the chances of heart disease, stroke and high blood pressure.

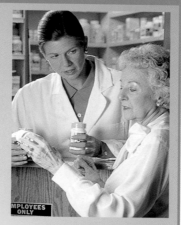

Drug treatment may be given if diet fails to control blood sugar levels. Drugs boost insulin secretion or help the body to absorb it more easily.

Hypoglycaemia is uncommon, but metformin can cause gastrointestinal side effects.

If oral treatments are not successful, insulin injections may be required.

Prognosis
In some people, diabetes mellitus leads to premature death, usually as a result of cardiovascular problems. The condition is now, however, easier to control due to effective drug treatments, and emphasis on leading a healthy lifestyle. The result is that individuals with diabetes are able to lead normal lives.

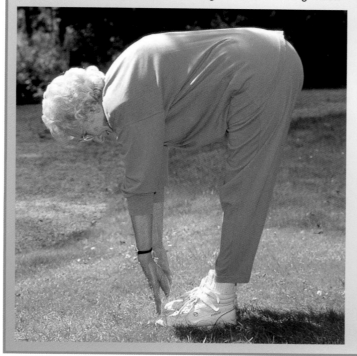

Malnutrition

Malnutrition is a major problem among older people. It results from decreased food intake or absorption, or changes in metabolism and may cause several conditions, including anaemia, fractures and frailty.

In the UK most older people are generally well-nourished, but a considerable number have an inadequate intake of essential nutrients, which may lead to illness and a decreased quality of life. There are also some groups of ageing people who are particularly likely to have a diet lacking in input appropriate to their energy and living needs.

BENEFITS OF A GOOD DIET
Inadequate intake of food and inappropriate diet can lead to illness; the subsequent complications can result in loss of the ability to live independently at home.

A good, healthy diet can help individuals to resist disease, minimize the ageing process and help retain a good quality of life into very advanced old age.

PROTEIN-ENERGY MALNUTRITION
Once past 65 years of age, humans are faced by many physiological challenges, one being the increased chance of developing protein-energy malnutrition. This condition is directly responsible for a number of the disease processes and functional impairments associated with old age.

Protein-energy malnutrition is a major problem although estimates of its prevalence vary. It is present to some degree in 15 per cent of older people living in the community and occurs in a severe form in 10–38 per cent of older hospital out-

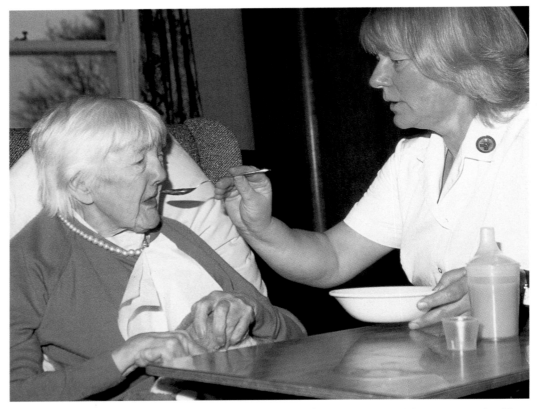

patients and 10 per cent of the house-bound. Although common, the condition is poorly recognized by family doctors and often inadequately treated when identified.

INSUFFICIENT DIETARY INTAKE
A national survey of older people's dietary intake has revealed that for many it is less than ideal, lacking several nutrients, including vitamin D in particular, potassium and magnesium. Food intake declines with ageing even in healthy people and ageing is associated with anorexia, weight loss and more subtle change in appetite, choice of food, patterns of eating and taste.

Decline in the volume of food intake is due in part to ageing

Malnutrition may occur in older people for a variety of reasons. Onset may be sudden following illness or result from a long period of inadequate eating.

people eating less overall, but more specifically to the consumption of less fat and protein. Smaller meals and fewer snacks are eaten by older people compared to younger.

Reasons for concern

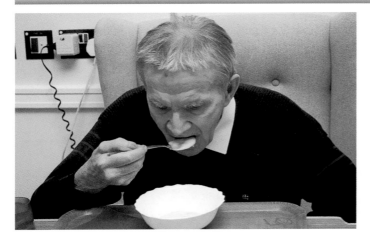

Whatever the cause may be, malnutrition in older people is a serious concern since it results in low body weight which, in senior years is related to early, perhaps even premature, death.

People weighing much less than the norm for their age are likely to die earlier than people of the same age who are of normal weight, as they are more susceptible to other illnesses.

Malnutrition in older people is a serious problem, as it leads to weight loss and reduces resistance to disease. It may even result in premature death.

HOW COMMON IS MALNUTRITION?
The prevalence of malnutrition rises steeply with age and doubles in frequency in those people aged over 80 compared to those aged between 70 and 80 years.

OTHER FACTORS
Age alone does not determine eating habits or predict nutritional status; several factors are involved in nutritional deficiency, including:
■ Disease
■ Social factors
■ Cultural responses.

Managing malnutrition

The report of the Department of Health working party on the nutrition of the older people recommends that the majority of people aged over 60 should adopt and maintain patterns of eating and lifestyle similar to those for maintaining health in the young. However, older people should reduce dietary intakes of fat and simple sugars and also increase their intake of starchy foods, non-starch polysaccharides and vitamin D.

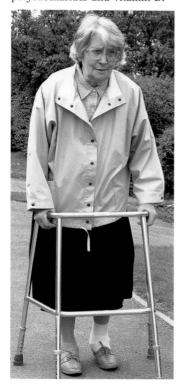

As people are less active in older age than in their youth, they require less energy-dense food. However, some sugar and fat intake is needed.

Meals consisting of fish, fruit, vegetables and wholemeal bread are recommended for people over 60. These products provide a balanced diet.

DIETARY ADVICE
It is recommended that senior citizens should:

■ Follow a diet with a variety of nutrient-dense foods such as milk and breakfast cereals. Dietary input should not be bulked up on energy-dense food requiring little preparation, such as cake and biscuits. With smaller appetites and meals, older people should not ignore energy-dense, protein-deficient food. Sugar and fat give energy rather than nutrition
■ Have the same intake of non-milk extrinsic sugars as the young
■ Have the same intake of non-starch polysaccharides as the young
■ Avoid foods with high phytate content such as raw bran
■ Utilize fibre-free beans and tomatoes, wholegrain breakfast cereals and bread for roughage
■ Increase dietary input of vitamin C gained from, for example, potatoes, fruit juices, dried fruit and assorted peppers
■ Increase intake of fresh vegetables, fruit and wholegrain cereals

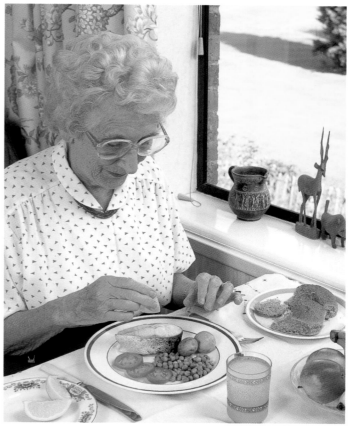

■ Increase intake of oily fish, such as mackerel, tuna, herring and sardines to reduce the risk of coronary thrombosis occurring. These fish constitute one of the few dietary sources of fat-soluble vitamin D
■ Follow low-fat diets which moderate plasma cholesterol blood levels and protect against coronary thrombosis and stroke at all ages
■ Avoid salt being added to food at the table and not rely on too many convenience foods because these have a high salt content, which may increase a person's blood pressure
■ Maintain low-fat-milk intake.

Dietary supplements

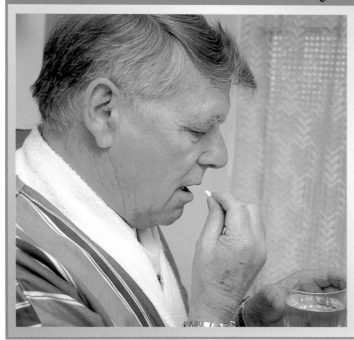

There is still debate about the benefits of diet supplements. However, for some people, such as those with heart disease, vitamins may be recommended.

There is much discussion and argument regarding appropriate supplementation of diet with vitamins and other nutrients.

■ Iron and vitamin C
Iron and vitamin C supplements may be added to the diet where individuals are deficient in vital nutrients or are in a vulnerable group. Vitamin C appears to have a protective health role and may prove a useful dietary supplement in the elderly.

There are dangers in ingesting large amounts of vitamins and professional advice should be sought before a long-term supplementation programme is undertaken.

■ Vitamin D
Vitamin D can be acquired from sunlight but may be supplemented in house-bound people and during winter. Older women are vulnerable to osteoporosis and calcium and vitamin D supplementation reduces fracture risk. Calcium alone has a more modest effect and vitamin D alone is ineffective. With 70 per cent of Britons over 60 years of age recording no outdoor activity in a one-month winter period studied, there is a case for supplementation with vitamin D and calcium for all older people during the winter months.

■ Vitamins B_{12} and B_6
Deficiency of vitamins B_{12} and B_6 are correlated with coronary heart disease and professional medical advice may recommend supplementation in vulnerable elderly people.

Causes of malnutrition in older people

Physical, mental and social problems faced by older people can cause reduction of food intake. Despite needing less food, people over the age of 60 require energy and nutrition to remain healthy.

People over retirement age are a very diverse group with radically different life experiences, lifestyles and cultural backgrounds that have shaped eating habits over a lifetime.

Quantity and content of food are both relevant to energy and nutritional needs. Low food intake not only leads to weight loss but increases the probability that the intake of key nutrients will also be diminished.

MEDICAL FACTORS

Some factors affecting diet and food intake are:
- General health
- Illnesses, such as hypothyroidism and dementia
- Physical mobility
- Mental capacity
- Gastric absorption
- Taste and smell sensitivity
- Emotional state
- Appetite
- State of teeth
- Condition of gums
- Over or under production of saliva
- Medication effects
- Ability to swallow
- Alcoholism.

INVESTIGATING MALNUTRITION

Doctors assessing elderly patients should:
- Note the dietary history
- Take blood samples
- Check body mass index
- Carry out a weight check
- Ask the patient to keep a diet record for several weeks.

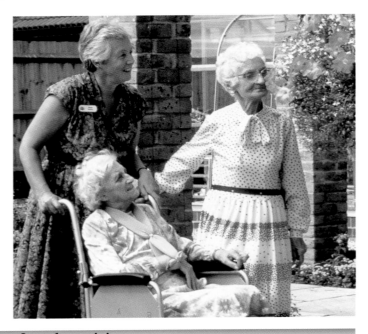

Impaired mobility in older people may be associated with reduced food intake. This often results in weight loss as well as insufficient nutrient consumption.

Physical causes of malnutrition

POOR DENTITION

A lack of teeth or loose teeth and painful gums will interfere with proper food intake by promoting an avoidance of hard foodstuffs, an over-reliance on soft and liquid preparations and a lack of roughage. Vitamin C and E levels have been shown to be lower in those without teeth.

Ill-fitting dentures may also create similar difficulties.

TASTE AND SMELL

Ageing brings a decline in taste and smell such that foods do not taste as appetizing, so less may be eaten. Decline in smell begins at about the age of 60 and taste sensitivity declines after 70. This

Poor dental health in older people can interfere with healthy food intake. In some cases, reduced consumption of citrus fruit can result in scurvy.

encorages an increase in the use of salt to season food, with repercussions for cardiovascular well-being. Loss of the smell function interferes with the maintenance of a healthy diet; people may consume less citrus food and low-fat products and more sweet foods.

ALTERED SALIVATION AND SWALLOWING

Many medications cause a dry mouth, making mastication (chewing) of foods more difficult. Some diseases, such as Parkinson's disease, cause excess salivation, which can interfere with normal eating. Narrowing of the gullet may make

Taste and smell sensitivity declines in older people, who may lose interest in food. Salt, added to food to enhance its flavour, raises blood pressure.

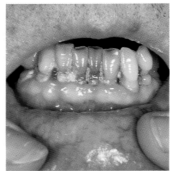

swallowing of dry foods and larger food particles difficult.

INADEQUATE ABSORPTION

Any failure in intestinal absorption can have serious consequences. Older people have a greater need for iron than the young, but the ability of gastric lining cells to secrete the acid required in absorbing nutrients declines with age – a condition known as hypochlorhydria.

Malabsorption diseases of the lower gut can also result in nutritional deficiency. Vitamin B_{12} absorption is increasingly impaired with advanced age.

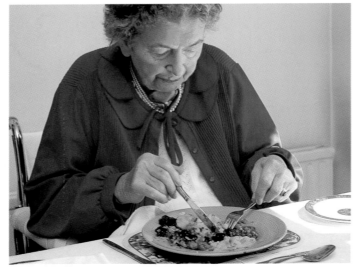

Chronic illness and malnutrition

Many chronic medical conditions are associated with loss of appetite, as are episodes of acute illness. Prolonged loss of appetite and weight loss require medical investigation to seek the underlying cause.

PSYCHIATRIC CONDITIONS

Clinical depression is a frequent cause of loss of appetite and weight loss in older people. Older people with depression are more likely to lose weight than younger people and the condition is more likely to be missed by physicians in older patients.

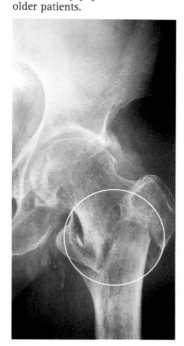

Clinical depression can lead to a loss of appetite, especially in older people. Subsequent weight loss can cause a variety of health problems.

Chronic alcoholism is particularly likely to result in inadequate food intake and weight loss in older people. Dementia is associated with weight loss, sometimes because the patient has forgotten if they have eaten or how to prepare appropriate food.

OSTEOPOROSIS

Osteoporosis is a significant factor in 90 per cent of fractures in older people. Broken hip and thigh bones are a dominant cause of morbidity and mortality. Vitamin D is important in bone metabolism as it is needed for the absorption of calcium, and older women often have low vitamin D stores, especially in winter.

MEDICATION EFFECTS

Many medications are associated with loss of appetite and malnutrition, such as:
- Antidepressants – can cause nausea and taste disturbance
- H² antagonists – reduce stomach acidity
- Digoxin – a heart preparation
- Anticancer drugs.

A common cause of fractured hips in the elderly (particularly in women) is osteoporosis. This X-ray shows a fracture of the femur, or thigh bone (circled).

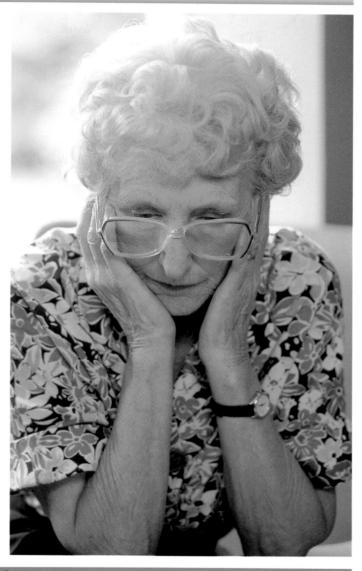

Social factors

Aside from medical reasons, malnutrition in older people may be caused by social factors, including the following:

■ Financial status

Retired people often have limited financial resources and may feel that they should buy fewer or cheaper foodstuffs which contain fewer nutrients.

■ Access to food stores

Many older people find it difficult to go shopping for food because they cannot get to the shops easily. For example, supermarkets are often on the outskirts of towns and are designed primarily for car owners.

Preparing food can be difficult for older people with impaired mobility. Arthritis sufferers may find it hard to open food containers when cooking.

■ Physical disability and loss of mobility

Physical disability has an important influence in the preparation of food. Disability compromises the ability to prepare cooked meals. Half of those over 65 suffer from a measure of arthritis and have difficulty opening cans, jars and bottles and may struggle with food preparation. Those with poor mobility may have difficulty getting to the shops.

■ Bereavement

Bereaved women may have a decreased motivation to prepare meals and men who are widowed may have inadequate cooking skills.

Older people living on their own may become depressed and lonely and consequently may develop nutritional deficiencies and lose interest in food.

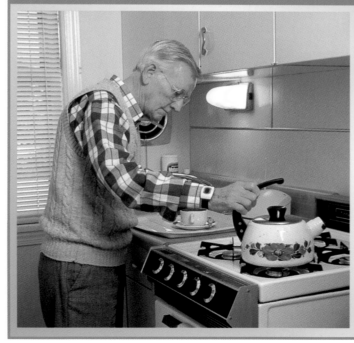

Chronic bronchitis

Symptoms

Chronic bronchitis is the term used to describe a persistent sputum-producing (productive) cough ('smoker's cough'), associated with a clinical condition referred to as chronic obstructive pulmonary disease (COPD). The cough is often worsened by exposure to cold air, sudden temperature changes, dust and cigarette smoke.

To fit the official medical definition of chronic bronchitis, the cough should be present for at least three months of the year for more than one year.

CLINICAL FEATURES

As well as a cough, people with chronic bronchitis may develop:
■ Breathlessness – in the early stages this may occur only on exertion; later it may become so severe that everyday tasks, such as getting dressed, become a major effort or impossible
■ An increased susceptibility to infections – colds and other respiratory infections increasingly tend to affect the chest, along with excessive sputum production, breathlessness and lung damage
■ Lethargy, sleepiness, poor concentration and a lack of general well-being.

Chronic bronchitis sufferers cough up excessive mucus secreted by enlarged bronchial mucous glands. This is often worsened by air conditions.

Lung tissue is badly damaged by emphysema, a condition that often goes hand in hand with bronchitis. As a result, severe breathlessness develops.

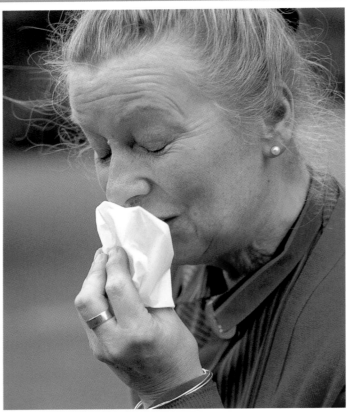

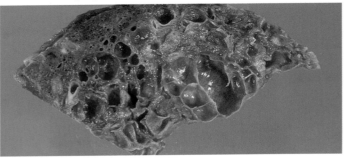

Incidence

Chronic bronchitis usually occurs in older people. It affects 17 per cent of men and 8 per cent of women between 40 and 64 years of age, most commonly those who smoke cigarettes.

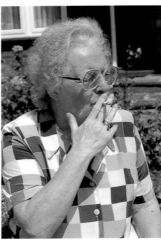

Chronic bronchitis is closely associated with smoking. The number of cigarettes smoked a day has an impact on severity.

Causes

The predominant cause of both chronic bronchitis and emphysema (see box) is tobacco smoke. Chronic bronchitis hardly ever occurs in non-smokers, and its severity is related to the number of cigarettes smoked each day. Atmospheric pollution and occupational exposure to dust are lesser causes, but aggravate the condition if it already exists.

In chronic bronchitis, the symptoms are caused by the following sequence of events:
■ Mucus-producing glands in the walls of the bronchi and trachea increase in size
■ These enlarged glands produce excessive amounts of thick, sticky mucus that is expelled as sputum
■ Increased sputum production clogs the airways
■ The bronchial walls become thickened and reduce the airflow further.

In advanced cases, the bronchi become inflamed, full of pus, ulcerated and scarred.

Emphysema

Most patients with COPD have both chronic bronchitis and emphysema.

Emphysema has several characteristics:
■ There is permanent lung damage in which the air sacs (alveoli) of the lungs become enlarged and lose their elasticity
■ The airflow in the lungs becomes increasingly impaired, causing breathlessness
■ Emphysema usually, but not always, affects cigarette smokers
■ Some people appear to be genetically predisposed to develop emphysema.

This X-ray of someone with emphysema shows a typical barrel-shaped chest. The ribs are widely spaced due to air trapped in their outer regions.

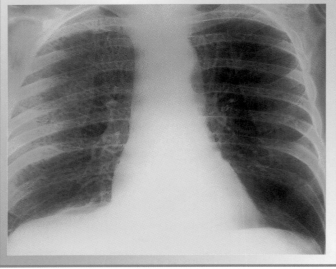

Diagnosis

The clinical picture of a long-term smoker, with a persistent, productive cough, suggests the diagnosis of chronic bronchitis. However, other causes of chronic cough and breathlessness, such as asthma, tuberculosis or lung cancer, must be excluded.

CLINICAL EXAMINATION
In chronic bronchitis, clinical examination may reveal:
■ Wheeziness
■ Crackling sounds or limited air entry to the lungs (through a stethoscope)
■ Rapid breathing
■ Difficulty in breathing – the muscles between the ribs, and the nostrils may be drawn in on inspiration and the lips may be pursed on expiration
■ Poor chest expansion on inspiration
■ Cyanosis – patients' skin may appear blue if they cannot inhale sufficient oxygen or if

lung damage strains the heart (cor pulmonale).

INVESTIGATIONS
Diagnoses are made using different techniques:
■ Chest X-ray – this is not always useful, as it may not be abnormal in the early stages of the illness
■ Blood tests – the haemoglobin level and packed red cell volume (PCV) in the blood may be increased, compensating for the low level of oxygen in the lungs
■ Electrocardiogram (ECG) – this may indicate strain on the right side of the heart, which pumps blood to the lungs
■ Lung function tests – these measure the airflow into and out of the lungs and the volume of air in the lungs.

Lung function can be measured using a vitalograph. The patient blows into a mouthpiece and a computer produces the results.

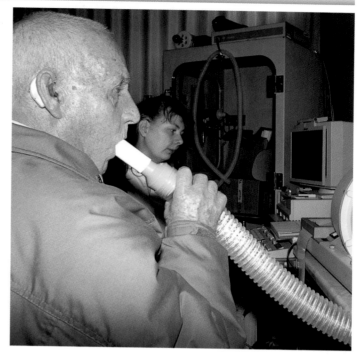

Prevention and treatment

Stopping smoking is of prime importance. Even with severe chronic bronchitis, this will improve the cough. Other

A nebulizer is used to deliver drugs directly to the lungs. Nebulizers convert a solution containing the drug into a fine mist which is then inhaled.

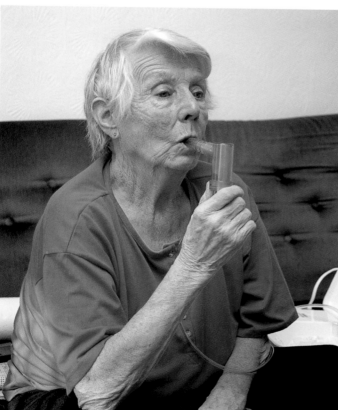

aggravating factors, such as pollution and industrial dust, should also be avoided.

DRUG THERAPY
There are several drug therapy options available:
■ Bronchodilators
Drugs that relax the airways, such as salbutamol or

ipratropium bromide, help some patients breathe better. They are usually most effective and are best tolerated if inhaled
■ Corticosteroids
These reduce inflammatory changes in the lungs. Not all patients respond to them, but if a trial period of treatment with oral prednisolone for 2-3 weeks decreases breathlessness, long-term treatment with inhaled steroids may be beneficial. The effective dose of inhaled steroids is lower than with oral drugs, so there is less risk of side effects
■ Antibiotics
Acute respiratory infections should be treated promptly with antibiotics to prevent further lung damage. Patients may be given a supply of antibiotics to keep at home so that they can start treatment if their sputum becomes yellow or green
■ Infection prevention
Yearly immunization against influenza is important for those with bronchitis, who are more vulnerable to infections
■ Oxygen therapy
This may be life-saving for patients suffering from acute worsening of their condition related to an infection. In severe chronic bronchitis, long-term oxygen therapy given virtually continuously, even when asleep, may lessen breathlessness and improve survival.

OTHER TREATMENTS
Other measures may also improve the condition:

Prognosis

At the start of the illness, the symptoms may be relatively minor, with patients coughing and producing a little sputum. If the patient stops smoking, the illness may not progress; the inflammatory changes in the airways may even return to normal.

With more severe chronic bronchitis and continued smoking, infections in the airways are common and may progress to infections in the lung tissue (pneumonia) and respiratory failure.

Smokers are more likely to die of chronic bronchitis and emphysema than non-smokers. About 50 per cent of severely breathless patients die within five years, but stopping smoking improves the outlook. The number of deaths increases with heavy atmospheric pollution.

■ Physiotherapy manoeuvres – help patients bring up sputum
■ Steam inhalations – thin the sputum, making it easier to cough up
■ Exercise training – patients may feel less breathless if they are take regular mild exercise
■ Assisted ventilation – patients whose condition is temporarily worsened by an acute infection may be helped by the use of a ventilator, if their breathing difficulties have become life-threatening.

Pneumonia

Symptoms

In pneumonia, the lungs become infected causing the alveoli (air sacs within the lung) to fill with white blood cells (which help to fight infection) and fluid.

The infection may affect only part of one lung, but in some cases, it affects both lungs. There are many different causes of pneumonia, some more serious than others.

TYPICAL SYMPTOMS
Pneumonia usually develops rapidly, often after a cold, with:
■ A high fever
■ Cough with yellow, green or blood-stained sputum
■ Rapid, shallow breathing
■ Chest pain that is worse after a deep breath or cough. This pain is due to pleurisy – an inflammation of the pleurae (the membranes covering the lungs).

Less commonly, pneumonia develops more gradually, with a dry cough, nausea, vomiting and diarrhoea. These symptoms may be associated with fatigue, muscular aches and headache.

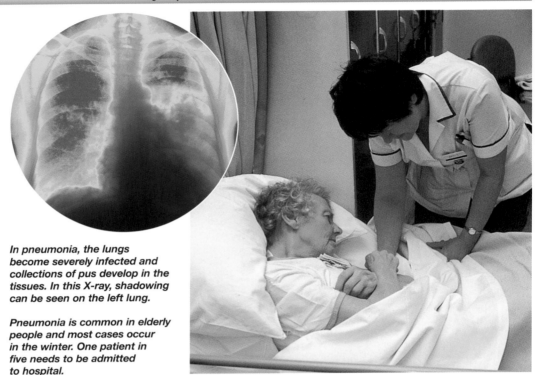

In pneumonia, the lungs become severely infected and collections of pus develop in the tissues. In this X-ray, shadowing can be seen on the left lung.

Pneumonia is common in elderly people and most cases occur in the winter. One patient in five needs to be admitted to hospital.

Causes

Most cases of pneumonia are due to infection by bacteria, and are only rarely due to a virus.

BACTERIA
There are many types of bacteria that can be responsible, but

Staphylococcus aureus is one of many bacteria that can cause pneumonia. This bacterium infects the air sacs in the lungs,

about half of all cases of pneumonia are due to a bacterium called *Streptococcus pneumoniae*. Typically, this follows parainfluenza virus infection (which causes the common cold). Other causes of pneumonia include:
■ *Mycoplasma pneumoniae* – mostly seen in younger people
■ *Haemophilus influenzae* – this tends to affect people with pre-existing lung disease, such as

chronic bronchitis and emphysema
■ *Chlamydia psittaci* – causes an unusual type of pneumonia, known as psittacosis, caught after contact with infected birds
■ *Staphylococcus aureus* – causes severe pneumonia, usually following infection with the influenza virus
■ *Legionella pneumophila* – this causes a rare form of pneumonia called legionnaires' disease, a

life-threatening condition that may spread through air-conditioning systems and shower heads
■ *Coxiella burnetii* (Q fever) and *Chlamydia* can be transmitted from infected sheep
■ *Pneumocystis carinii* occurs in people with a weakened immune system, most commonly those with HIV (the virus that causes AIDS)
■ Tuberculosis.

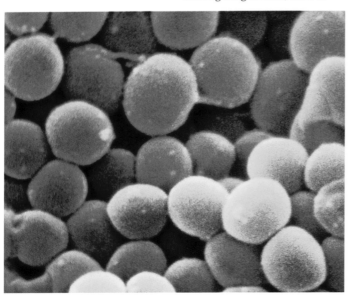

Incidence

Pneumonia causes about 27,000 deaths in the UK each year.

In the past, tuberculosis was a common cause of pneumonia in the UK. Worldwide, there are still around 23 million deaths from tuberculosis every year. There has been a rise in the number of cases in the UK in the last decade, which may be related to:
■ People coming to live in the UK from areas of the world where tuberculosis is more common
■ Poorer social conditions and homelessness
■ HIV infection
■ Drug abuse.

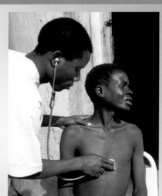

A doctor examines a TB patient in Mozambique. TB is still a major cause of death in the developing world.

Diagnosis

The patient's clinical history is important, as pneumonia often occurs a few days after a cold. Physical examination includes observing the breathing rate, which is often fast and shallow. Tapping the chest reveals that the affected part of the lung sounds dull, because the lung is filled with mucus.

Fluid conducts sound better than air, so the sound of the patient speaking will be louder on the side of the infection when heard through a stethoscope.

FURTHER INVESTIGATIONS
Other tests include:
■ Chest X-ray to confirm the presence of infection
■ Microscopic examination of a sputum sample to identify the bacteria responsible for infection
■ Blood tests to measure the white cell count
■ More specific tests that detect antibodies produced in response to a specific organism
■ Arterial blood test to measure circulating oxygen levels

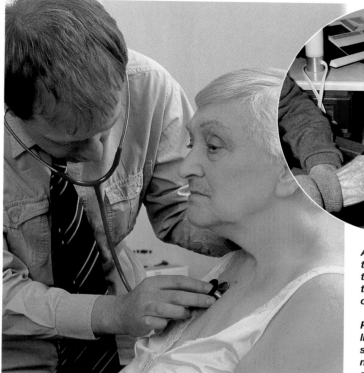

A pulse oximeter may be used to confirm low oxygen levels in the tissues. A sensor is attached to the finger and a digital read-out is obtained.

Pneumonia can be detected by listening to the chest with a stethoscope. If there is fluid or mucus in the lungs, crackling and wheezing can be heard.

Treatment

Pneumonia is usually treated with antibiotics, but these are effective only if the pneumonia is due to a bacterium – they are ineffective against viruses.

ANTIBIOTICS
The choice of antibiotic depends on the type of bacterium. To avoid delay, treatment is usually started before the results of any tests are known and is altered appropriately once the results are available. The choice of drug also depends on many other factors, such as:
■ Whether the patient has an allergy
■ Whether there is kidney or liver damage present
■ Whether the patient is pregnant or breast-feeding.

Most patients can be treated at home with a seven-day course of a single antibiotic. Patients who have contracted a severe form of pneumonia, or who are very frail, may need more than one type of antibiotic.

OTHER TREATMENT
In some cases, hospital admission may be necessary to administer oxygen and intravenous antibiotics.

Physiotherapy can help to loosen mucus, encourage coughing, and therefore make breathing easier. Pain relief may be required if a person has pleurisy.

If pneumonia is severe and the patient is very ill, admission to hospital may be required. Oxygen and intravenous antibiotics are administered.

Prevention

To prevent pneumonia:
■ BCG immunization against tuberculosis is advised
■ Lung function checks in immunosuppressed patients are needed
■ Smoking tobacco or drinking alcohol to excess should be avoided
■ Vulnerable groups are given flu vaccinations
■ Care should be taken when handling certain animals.

Prognosis

In the past, pneumonia was a common cause of death in young adults.

Nowadays, due to more effective antibiotics, young, previously healthy people with simple pneumonia tend to recover completely within two to three weeks.

SEVERE PNEUMONIA
In some cases however, pneumonia may be fatal – either because the patient is already frail, or because the pneumonia itself is very severe, such as in *Pneumocystis carinii* pneumonia.

Atypical pneumonias, including legionnaires' disease, can be very severe and more difficult to diagnose initially.

The emergence of new strains of tuberculosis that are resistant to the drug therapies currently available has also made it increasingly difficult to treat some patients with pneumonia.

Treating pneumonia

Doctors treating pneumonia have a wide range of technology at their disposal. These include diagnostic tests and microbiological studies to isolate the particular cause in each case, highlighting the most appropriate treatment.

In cases of mild pneumonia, the symptoms provide a sufficient diagnosis, and treatment is generally started immediately.

In patients in whom there is doubt about the diagnosis, a chest X-ray should be taken. This will show the characteristic appearance of lung consolidation. The extent of the consolidation (white shadowing on the normally dark lungs on X-ray) is useful to assess the severity of pneumonia; the pattern of consolidation may also suggest a likely cause (pneumococcus as oppose to mycoplasma, for example).

SAMPLE TESTING

A specimen of sputum should ideally be sent for culture before any treatment. Some of the common bacterial causes of pneumonia can be cultured (grown) from the sputum in the laboratory and identified. In addition, the sensitivity of these organisms to antibiotics can be tested. These tests, however, take several days to be performed, and so initial treatment is often 'blind'.

In more severe pneumonias, the organisms may be cultured from the bloodstream if suitable samples are taken. Many of the causative agents of pneumonia, however, are either difficult or impossible to grow from

The so-called 'rusty' sputum produced by a patient with acute pneumococcal pneumonia is typically purulent (containing pus) and blood-flecked.

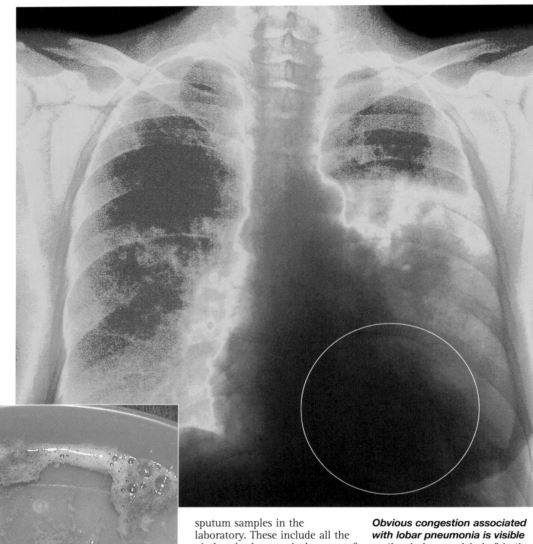

sputum samples in the laboratory. These include all the viral and other atypical causes of pneumonia. The diagnosis of these types of pneumonia often relies on blood tests. When we are infected by an organism, our body produces specific

Obvious congestion associated with lobar pneumonia is visible as the dark mass (circled) in the lower lobe in this coloured, computer-enhanced chest X-ray.

antibodies against it. This response does not occur immediately but can be measured some time after the infection (usually four to six weeks). These paired serology samples (one taken during the illness and the other four to six weeks later) are used to detect a rise in antibodies and thus suggest the infecting organism.

In routine hospital practice, such testing is used to diagnose Legionnaires' disease, viral pneumonias, mycoplasma pneumonia and other atypical (less common) organisms.

Causes of pneumonia

Infective
There are several pathogens and infective agents that may cause distinct types of pneumonia:
■ Bacteria
■ Viruses
■ Fungal organisms
■ Chlamydial organisms
■ Mycoplasmal organisms
■ Protozoal organisms

Non-infective
Pneumonia may arise in patients exposed to external disease-causing agents:
■ Chemicals or radiation
■ Allergic reaction
Alternatively, lipid pneumonia may result from lung damage caused by tumour or accident. Food or fluid in the lung leads to aspiration pneumonia.

In immunosuppressed hosts
If a patient's immune system is limited (in AIDS, for example), they become susceptible to pathogens that are not normally harmful in healthy humans. These 'opportunistic' agents may be certain:
■ Bacteria
■ Viruses
■ Fungi

Managing pneumonia

Advances in antibiotics and medical care mean that most forms of pneumonia can be controlled and treated, usually leading to a complete recovery.

The treatment of pneumonia depends upon the underlying cause and the severity of the pneumonia. Various bodies, including the British Thoracic Society, have published guidelines on the management of pneumonia.

Most patients who develop pneumonia have a mild form of the disease and consult their GP. They may have a very mild fever and minimal breathlessness, with no underlying systemic or lung disease. They require no further investigations and are usually treated with broad spectrum antibiotics to combat the infection, often including penicillin. These patients will usually recover well, and there is a very low incidence of short or long-term consequences.

In patients with more severe disease, further investigations, including chest X-ray and sputum culture, should be performed, and patients should take a course of antibiotics to cover the common bacterial and atypical pneumonias. For some of these patients, hospital admission may be considered necessary. The most common infective organisms and the appropriate antibiotics for them are listed below.

HOSPITAL TREATMENT
In the most severe cases admitted to hospital, treatment with oxygen supplements, intravenous antibiotics and physiotherapy is needed. In a small number of patients who have severe pneumonia, assisted ventilation using a

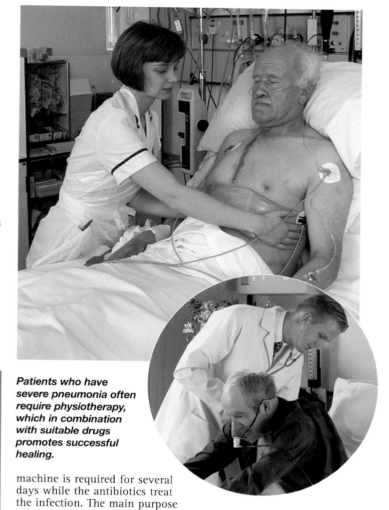

Patients who have severe pneumonia often require physiotherapy, which in combination with suitable drugs promotes successful healing.

Antibiotic treatment

The administration of the appropriate antibiotic targeted against the specific infective organism in each case of pneumonia will usually bring about a complete recovery. The most common antibiotics used are:

- **Penicillin**
  Active against bacteria such as *Streptococcus pneumoniae* (pneumococcus), *Haemophilus influenzae*, *Staphylococcus aureus* and *Legionella pneumophila*.
- **Tetracycline or erythromycin**
  Used when infection is with organisms that do not respond to penicillin (in cases of 'atypical pneumonia'), such as *Mycoplasma pneumoniae*, *Chlamydia psitacci* or *Coxiella burnetii*

Generally, when the pneumonia has a viral cause, it is treated by other means – clinical supportive care, for example. However, there is often a concurrent bacterial infection, which should respond to antibiotic therapy.

machine is required for several days while the antibiotics treat the infection. The main purpose of the ventilator is to increase the amount of oxygen transported from the inspired air into the bloodstream.

If a patient does not respond to an antibiotic given 'blindly' (that is, before tests), this suggests that the organism is not sensitive to that particular antibiotic. Every effort must

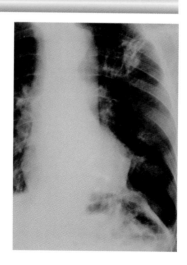

Those with severe pneumonia and damaged lungs often need to be given additional oxygen to aid their breathing.

then be made to identify the organism so that an alternative and more appropriate antibiotic may be prescribed to the patient.

Complications

Since the advent of effective antibiotics such as penicillin, the incidence of complications associated with pneumonia has reduced considerably, but they can still occur. Complications tend to occur in patients with more severe forms of pneumonia who have delayed starting antibiotics for whatever reason, whether due to late diagnosis, or failure to take the drugs prescribed.

In some circumstances, a cavity within the pneumonia-affected area may form due to destruction of the lung tissue. This is a lung abscess, and is treated with prolonged

intravenous antibiotics, surgical drainage, or both. Such abscesses are easily visible on a chest X-ray.

It is quite common for fluid to accumulate outside the lung in the pleural space around the lung. This is called a parapneumonic effusion and is usually not treated unless the fluid itself becomes infected, forming pus. This condition is empyaema, and it is diagnosed by aspirating some of the fluid through a hollow needle inserted between the ribs. Treatment is by drainage of the fluid and prolonged use of antibiotics. In chronic cases, the inflamed

capsule (membrane sheath) surrounding the empyaema needs to be surgically removed in a procedure known as decapsulation.

In some circumstances after a severe pneumonia, the lung heals to produce a scar which distorts the airways to cause bronchiectasis. This condition predisposes the sufferer to further multiple infections, but is now fortunately rare.

A lung abscess occurs when the tissues have been destroyed by pneumonia. It is visible on this X-ray as the cloudy mass in the left lung.

Gout

Symptoms and causes

Gout is the excess accumulation of monosodium urate crystals in body tissues and joints. These crystals are the by-product of the body's purine (nitrogen-containing compound) metabolism.

High levels can result from a high purine intake – such as a protein-rich diet – or from the body's own overproduction of urate. This tendency is inherited and present from birth.

URIC ACID

Uric acid is excreted from the body through the bowel and kidneys. Certain drugs, such as low-dose salicylates (aspirin) and diuretics, interfere with this process and raise urate levels. Crystals of monosodium urate are deposited into the joint causing intense irritation and pain. The joint becomes hot, red and swollen.

Classically, the big-toe joint is affected, but ankles, knees, elbows and the joints of the hands and feet can be involved. Only the large hip and shoulder joints tend to be spared.

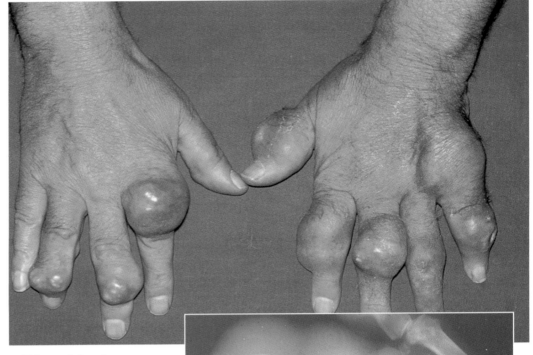

▲ *This man's hands are seriously affected by gout. Uric acid crystals in the blood have been deposited in the tissues, causing swelling and pain.*

▶ *An X-ray reveals the extent of damage to the finger joints. The hard crystals irritate the joint, causing an intense, painful inflammatory reaction.*

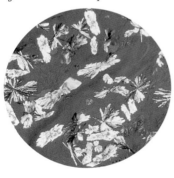

◀ *Tophi – hard, crystalline deposits of uric acid in the joints, skin and cartilage – can be seen under a microscope. Tophi are a characteristic feature of gout.*

Predisposing factors

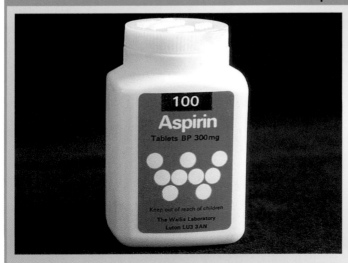

Men are eight times more likely to be affected than women, who are rarely affected before the menopause. The commonest age for a first attack is between 30 and 60. Other risk factors include:
■ A high alcohol intake. In itself, alcohol does not cause gout, but it will provoke attacks in those who are affected
■ A high protein diet
■ Obesity

Although aspirin is a non-steroidal anti-inflammatory drug, it is not used to treat gout as it slows excretion of uric acid. This may exacerbate symptoms of a gout attack.

■ Certain races, such as the Maoris and Polynesians, have higher blood levels of uric acid and are more susceptible to gout
■ Disorders that cause a high cell turnover, such as polycythaemia (increased red cells), lymphomas and various other cancers
■ A family history of gout
■ Diuretics or low-dose salicylates
■ Kidney disease.

Gout sufferers are more likely to have lipid disorders and high blood pressure. Twenty-five per cent of patients have had an episode of renal colic due to the presence of uric acid crystals before their first attack of gout.

Treatment

In an acute attack, non-steroidal anti-inflammatory drugs (NSAIDs) are very effective at dissolving away the intra-articular crystals. They should be given in high doses early in the attack; most gout sufferers will keep a ready supply in hand. For those who are unable to take NSAIDs, colchicine, one of the oldest known drugs, is also very effective.

DRAWBACKS

The main disadvantage of colchicine is that it has a very narrow therapeutic range, so side effects are common. The salicylates in low dose will aggravate gout; although in high dose they are therapeutic, they are probably best avoided.

Paradoxically, on initial dose, allopurinol, the usual preventative treatment for gout, can actually provoke an attack.

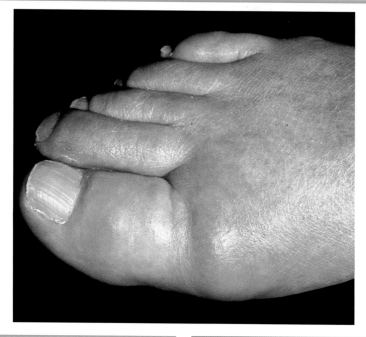

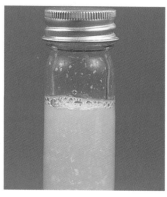

Pus, a fluid containing dead white blood cells, may be found in joints affected by gout that have become infected.

Gout commonly affects the joint of the big toe, causing acute pain. Treatment is with high doses of NSAIDs at the beginning of an attack.

Diagnosis

A classical history in a patient with predisposing factors and an elevated level of uric acid will confirm the diagnosis. If there is doubt, the presence of monosodium urate crystals in a synovial fluid aspirate is diagnostic.

In chronic gout, the joint can be destroyed, and X-rays reveal the typical changes. Similarly, urate is deposited in the tissues in the form of gouty tophi, around the joints, bursae and tendon sheaths and in the cartilaginous helix of the ear.

DIFFERENTIAL DIAGNOSIS

An acute attack can last a few hours to a few weeks. Acute gout can be very similar to septic arthritis and may warrant admission to hospital to exclude this more serious condition. Similarly, inflammatory arthropathies may begin with a mono-arthritis similar to gout.

An acute attack of gout may appear similar to septic arthritis (below). A positive diagnosis may be made after blood testing and X-ray.

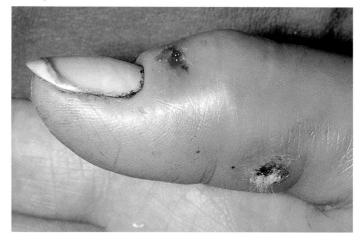

Prevention

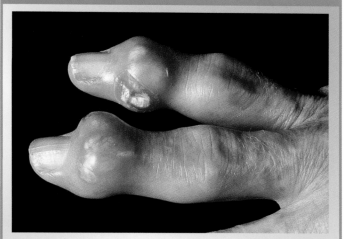

An elevated uric acid level alone is not an indication for drug treatment. The vast majority of patients with raised uric acid will remain asymptomatic throughout their lives. Some will suffer from intermittent attacks only and will benefit most from taking high-dose NSAIDs and following preventative advice, rather than life-long preventative medication.

High-purine foods, dehydration, especially in hot weather, and unaccustomed strenuous exercise should be avoided. Diuretics and low-dose aspirin should only be prescribed with caution.

Drug prevention should be aimed at those at risk of the long-term complications of gout, such as arthritis, and the rare complication of chronic renal disease. Those most at risk are young patients with high levels

Tophaceous gout is painful and disfiguring. As gout cannot be cured, prevention of the condition is important. This will involve drug treatment and dietary advice.

of uric acid, sufferers with evidence of chronic tophaceous gout, those who have frequent attacks of acute gout and people with renal disease.

Allopurinol is one of the commonest preventative drugs. It is very effective and safe even when taken long-term. Some patients suffer from rashes, but these improve when the drug is withdrawn.

The drug inhibits the enzyme xanthine oxidase, which converts xanthine into uric acid. Other preventative drugs are probenecid and sulphinpyrazone, which promote the excretion of uric acid through the kidneys.

Incidence

Gout is a relatively common condition affecting one per cent of the population. It causes excruciating pain in the joints. Historically, it affected the better-off in society (who ate more purine-rich foods), and whose lives were often ruined by the recurrent attacks and destruction of the joints.

Today, the acute pain that the condition may cause can be treated effectively with anti-inflammatory drugs or prevented completely with urate-lowering drugs.

Exercise in the elderly

Regular, sustained exercise can be of enormous benefit to the elderly. It exerts a powerfully protective influence, minimizing risks of cardiovascular disease, stroke and depression.

It is now widely recognized that consistent daily physical activity contributes to general good health. Conversely, the inactivity of a sedentary lifestyle can hasten the onset of heart, lung and bone disease, having a detrimental effect on both quality of life and longevity.

BENEFITS AT ALL AGES
Young people participate in physical exercise to increase fitness and gain sporting achievements, while for those in middle age it is often a source of leisure and pleasure. The elderly, however, have come to recognize it as an essential means of maintaining wellbeing and sound health.

Research initially suggested that physical exercise was helpful for people until their 60s, but new investigations have revealed its importance into very old age. Regular walking and activities such as swimming are enormously beneficial.

Aerobics classes combine an opportunity to improve fitness with a social activity. Both aspects contribute positively to feelings of health and wellbeing.

The heart and the lungs are strengthened through cardiovascular workouts. Within a matter of weeks, the benefits become apparent.

Effects of ageing and inactivity

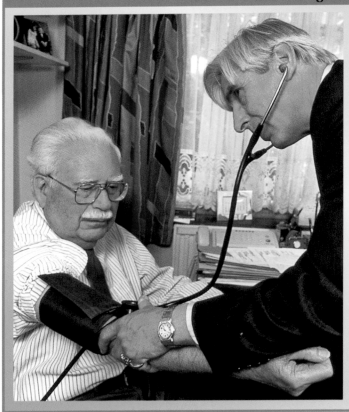

Those who have led sedentary lives are more at risk of heart disease in old age. High blood pressure may indicate a need for lifestyle changes.

Ageing affects many parts of the body, including the:
■ Heart and circulation – the heart loses muscle mass and its elastic fibres become replaced with fibrous tissue. There is a lower reserve for coping with the demands of living and any illnesses, while a diminished cardiac output is less able to meet body requirements
■ Lung capacity – the lungs lose elasticity and functional capacity. Breathing becomes more difficult generally, and any sudden physical demands may cause breathlessness. It also increases susceptibility to lung infections
■ Skeletal structure – long bones and vertebrae tend to thin and joints become less resilient. In people over 65 years of age, falls are common, and 15 per cent cause serious injury. Hip fractures are common due to osteoporosis (thinning of the bone)

■ Muscle mass – muscle mass is replaced with fibrous tissue and fat in old age. This creates a tendency to obesity, which in turn creates joint and blood pressure problems, and these may lead ultimately to heart failure, stroke or coronary artery disease.

Physical inactivity
Studies suggest that 70 per cent of men take insufficient exercise, and it is believed that the figure for women may be even higher.

Inactivity tends to worsen the problems of old age, because it:
■ Plays a crucial role in the development of obesity
■ Is thought to contribute to the onset of non-insulin dependent diabetes
■ Leads to adiposity (the accumulation of fat), which doubles the risk of coronary heart disease and is also a major risk factor for stroke
■ Is detrimental to all the structures in and around the joints, which are designed to move regularly rather than to remain static.

Taking exercise in old age

Long-held exercise habits should be maintained for as long as possible. Longevity and good health increase in proportion to the regularity and duration of the exercise undertaken.

FITNESS INITIATIVES
New government guidelines are encouraging family doctors to promote physical exercise in both the fit and the unfit. The aim is to reduce the incidence of coronary artery disease, stroke, diabetes, high blood pressure and mental illness.

The British Heart Foundation recently started a five-year initiative, 'Walking the Way to Health', to encourage people to walk more in their local area.

MODERATE EXERCISE
Moderation is the key concept for the elderly when taking exercise.

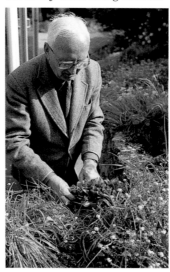

There is a wide scope of physical activity involved in gardening. It ranges from gentle watering to the hard labour of digging over a vegetable patch.

Exercise needs to be regular and sustained, but not vigorous or strenuous, to be of benefit.

Older individuals should not suddenly take up an ambitious exercise programme if they have been sedentary for a number of years. A gradual exposure to increasing activity is the wisest course, following a general health check-up by a doctor.

EXERCISE PROGRAMME
All exercise programmes should be tailored to age, needs, existing infirmities and medical state. From a sedentary lifestyle, the elderly should start by extending the limited exercise acquired through everyday activities, such as lengthening a walk to the shop into a walk around the park.

A slow, steady addition of exercise to existing lifestyle will gradually increase fitness without any adverse effect on the elderly individual. General health checks should be undertaken as muscular use increases within the programme.

Exercise should take place for an average of 30 minutes per day, at least five days per week. The individual should aim to become slightly out of breath and well warmed up.

PRECAUTIONS
Inactive people should start with minor exercise and gradually

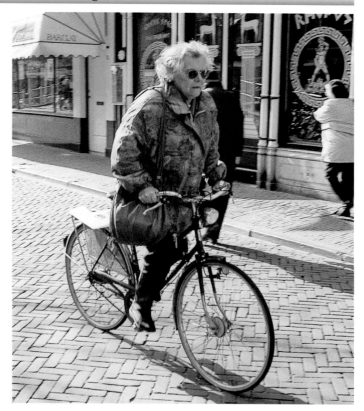

Everyday tasks such as riding a bicycle to the shops may be extended into longer periods of physical activity. The aim is to exercise for 30 minutes each day.

increase the duration, frequency, and intensity. Very vigorous exercise is not recommended in older people, as it may result in sudden unexpected death through cardiovascular causes (such as a heart attack). This is particularly true where exercise is a new element in someone's lifestyle.

Those with heart or lung disease or any form of chronic illness should consult a doctor before embarking on regular

exercise. Those with heart disease should be particularly careful, exercising within the limits of their angina or breathlessness. They should avoid exercising outside in very cold weather and stop if they experience any chest pain.

Physical activities

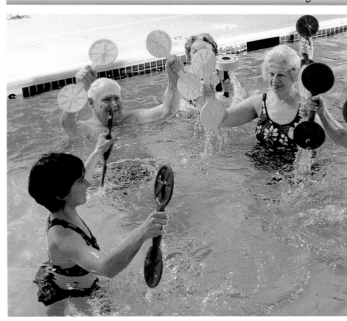

Swimming and water aerobics are both useful forms of exercise for the elderly. The limbs are supported and the joints do not have to bear any weight.

With all exercise programmes, the secret to increasing general health is to practise regularly; a daily short spell is more beneficial than an occasional vigorous outburst. Regular, frequent aerobic exercise of moderate intensity is the goal.

PHYSICAL ACTIVITIES
Examples of physical activities appropriate for elderly people include the following:
■ Gardening for 45 minutes
■ Walking a mile in about 20 minutes
■ Bicycling five miles in over 30 minutes
■ Swimming for 20 minutes

■ Doing water aerobics for 30 minutes
■ Walking up and down stairs for 15 minutes
■ Washing windows for 45 minutes.

SWIMMING
Swimming is a particularly useful form of exercise for the elderly. The limbs are supported by the water and joints are no longer weight-bearing.

The enjoyment of the exercise and the physical activity combine to produce a feeling of wellbeing which makes swimming especially worthwhile.

It is not necessary to be a good swimmer to benefit from water activity, as breast stroke or a 'doggy paddle' bring similar results. A 20-minute swim can renew the psyche and ease the stiffness of arthritic joints.

Benefits of exercise in old age

The likelihood of the elderly being affected by diabetes, propensity to falls, heart attacks and strokes has been shown to be dramatically reduced by a programme of exercise.

The inevitable physical decline caused by the ageing process can be slowed by moderate but regular physical exertion.

When exercise is practised on a daily basis, it can bring rich health rewards. Improvements in mindset, motivation and mobility can help to ensure quality and length of life for all those entering or already enjoying retirement.

WEIGHT LOSS

In old age, body muscle is slowly replaced with fat. This process cannot be halted, but it can be decelerated by exercise.

The calories burned by exercise also help to redress the accumulation of fat around the abdomen that is an inevitable consequence of advancing years.

PROTECTION FROM DIABETES

Exercise has been shown to play an important role in limiting the complications of diabetes mellitus, and to exert a protective influence on those at risk of developing non-insulin dependent diabetes.

EASING BONE DISEASE

Long bones and joints can be maintained at optimal fitness by sustained daily exercise.

Osteoporosis, which affects five per cent of the population, is a form of bone atrophy in which the bones thin to such an extent that fractures easily occur. Painful crush fractures of vertebrae are common.

Studies have shown that weight-bearing exercise works to counteract the thinning effect, achieving greater bone mass and lessening the risk of fractures considerably.

Exercise may also be beneficial in reducing pain from osteoarthritis.

REDUCING RISK OF FALLS

Exercise improves balance and gait, increases muscle strength and endurance and enhances joint mobility, all of which reduce the risk of falls.

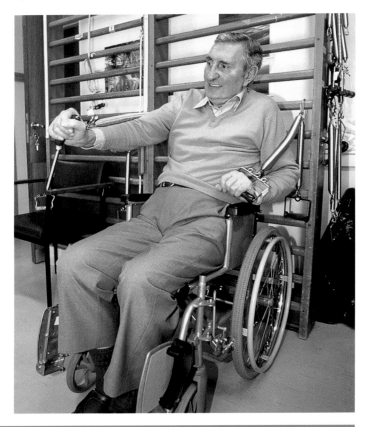

With commitment, even being wheelchair-bound need not impede an exercise programme. Individual areas of the body can be worked one at a time.

Cancer and exercise

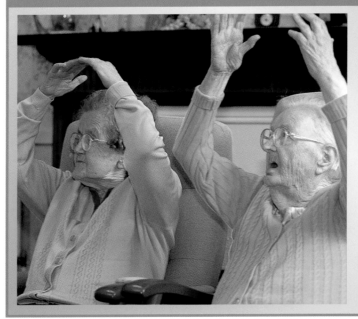

Research over the last 15–20 years suggests that workers in highly active professions are at 40–50 per cent less risk of developing cancer than those in sedentary professions.

Within the general population, three to four hours of aerobic exercise each week seems to reduce risk (particularly of colon cancer). Activities such as swimming, cycling or gardening, even when taken up only during retirement, can reduce risk levels.

Possible cause

The relationship between exercise and cancer has not yet been

Exercise seems to be useful both in preventing cancer and in minimizing the side effects of cancer treatments such as radiotherapy and chemotherapy.

definitively determined. One hypothesis is that exercise decreases the production of prostaglandins (hormone-like substances that control cell functions such as cell growth). It is thought that this may prevent the vigorous growth of cancerous cells.

Combating fatigue

Exercise has been shown to help combat fatigue associated with radiation and chemotherapy treatment. Generally, tiredness prevents activity, which reduces strength further, resulting in increased fatigue.

Exercise, on the other hand, helps keep energy levels high, maintains functional capacity during treatment, protects against cachexia (muscle wasting) and improves immune function.

Preventing cardiovascular problems

Physical exercise offers considerable potential benefits in the prevention of cardiovascular disease. Heart muscle and lung tissues can maintain optimal function through to old age if physical activity is maintained.

However, exercise must be regular and sustained to be effective against developing heart disease; high levels of exercise in adolescence will not, alone, prevent cardiovascular problems in old age.

A STRONGER HEART

Regular exercise at any age strengthens the heart, making it more efficient. It pumps more blood, increasing stroke volume, which ensures that blood is circulated efficiently to every part of the body. Cholesterol levels are reduced and blood pressure is lowered.

Regular exercise reduces the risk of a heart attack, and also the risk of death following a heart attack. People who do not exercise are three times more likely to die after a heart attack than those who do. Lack of physical activity also triples the likelihood of suffering a stroke.

REDUCING BLOOD FATS

A moderate amount of regular exercise has a positive effect on the blood lipids (fats) which play a large part in heart and artery disease. It helps to reduce the dangerous fats and produce a favourable lipid profile, which decreases the possibility of cardiovascular disease.

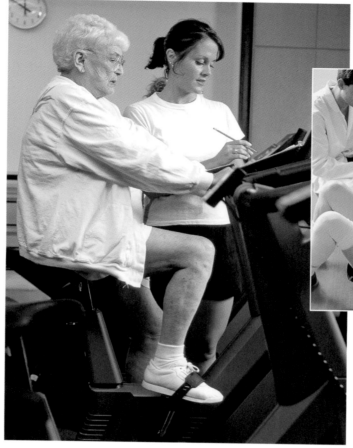

A qualified trainer is able to focus on specific muscle groups. This allows for safe exercise, in which weak points are protected, while other areas are worked.

Cycling is of particular benefit to people with ankle swelling. The repetitive movement of the legs forces fluid out of the tissues into the bloodstream.

ANKLE SWELLING

Repetitive leg movement and exercise massages the leg veins and moves peripheral blood through the valves. This prevents stasis of blood in the veins and the ankle swelling associated with old age and immobility.

Regular exercising helps to alleviate this problem as leg muscles force the fluid out of the tissues and back to the heart.

INCREASED LONGEVITY

Regular activity can increase longevity significantly in people over 60 years age, either with or without heart and artery disease.

The National Health Service recommends that all adults undertake moderately intense physical activity five days a week. Brisk walking, cycling, swimming, dancing and gardening are useful both for maintaining good health and for successful rehabilitation after a coronary thrombosis or other cardiac event has occurred.

Improving mental health

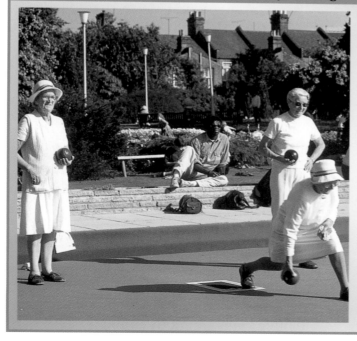

Exercise benefits both mind and body. There is now sound evidence of a positive association between regular physical activity and reduced rates of age-related mental disorders.

Improving mood

Regular physical activity appears to improve mood and decrease stress or anxiety.

This is thought to be due partly to the production of natural body chemicals called endorphins, which are released during strenuous exercise. These are morphine-like substances that produce feelings of pleasure and wellbeing, and have a similar effect to antidepressants.

While all sports can increase feelings of wellbeing, the social aspect of team sports holds a special appeal for elderly people living alone.

Increasing confidence

Regular exercise can bring about improvements in certain debilitating conditions and decrease feelings of fatigue. As strength begins to return, many older people feel able to accomplish more; their self-confidence and self-esteem are enhanced and life seems to have more opportunities for enjoyment.

Social benefits

There may also be social benefits to an exercise programme. Many old people are isolated, often living alone with scant social contact. Since most physical activities, such as bowling, take place in a social situation, they present opportunities for new social contacts.

Taking part in team sports can also foster mutual respect and support among elderly people as a group.

Maintaining health in old age

Staying healthy is essential to a good quality of life at any age.
Although nothing can halt the process of ageing, a healthy lifestyle
can prevent a number of illnesses common in older people.

One of the most important factors that determines a person's health in later life is their genetic inheritance – the genetic blueprint that has been handed down to them by their ancestors. Genes determine both the rate at which a person ages and the diseases that they are prone to develop.

LIFESTYLE FACTORS

The state of a person's health also depends on the environment in which they live and the lifestyle that they adopt.

There is good evidence that cultivating healthy habits can increase a person's well-being in later years and add to their enjoyment of life. It has been estimated that as many as half of all premature deaths may be attributed to unhealthy lifestyles.

DIET

It is particularly important for older people to consume the right amount of energy to keep the body within healthy weight limits for their height and build.

The rate at which the body processes food and drink declines with age, so keeping the same body weight requires a gentle reduction of calorie intake. Being overweight is unhealthy, and is associated with a number of conditions,

While genetics are an important factor in ageing, lifestyle plays a significant role. A balanced diet helps protect against a number of age-related diseases.

Excessive amounts of alcohol can be detrimental to health. In moderation, however, alcohol may actually help to prevent arterial disease.

including diabetes, stroke, coronary heart disease, arthritis, high blood pressure, gallstones, cancer, chest diseases and varicose veins.

People need to eat a balanced diet that contains adequate amounts of protein, carbohydrates, fats, minerals and vitamins. Fat in the diet should be reduced in later life since this may lead to the development of

atherosclerosis, in which the arteries become narrowed and inadequate supplies of oxygen are delivered to the organs. In the long term, this process may result in a heart attack.

HEALTHY BOWELS

Older people need to counteract their tendency towards constipation by increasing the amount of fibre included in their diet. High-fibre foods include cereals, wholemeal bread, pasta, rice, pulses (such as peas, beans and lentils) and most fruit and vegetables.

Eating plenty of fruit and vegetables is also important because these contain hundreds of disease-fighting phytochemicals that have evolved to give plants an in-built protection against the damaging effects of sunlight and atmospheric oxygen.

When consumed by humans, these phytochemicals are

Smoking has a harmful effect on the body at any age. In older people, smoking exacerbates the ageing process, causing a number of diseases.

thought to strengthen the body's defence against cancer-causing agents.

Research has consistently shown that people who eat a lot of fruit and vegetables are about half as likely to develop cancer as those who eat very little.

SMOKING

It is never too late to give up smoking. The risks of heart and blood vessel disease fall the moment the last cigarette is stubbed out. After 10 years of abstinence, the chances of developing lung cancer approach those of a non-smoker.

Even people who are over 80 years old when they give up smoking feel the benefits of a clearer chest, and as a result, recover more quickly from coughs and colds.

ALCOHOL

As people age, their tolerance of alcohol becomes reduced. This is because alcohol is metabolized more slowly, causing it to have a more toxic effect on the brain tissue. For this reason, older people are more vulnerable to the ill-effects of excess alcohol.

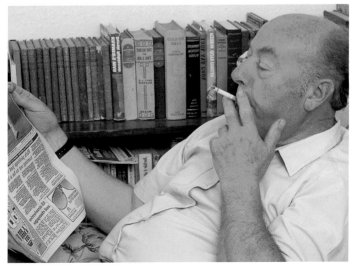

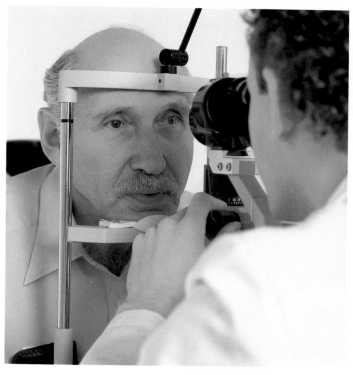

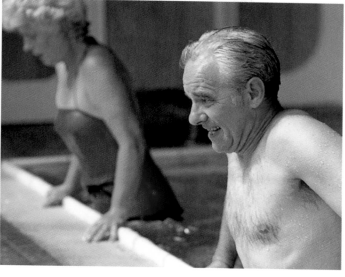

The eyes are prone to degenerate with age. Regular screening will enable visual disorders, such as glaucoma, to be detected as early as possible.

Exercise helps to maintain both physical and spiritual health. Swimming is particularly good for arthritis, since the water supports the body's weight.

SIDE EFFECTS

Consequently, older people who drink large quantities of alcohol run a greater risk of liver damage, bleeding from the stomach lining (chronic gastritis), painful legs from nerve damage, high blood pressure, vitamin deficiency, sexual impotence and depression.

BENEFITS

However, alcohol taken in moderation can confer benefits on older people. At least 20 studies have shown that people who have one or two drinks a day are less likely to have a heart attack than people who drink no alcohol at all.

It seems that small amounts of alcohol increase blood levels of the 'good' high-density lipoprotein (HDL) cholesterol. Unlike low-density lipoprotein (another form of cholesterol), HDL seems to have a protective effect against atherosclerosis.

EXERCISE

Adults who exercise regularly are less likely to become ill or to die prematurely. Exercise increases stamina of the heart and lungs, strengthens the muscles and bones, and improves balance and suppleness of joints. This helps to maintain mobility and independence well into old age.

People are never too old to exercise – useful exercises can be performed even while sitting in a chair. Good exercises for older people include swimming and walking. Swimming is particularly suitable for those with arthritis as the water supports much of their body weight. It also helps to strengthen the supporting muscles of the back, improves spinal mobility and relieves back pain.

For elderly people who can be prone to depression, exercise can improve self-esteem and decrease feelings of anxiety. It has even been shown to lift mild depression.

INHERITED DISEASE

Routine screening tests make it possible for certain medical problems to be detected at an earlier stage, when they can be treated more easily. People with a family history of certain diseases can therefore be targeted. For example, it is recommended that, after the age of 50, anyone with a family history of intestinal cancer should have an annual test for blood in their faeces, and after the age of 40, anyone with a family history of glaucoma should have the fluid pressure of their eyes measured at two-yearly intervals.

SCREENING TESTS

Doctors often carry out blood pressure measurements on older people coming to their surgeries with non-related conditions.

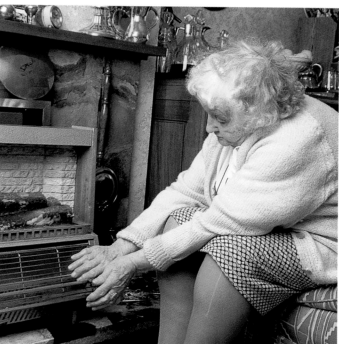

Unfortunately, however, many screening tests are not routinely offered to older people. For example, women over 65 are not automatically invited for mammography (breast screening), and women over 64 do not routinely receive cervical screening in the form of smears. However, if a woman in this age group is anxious, she is entitled to request these tests.

ENVIRONMENT

To keep healthy, older people need to pay particular attention to their environment. It is important that the home is safe and hazard-free; it should also be kept at a suitable temperature.

People's perceptions of body temperature become blunted with increasing age and, as a result, they may be unaware that they are becoming dangerously cold.

One sensible approach is to purchase a room thermometer and try to maintain living room and bedroom temperatures above 20°C (68°F).

In addition, older people need to control their environment more carefully than a younger person would need to. Elderly people should avoid extremes of temperature, since their impaired ability to regulate body temperature makes them more prone to heatstroke, as well as to hypothermia.

Older people are less able to regulate their body temperature. To prevent hypothermia, it is important that heating and clothing are adequate.

Enjoying retirement

Most people look forward to the day when they will no longer have to work. When retirement does arrive, however, it can be a daunting prospect, although most people adapt easily.

With increasing life expectancy, people retiring today can expect to spend nearly as long in retirement as they did at work. It is very important, therefore, that provision is made for this stage in life, so that it can be a time of enjoyment and new opportunities.

For many people, retirement is the first time they have ever really been able to indulge themselves without being weighed down by responsibilities such as child-rearing or having to earn a living. While this can be an enjoyable time for many people, some find that, having longed for retirement, when it actually arrives, it is not all they imagined.

PERIOD OF ADJUSTMENT

Attitudes towards retirement tend to vary. Some people feel ready to embrace the challenges of retirement, while others dread leaving work for fear of the loss of income and social status that this may bring. The absence of a rigid daily structure can also be a daunting prospect for many.

Some people choose to wean themselves off work gradually by working part-time for a while before leaving the company altogether. This allows time to develop new interests and hobbies, providing an incentive to leave work.

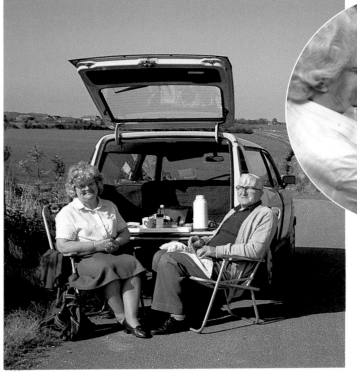

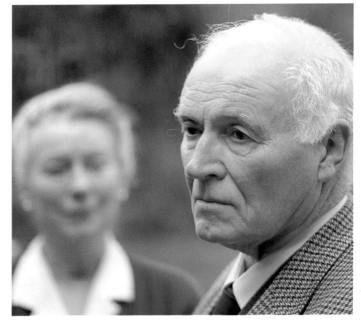

RELATIONSHIPS

Retirement brings profound change. In particular, it may sometimes put stress on relationships. Couples who have been together for many years may find that their relationship comes under strain when they are suddenly thrown together for 24 hours a day.

It can be a shock for both partners, if they have been used to leading separate lives, to find that they no longer really know each other. In addition, spending too much time together can cause some couples to feel claustrophobic, to the extent that a partner's presence and personal habits can be irritating. Some individuals also resent their loss of independence.

Many couples, however, find that retirement offers them the opportunity to reacquaint themselves with each other by spending quality time together, pursuing shared interests.

FINANCIAL PLANNING

With the loss of their salary, many retired people find that they have very little disposable income, since the greater part of their money is invested in their home. In order to enjoy

Some people experience a sense of loss after retiring. It can be difficult for couples who have led separate lives to adjust to spending more time together.

Retirement offers people the chance to pursue new interests. They may have always wanted to take up painting, for example, but never had the time.

Most people look forward to the freedom that retirement brings. Couples, in particular, can benefit from spending more quality time together.

retirement, therefore, careful financial planning is required from early on in a career.

Some couples find that the drop in their income after retirement is often balanced by the fact that their expenses decrease as well.

A retired couple no longer has to bear the costs of bringing up children, commuting to work, lunches away from home, or clothing for work. In addition, their housing costs are reduced as mortgages tend to be paid off by this time in life.

SETTING NEW GOALS

Careful planning is also necessary to ensure a fulfilling lifestyle. Individuals should set goals for themselves, to replace those no longer presented by work. Without such goals, there may be a tendency to while away the days achieving nothing in particular.

This lack of achievement can lead to a loss of confidence and a lowered self-esteem. Achieving personal objectives, however, can be extremely fulfilling and may motivate individuals to further action.

Some people see retirement as an opportunity to make a life change. Many use this time to travel abroad and enjoy stimulating holidays.

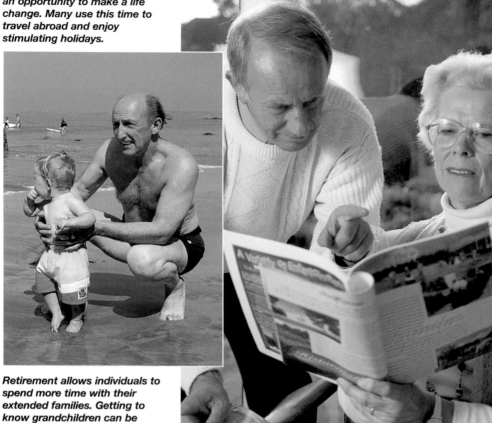

Retirement allows individuals to spend more time with their extended families. Getting to know grandchildren can be particularly rewarding.

FURTHER EDUCATION
Further education is one way to set new goals and challenges. People who have never been to university can use retirement to catch up on the education they missed out on when they were younger.

Others who have studied exclusively arts or sciences, but had a hankering after the other, can use retirement as an opportunity to enter a completely different area. Some people choose to go to adult education classes, or they may prefer to study by correspondence – an Open University course, for example.

Retirement also offers the opportunity to take up new hobbies. Individuals may find that they finally have the time to nurture long-cherished ambitions, such as creative writing or painting.

SOCIAL DEVELOPMENT
Joining a club or a society is one way of pursuing a hobby and, at the same time, meeting people with similar interests.

Retired people may also find that, after years of commuting to work, they can now become more involved in the life of the local community. This helps to increase social networks, allowing new friendships to be

established. Social interactions become increasingly important when a person is not working alongside colleagues on a daily basis, particularly for those who live alone.

Another way to remain active in the community is through charity work. Working as a volunteer can enable a person to put the skills they have acquired at work to good use and can also be helpful in easing the transition from full-time work to retirement.

LIFE CHANGES
Some people see retirement as the opportunity to make bold life changes. This may be the ideal time to move to that long-dreamt-of cottage in the country or even to a villa in the sun. An increasing number of people are choosing to live abroad after retirement, since a warmer climate can often bring a better quality of life.

Retired people also have the advantage of having the freedom and flexibility to enjoy off-peak travel and to take longer holidays.

Retirement offers people the chance to get fit through healthy pursuits and exercise. Keeping fit is important if a person is to enjoy their retirement to the full.

People in retirement often have priorities for holidays that are different to those of working people. They may prefer a stimulating activity programme, such as a golfing holiday, a cycling break or a safari, rather than the relaxing vacations favoured by people who work.

CHANGING FAMILY ROLE
Another advantage of retirement is that it offers people the opportunity to spend more time with friends and family. One of the great joys of this is having more time to spend with grandchildren.

Being a grandparent can give a new meaning to life. It offers people both a stake in the future and the pleasure of reliving earlier experiences through the children, reminiscing about their own grandparents, parents and children. It can also be a liberating experience, since it allows grandparents to spend quality time with their grandchildren, without having to bear the responsibility for their upbringing.

MAINTAINING HEALTH
Retirement offers people the opportunity to be fitter than they have been in years, and positive benefits can be reaped from healthy lifestyle changes, regardless of a person's age.

Everyone can benefit from exercise, provided it is gentle and safe. Some forms of exercise, such as squash, jogging or aerobics may prove to be too strenuous for the unfit, but walking and swimming offer an ideal all-round form of workout.

Maintaining health through careful exercise and diet is essential if a person is to make the most of their retirement.

If an individual is healthy and active, there is no reason why retirement cannot be one of the most fulfilling and enjoyable times in his or her life.

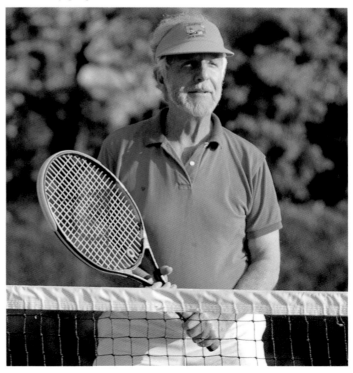

Sex and the elderly

As people age, they experience physical and mental changes that may lead to reduced sexual desire and performance. However, most couples learn to adapt successfully to their changing needs.

Although sexual desire and performance tend to decline with age, most elderly people are still interested in sex. Studies show that more than half of all adults over 60 are still sexually active.

LACK OF DISCUSSION
Sex and sexuality in older people are, however, sensitive and often taboo issues that are rarely discussed openly. This can have an unnecessarily detrimental effect on the physical and emotional well-being of a sizeable proportion of the population.

Fortunately, this situation is changing, and these issues have an increasingly higher public profile thanks to demographic changes and headline-grabbing developments such as Viagra.

SEXUAL CHANGES
Both men and women undergo real physical and mental changes that affect sex and sexuality throughout their lives, a pattern that continues through middle and old age. Age-related sexual problems may occur as a result of these changes, but elderly people can benefit enormously, both physically and emotionally, from advice about overcoming such difficulties.

MALE CHANGES
Several factors determine male libido (sex drive), including physical fitness, testosterone (male sex hormone) levels and mood, all of which decline with age. As well as adversely affecting libido, testosterone reduction also leads to reduced genital sensitivity and mild depression. Eventually, men may find it increasingly difficult to achieve and sustain an erection, and to reach orgasm.

FEMALE DEVELOPMENTS
Physical changes in women are more marked due to the menopause, which results in falling levels of both oestrogen and testosterone. Resulting sexual changes can include reduced libido, vaginal dryness and pain on intercourse, and reduced orgasmic sensitivity.

Contrary to popular stereotypes, older people do not lose interest in sex. Indeed, research indicates that the majority of elderly people are sexually active.

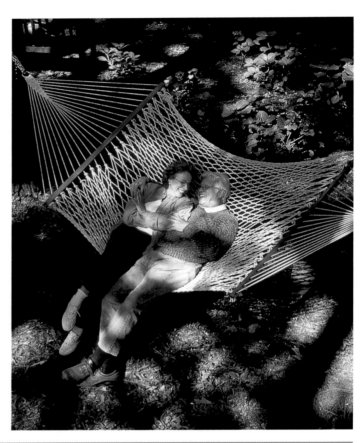

Maintaining sexual activity

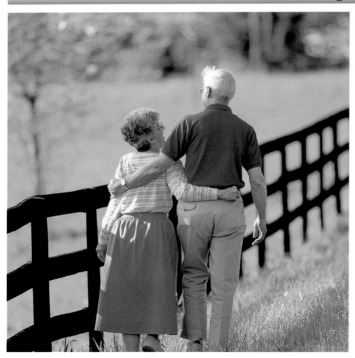

By the time they reach old age, many people will have adapted successfully to the effect of physical changes on their sexual development. Couples often become more relaxed and content, developing greater intimacy as their relationships mellow with age, which makes up for reduced sexual activity.

SELF-HELP MEASURES
Specific measures can also be taken to combat or accommodate sexual decline, helping older people to maintain an active and satisfying sex life. These relate to:
■ Time – men in particular can use unavoidable changes such as reduced genital sensitivity, and taking longer to reach orgasm, to become better lovers

Even light exercise, such as regular walks, can help to overcome sexual problems. Self-image and vitality are also boosted, increasing sex drive.

■ Foreplay – both men and women may need a longer period of foreplay before intercourse
■ Focus – couples may need to shift the focus of sex to non-penetrative techniques, such as oral sex, mutual masturbation and massage, which do not rely on lubrication or erections
■ Lubricants – these can be useful to overcome dryness and pain on intercourse
■ Fantasy/role play – these are useful techniques for increasing arousal and maintaining interest between long-term partners
■ Physical fitness – this is related to libido and performance. Lifestyle changes such as giving up smoking and adopting a healthy diet, together with even a mild exercise regime, can produce dramatic sexual improvements. They can also boost sex drive by positively affecting self-image and vitality.

Illness-related sexual problems

Ageing brings an increased incidence of disease and disability, which can affect sex drive and performance. Older people are often too embarrassed to report sexual difficulties to their doctor, and therefore suffer unnecessarily from problems that can be overcome.

SOURCES

Common sources of sexual problems in older people include:
■ Diabetes, prostate problems, cardiovascular disease and smoking – diabetes and prostate conditions can affect the nerves that serve the genitals, while cardiovascular disease, smoking and diabetes can affect the blood vessels supplying the genitals
■ Arthritis – this can make any activity, including sex, both difficult or painful. Side-by-side positions can ease discomfort, and pillows can be used to provide support and cushioning for painful or stiff joints. Partners may need to shift the focus of sex away from intercourse to relaxed techniques such as massage
■ Disability – disability and sex is an issue that remains taboo.

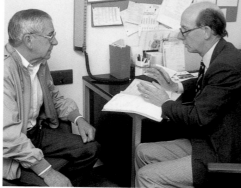

▶ *Physically handicapped people can still enjoy an active sex life. They may, however, need to look at other means of deriving sexual pleasure.*

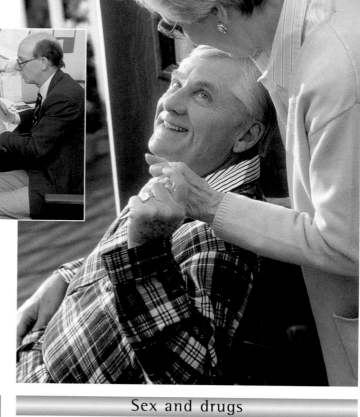

▲ *Elderly people may not discuss problems with their doctor due to embarrassment. However, many difficulties can be treated successfully.*

However, disabled people, both old and young, have sexual needs and drives. Disabled people may need to shift the emphasis away from intercourse, and to explore alternative sexual techniques.

Depression and sex

Depression is a major cause of loss of libido in men and women, and can affect performance, causing impotence, inorgasmia (difficulty in reaching orgasm) and pain on intercourse.

Causes

Common causes of depression include illness, disability, surgery, hormonal changes such as menopause, and life events such as the death of a spouse. Older people are more

vulnerable to all of these, and should be aware of the role that depression can play in causing sexual problems. Treatment for depression can thus also help to overcome sexual difficulties, although some antidepressants can also affect libido.

Having an operation can be a stressful and depressing experience. Many elderly people lose interest in sex completely at this time.

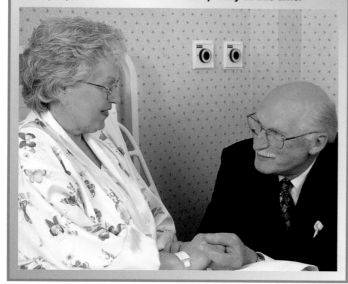

Sex and drugs

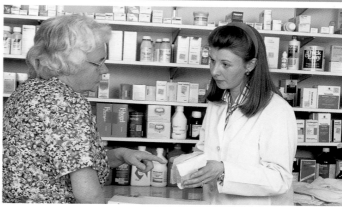

Many medications have sexual side effects, affecting libido and performance. Older people are often reliant on heavy medication regimes, and are therefore more vulnerable to these side effects.

Being aware of side effects can help older people to overcome feelings of shame and inadequacy about sexual dysfunction, while side effects can often be reduced by changes in dosage or type of drug. Classes of drugs that can cause sexual problems include:
■ Antidepressants – these can reduce libido and cause problems such as delayed ejaculation/orgasm. On the other

Some classes of drugs may have a detrimental effect on libido and sexual performance. These include antidepressants and cardiovascular drugs.

hand, successful treatment for depression can alleviate sexual dysfunction
■ Anti-Parkinson drugs – L-dopa, the primary drug therapy for Parkinson's, has been linked with increased sexual desire
■ Cardiovascular drugs – cholesterol-lowering drugs, antihypertensives and diuretics can all cause reduced libido, and some may cause vaginal dryness, erectile dysfunction and delayed ejaculation/orgasm.

Managing sexual problems

Sexual difficulties can be treated successfully in a number of ways. These include the drug Viagra, which has revolutionized the sex lives of millions of men.

New drugs have had a radical impact on the treatment of sexual difficulties, changing the sexual outlook for a whole generation. The most important drugs are Viagra and hormone treatments including HRT, testosterone and DHEA.

VIAGRA

Viagra is the brand name for sildenafil citrate, the first of a new class of drugs for treating erectile dysfunction (impotence). It has been a huge success: by June 2000 in the United States alone, Viagra had been dispensed more than 22 million times to more than seven million patients by more than 290,000 doctors. It is estimated that, worldwide, four Viagra tablets are dispensed every second.

HOW IT WORKS

Viagra is taken 30-60 minutes before intercourse, and works by preventing the breakdown of nitric oxide in the penis. Nitric oxide relaxes smooth muscle in the penis, allowing blood to flow in and cause an erection. Viagra does not directly affect the penile smooth muscle, however; it works only in conjunction with sexual stimulation, which itself elevates levels of nitric oxide.

Side effects, which are generally mild and short-lived, include headache (in 16 per cent of people), flushing (10 per cent), indigestion (7 per cent) and visual effects (3 per cent). Viagra should never be taken in conjunction with nitrates (often prescribed for heart problems).

CONCERNS

Viagra has been hailed as a panacea for male sexual problems. However, it does not directly affect libido and there is concern that it is being over-prescribed and used by people who do not need it – for instance, by those whose erectile dysfunction is psychological rather than organic in origin.

On the other hand, many older men, and their partners, benefit from the increased confidence and relief from impotence-related anxiety that Viagra brings, which increases libido indirectly.

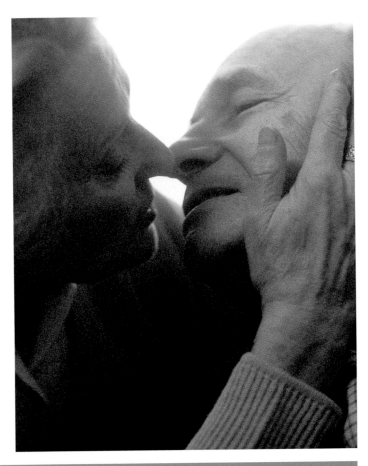

Viagra has been very successful in the treatment of erectile dysfunction. Many men who were burdened by impotence are now free to enjoy fulfilling sex lives.

Erectile assistance

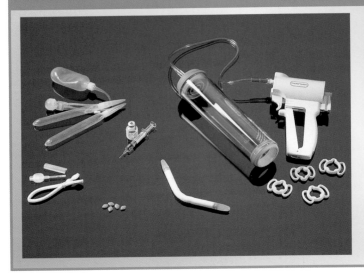

A variety of treatments exist for erectile dysfunction. These include flexible and inflatable penile implants, vacuum pumps, injections and drugs.

Erectile dysfunction can also be treated mechanically, by means of:

■ Implants – a common cause of erectile dysfunction in older men is nerve damage sustained during prostate operations; this can be remedied by an implant.

One form of implant is a bendable rod in the penis, which is bent upwards for intercourse. The drawback is that the penis is permanently erect. Another type of implant is an inflatable sac, which can be inflated via a pump in the scrotum to produce an erection

■ Vacuum devices – prior to Viagra, a common therapy involved a vacuum pump sheath that fitted over the penis. Air is pumped out of the sheath to create a vacuum that draws blood into the penis, giving an erection

■ Rings – an elastic ring around the base of the penis can help to prevent venous leakage. If blood leaks too easily out of the penis, it becomes difficult to sustain an erection

■ Injections – effective anti-impotence drugs, which were available before Viagra, can be injected directly into the penis.

Hormonal treatments

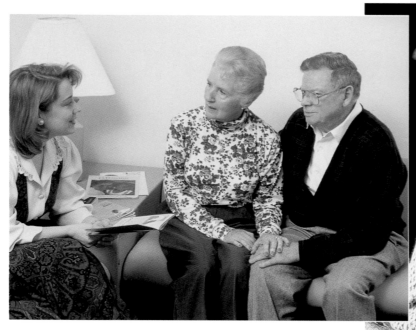

In some people therapy with a specialized counsellor may be appropriate. This is useful when sexual problems appear to be psychological in nature.

A number of hormonal treatments may be used in the management of sexual problems.

HRT
Supplements of oestrogen, and sometimes other female hormones such as progesterone, can alleviate many of the effects of the menopause. In particular, sexual problems such as dryness and loss of orgasmic sensitivity, may be helped by hormone replacement therapy (HRT), although women vary widely in their response to HRT.

Some women report increased libido, although this may be an indirect benefit of HRT, which

Sexual desire and performance may be boosted by the use of hormonal supplements. These include oestrogen, testosterone and DHEA.

can help women to feel healthier, happier and more attractive, and therefore sexier.

Oestrogen creams and ointments can also be used topically to treat vaginal dryness and pain on intercourse.

TESTOSTERONE
Research has increasingly underlined the role of testosterone in determining libido in both men and women. Previously, testosterone replacement therapy (TRT) was used only to treat men with abnormally low levels of the hormone, but there is increasing interest in the use of

supplements for healthy older men and women.

It is claimed that supplements boost both libido and performance. There are, however, concerns about the long-term effects of TRT, including the increased incidence of prostate enlargement, heart disease, stroke and masculinization in women.

Testosterone supplements can be administered:
- Orally
- By injection (usually once a week)
- Through skin patches
- By topical application in the form of gels or ointments.

Sex therapy

The proportion of erectile dysfunction cases that have psychological causes is still in dispute. However, there is no doubt that not all impotence is organic in origin.

Sex therapy is a form of psychotherapy that combines counselling and cognitive-behavioural therapy (a therapy aimed at changing a person's way of thinking). This type of therapy is an effective treatment for non-organic impotence and, moreover, has no side effects or health risks.

DHEA

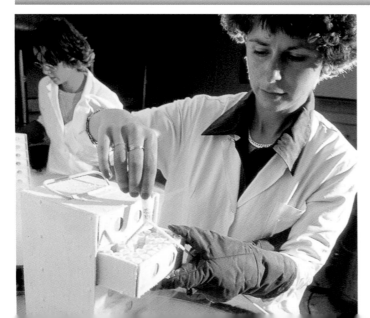

Medical research indicates that DHEA supplements may improve sexual performance and desire. A doctor should be consulted before taking DHEA, however.

Dehydroepiandrosterone (DHEA) is produced in the body as a precursor to several steroid hormones, including testosterone and oestrogen. Levels of DHEA in the body fall from the age of 30 onwards; by the age of 80, production has dropped by 90 per cent.

SUPPLEMENTS
Some studies appear to show that DHEA supplements have rejuvenating effects on the body

and, in particular, boost sex drive, performance and satisfaction. As a result, over-the-counter DHEA supplements have become very popular, but in practice the medical evidence is not clear-cut.

SIDE EFFECTS
Moreover, DHEA may have serious side effects, including liver damage, increased incidence of hormone-dependent cancers (such as breast cancer) and masculinization (in women).

Medical advice should always be sought before taking DHEA, and all hormonal supplements should be treated with caution.

Travel-related illness in elderly people

Elderly people are at a higher risk of developing complications associated with travel. There are many health considerations for this group, and therefore preparation before travelling is vital.

One in five people in the UK is over 65 years of age, with the majority retired from active work, but healthy and fit to travel the world.

ELDERLY TRAVELLERS
With the development of tourism, travel has become less expensive and far more accessible than in previous years, and this is reflected in the increasing number of elderly people holidaying abroad.

The majority of these travellers return home safely, but some succumb to travel-induced illness or injury, which could be avoided with foresight.

EFFECTS OF AGEING
In general, ageing is associated with a general decline in an individual's physical and mental state. A number of organs in the body may gradually deteriorate, causing:
- Loss in kidney function
- Reduced lung efficiency
- Decreased heart efficiency
- Gradual degeneration of the brain leading to dementia.

HIGH-RISK GROUP
In addition to the general effects of ageing, elderly people are likely to suffer from chronic illness, such as diabetes and heart problems. This means that they are at greater risk of developing travel-related illness.

Awareness of the effects of ageing on the intercontinental traveller, the health risks of travel and available preventive measures is invaluable. It can make the difference between safe, healthy travel and unwanted illness, accident, and emergency care.

PRECAUTIONS
Older people should be aware that they are vulnerable to a number of conditions when travelling. While this should not prevent people travelling, taking some precautions is advised before going abroad.

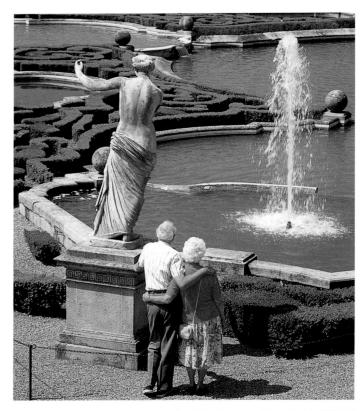

The number of people travelling during retirement has increased in recent years. Preparation before travelling can help to avoid travel-related illness.

Risks associated with travelling

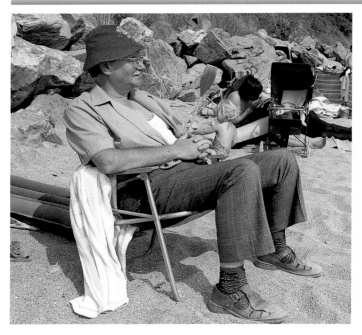

Sitting in the sun for long periods of time can cause dehydration. Elderly people can lose fluid rapidly in the heat and are advised to drink plenty.

International travel can exacerbate the effects of ageing, bringing added health risks from infection, trauma and environmental factors.

EFFECTS OF TRAVEL
The risks associated with travel that can worsen the effects of ageing include:
- Temperature extremes – high temperatures can cause hyperthermia (body over-heating), heat exhaustion and dehydration. Low temperatures bring about hypothermia and the effects of exposure. Excess humidity can cause an upset in body temperature control
- Air travel – may cause hypoxia, dry air effects and slowing of the blood circulation in the legs due to enforced immobility (which may cause deep vein thrombosis)
- Mountain sickness and hypoxia (low oxygen levels in the body) due to high altitude
- Accidents, such as falls, due to loss in balance on unfamiliar and uneven surfaces
- Diarrhoea and vomiting accompanied by dehydration
- Motion sickness caused by sea, land and air travel – this may be associated with a rigid neck, which affects the ability to compensate for movement
- Jet-lag – occurs more quickly when changing time zones because an elderly person's body clock adapts less easily
- Travel fatigue – physical stress from walking and carrying luggage. Travel delays can also be exhausting.

Preparation for travel

Age is not the arbiter of ability to travel and retain good health. Older people should satisfy their desire to travel, but should do so with more caution than younger people. Simple precautions, forward thinking, appropriate route planning and choice of final destination can all ensure healthy and safe travel.

HEALTH CHECK

A pre-travel health check at a travel health clinic or by a health professional with appropriate expertise is advisable for long-haul trips. Travel health counselling should include advice on:

■ Appropriate vaccinations – if an individual was born before 1930, they may not have been immunized against certain diseases, such as diphtheria
■ Malaria prophylaxis and protection from mosquito bites
■ Medication for motion sickness
■ Changes to drug medication because of time zone changes with travel
■ Coping with jet-lag and travel fatigue
■ The hazards of air travel, particularly avoidance of deep vein thrombosis
■ Effects of high altitude and prophylaxis
■ Coping with travellers' diarrhoea and dehydration
■ Management of any functional disability
■ Chronic illness and its effects on travel.

MEDICATION

The older traveller is more likely to be suffering from a chronic illness and be on medication than a younger person. This does not normally prevent travel, but it

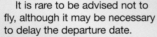

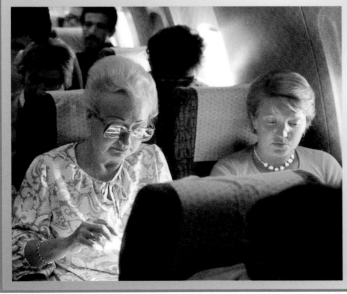

Before travelling a long distance, it is advisable to have a health check. Experts can give practical advice on travel and health.

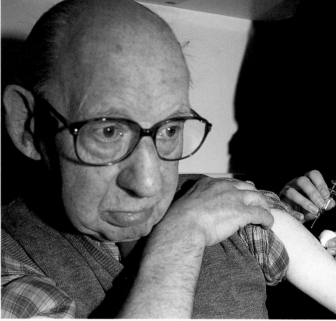

may require additional preparation and precautions.

Failure to take appropriate medication may lead to illness, and so travellers are advised to take medication as usual on the day of travel and to carry their drugs with them in hand luggage. They should also ensure that they carry sufficient medication for the duration of the holiday with a 10 per cent

People visiting countries in Asia, Africa, South America and Eastern Europe should be vaccinated. This is to protect them against tropical diseases.

allowance for unexpected delay as it may not be stocked abroad.

It is also advisable to carry a list of drugs routinely taken in case an individual has to consult a doctor while away.

Air travel and health hazards

Travelling for many hours at 560km/h (350 miles per hour) at high altitude in a cramped environment is not without health hazards.

Airlines operate systems encouraging those with health problems to complete a form advising of their condition. Five per cent of travellers are given 'invalid' status for travel. This usually means that customer assistance will be provided.

It is rare to be advised not to fly, although it may be necessary to delay the departure date.

Exclusions from air travel

Airlines refuse to carry the following categories of traveller:
■ People who have had a stroke or coronary thrombosis within three weeks of intended travel
■ People who are very anaemic
■ Those with angina or breathlessness while at rest
■ People who have had a stomach or intestinal bleed within the previous three weeks, or undergone abdominal surgery within that period
■ People with existing deep vein thromboses.

Deep vein thrombosis

Sitting for a long time in coaches or aircraft can cause pooling of blood in leg veins. This may cause a clot to form in a vein, which can occasionally reach the lung (pulmonary embolism). This condition is potentially fatal.

There is risk of deep vein thrombosis while travelling in an aircraft. This risk can be reduced by moving about regularly and taking aspirin.

Older people often sit immobile on long-haul journeys and they may have a predisposition to blood clotting.

Precautions

Exercising the limbs and thinning the blood decreases the risk of blood clots forming. It is particularly important to exercise calf muscles on long journeys when in restricted seating.

Taking a junior aspirin just before a lengthy flight can help to prevent the formation of a blood clot. One cod liver oil capsule per day for one week before a long flight is also thought to be helpful.

Wearing elasticated stockings for the journey improves the return of blood from the legs and feet to the heart along the veins (venous return).

Enjoying travel

Most older people who wish to travel abroad will be in good health during their holiday and while travelling, especially if they take sensible precautions in view of their health considerations.

Sleep patterns in the elderly

The established sleep patterns of adult life can become badly disrupted during old age. Anxiety, illness and an alteration in daily lifestyle can lead to debilitating insomnia.

Age is the major determinant of the amount of sleep people need. Across the human lifespan this amount changes dramatically.

Newborn babies sleep for 16 to 18 hours in each 24-hour period, decreasing gradually to 12 hours by the age of four or five. By the teenage years, this settles into an eight-hour sleep period which continues throughout adult life, except when interrupted by illness or the care of a dependent.

SIGNIFICANT CHANGE

Elderly people experience a number of changes in their pattern of sleep.

While the total time spent asleep seems to remain the same, at between seven and eight hours, the overall quality may be deficient for a number of reasons.

QUALITY OF SLEEP

There are two basic kinds of sleep: rapid eye movement (REM) sleep and non-REM sleep.

During REM sleep, electrical activity increases, dreaming occurs and blood flow to the brain is increased. The pattern of electrical activity in the brain is similar to that of someone who is awake. The muscles of the body are largely rendered inactive, which prevents people from acting out their dreams.

Non-REM sleep falls into four categories. Stages one and two consist of relatively light sleep, from which it is easy to awaken.

In stage three, the sleep deepens, and by stage four the brain wave activity shows even slower, deeper and more regular waves. This is the most refreshing and rejuvenating level of sleep, from which it is difficult to awaken.

We fall asleep by entering stage one of non-REM sleep and work through to stage four. After 70 to 90 minutes, the body goes through a 10–20 minute period of REM sleep before restarting the cycle.

As the night progresses, the periods of REM sleep become

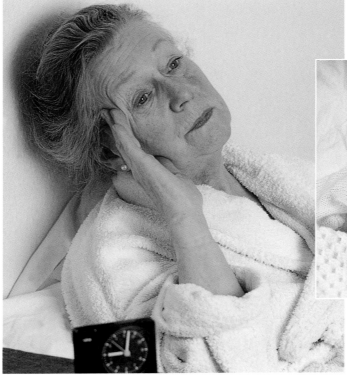

◀ As we get older, sleep can become problematic. Elderly people may find it more difficult both to fall asleep and to stay asleep.

▲ Sleep patterns are strangely similar at either end of the lifespan. Both babies and older people spread sleep in small chunks over a 24-hour period.

longer and the brain moves only between stages one and two of non-REM sleep. It seems that two or three incursions into the deeper stages of sleep are sufficient for the body's needs.

Researchers have discovered that the proportion of REM to non-REM sleep remains steady during adulthood, but then declines among people in their eighties, with fewer periods of deep stage four sleep occurring.

This means that while the total sleep periods may add up to eight hours, the quality may not be as refreshing, and may leave the elderly person feeling as though they need more sleep.

FALLING ASLEEP

Young adults take an average of 10 minutes to fall asleep. From

Electrodes can be attached to a patient to measure the electrical activity in the brain during sleep. This enables researchers to monitor the stages of sleep.

the age of around 60, this figure starts to get higher, until at ages above 70 it may take up to half an hour to go to sleep.

Coupled with the fact that elderly people wake more frequently, this longer drop-off period can become a significant problem. The insomnia itself can

cause or aggravate depression; long periods spent awake in bed at night can all too easily become periods of time spent dwelling on problems.

This in turn can deepen any existing anxiety or depression and cause further sleep problems.

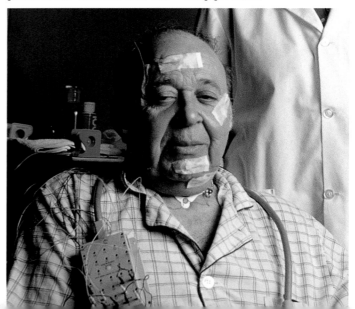

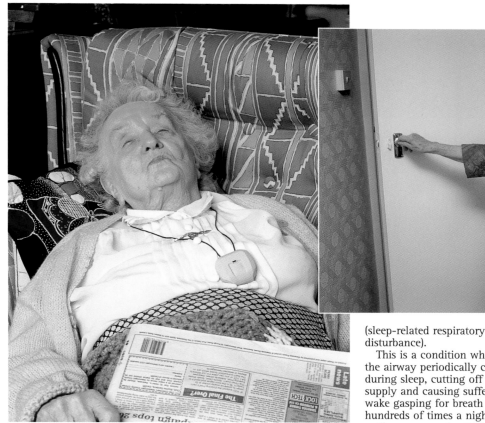

FREQUENT WAKING

Elderly people may wake several times during the night, for a number of reasons. One factor is that the older age group tend to suffer from many more medical conditions than younger people.

These conditions may result in a frequent need to wake in order to urinate (particularly prostate problems in men or stress incontinence in women). In addition, the chronic pain of an existing condition (such as osteoporosis or arthritis) may lead to sleep disturbances.

The incidence of anxiety and depression may also be higher than average for this group, as they are likely to have suffered bereavement and may be depressed or anxious about their living circumstances. This can cause sleep disruption, with very early morning waking patterns.

Older adults are also more likely to be woken by a condition known as nocturnal myoclonus, or restless legs. This forces the sleeper's leg muscles to twitch involuntarily every 20 to 40 seconds or so, making sleep difficult.

LENGTH OF SLEEP

For elderly people, sleep no longer occurs over one extended period. They tend to wake during the night, sleeping in two or more stretches, then supplement their five or six hours of sleep with naps during the day. This

Napping during the day can aggravate existing sleep problems. Studies suggest that while naps relieve tiredness, they disrupt night-time sleep.

condition can lead to a vicious cycle as more and more naps are taken to relieve a feeling of tiredness, so causing night-time sleep to be further disrupted.

SLEEP APNOEA

Studies suggest that among supposedly healthy adults aged over 60, one-third are woken at least five times an hour by a condition called sleep apnoea

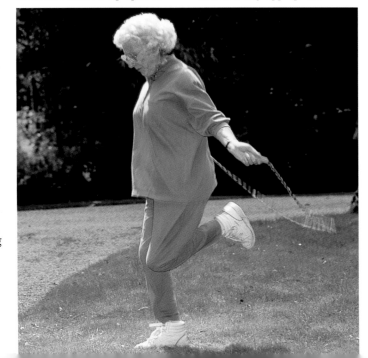

(sleep-related respiratory disturbance).

This is a condition whereby the airway periodically collapses during sleep, cutting off the air supply and causing sufferers to wake gasping for breath hundreds of times a night.

Sleep apnoea drastically interrupts the sleep cycle, taking the sleeper back to an almost awake condition and preventing them from ever reaching the deepest and most refreshing stage four sleep.

Interestingly, sleep apnoea tends to occur at opposite ends of the human lifespan, in both newborn babies and older adults.

IMPROVING SLEEP

The following routines have been found to be beneficial in securing longer and more restful sleep in the elderly:

■ Ensuring that adequate pain relief and any appropriate

Waking in the night is a common problem for the elderly. Health disorders, such as painful arthritis or prostate conditions, can disrupt sleep.

medications for existing diseases or conditions have been taken before retiring to bed
■ Following guidelines for increasing general health through diet to avoid problems such as constipation
■ Maintaining a reasonably high level of activity during the day
■ Keeping daytime naps to a minimum (in some cases avoiding them altogether)
■ Getting up at a regular hour every morning
■ Going to bed late every day – around 10 or 11 pm
■ Maintaining a comfortable temperature in the bedroom
■ Avoiding coffee or tea in the evening, and drinking a warm milky drink before bed
■ Performing a relaxing activity before going to bed, such as watching television or reading
■ Dealing with stress in a positive way, perhaps through discussion with a counsellor, to prevent anxiety and depression building up
■ As a last resort, hypnotics (sleeping pills) may be prescribed. Since these can set up a cycle of dependence and become less effective with continued use, they should be used with caution. They can also increase problems of confusion and unsteadiness, particularly in the elderly.

The best way to achieve beneficial sleeping patterns is to follow a healthy lifestyle. Light exercise, a healthy diet and calm evening activities can all help.

Health screening for elderly people

All people over 75 years of age should be offered an annual health check by their GP. This service means that a high proportion of problems can be identified – and treated – early on.

Health screening is an attempt to identify diseases in groups of people believed to be at special health risk and who are either already suffering from, or are likely to develop, an illness. The elderly comprise one such group.

Screening usually involves patients undergoing a test or a standardized procedure. The aim is to try to detect illness risk factors with the intention of implementing early preventative treatment.

NATIONAL SCREENING

National screening is usually organized by the Government, but many smaller projects are developed by elements of the NHS such as hospitals, the hospital trusts or community health professionals.

An assessment exercise has been decreed by the Government for all people over 75 years of age, in which GPs must identify people over this age on practice lists and offer each one the opportunity to participate in a simple health assessment. Individuals are free to decline the offer, of course, but this response will be recorded by the GP and a further offer made a year later.

PARTICIPATION

Seventy per cent of the population will now live to over

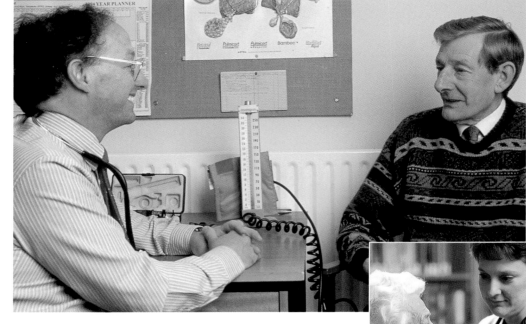

There are changes in the physical and psychological well-being of people as they age. It is therefore important that regular health checks are available.

65, and 30–40 per cent will live over 80 years, and today illness among the elderly accounts for a high percentage of GP workload. Screening assessments for over-75s have therefore become an integral part of GP care.

The terms of service for all general practitioners stipulate that all patients over the age of 75 should have their medical needs assessed.

Many family doctors are encouraging people in this age group to participate in screening programmes, and anyone over the age of 75 can insist on their right to an annual health appraisal in their family practice.

Performing the consultation

The person who carries out the assessment may be the patient's family doctor, but the task may be delegated to other members of the primary care team.

In different practices, this means that the assessor may be the practice nurse, the community nurse, the health visitor or a nurse employed to carry out these assessments.

AIMS OF THE CONSULTATION

During the consultation, the appointed doctor or nurse will assess several aspects of the patient's general state

and their circumstances. These aspects include:
■ Neurological/sensory function
■ Mobility
■ Mental condition
■ Physical condition, including state of continence
■ Social environment
■ Use of medicines
■ Any medical conditions affecting the person's current health.

An annual health check allows older people access to professional medical support and advice. Any special needs can also be identified.

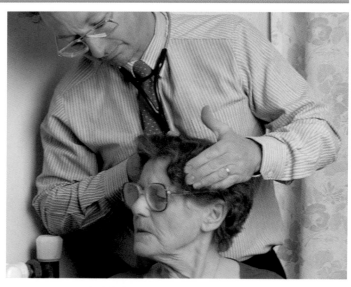

What does the consultation involve?

The consultation covers the whole range of the individual's circumstances in an attempt to identify areas of special need. The doctor will:

■ Take a history of previous illness and record any current symptoms
■ Check on any prescription and over-the-counter medicines being taken. The doctor or nurse may want to see drug containers to confirm the dose

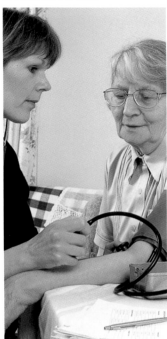

Part of the check-up will involve a review of any medication that the person is currently taking. It is important that the correct doses are adhered to.

■ Note the social circumstances, including whether the person is living alone and, if so, whether neighbours are helpful
■ Note any NHS and social work services used by the person.

REGULAR TESTS
If necessary, a physical examination will be performed. Other tests include:
■ Blood pressure check
■ A blood test as part of a routine screen to check that the liver and kidneys and blood system are functioning normally. A more targeted screen for older people includes tests for anaemia, thyroid disorder, rheumatism and prostate problems
■ Specific blood tests for cholesterol and blood fats.

Most of these tests can be carried out on blood obtained from one venous sample, usually taken from the arm in front of the elbow; it is an almost painless procedure.

Blood pressure is an important indicator of general health, and it will be checked regularly. Any abnormalities could be a sign of underlying disease.

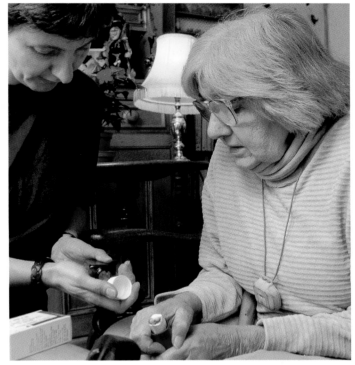

■ Lung function check to exclude or confirm bronchitis. This usually involves the use of a peak flow meter, a simple instrument that measures the rate of airflow when a patient blows strongly into a mouthpiece
■ Electrocardiography, if the doctor is concerned that there might be a problem with heart

function. An ECG machine can be used to record defects in heart muscle activity
■ Weight checks to compare the patient's weight with the ideal weight. Impaired mobility in older age is often associated with excess weight. Excess or low weight is associated with nutritional intake, and details of diet should be discussed.

Memory tests

A simple memory test should be part of every over-75 health check. Early diagnosis of dementia is now important for new drugs in use, or soon to be launched. This can bring some improvement in memory for people who are identified as being in the earliest stages of Alzheimer's disease. If the reason for the test is explained, few people object to being asked to complete a simple questionnaire.

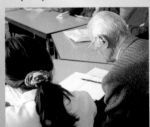

Alzheimer's disease affects up to one third of people over the age of 85. A simple memory test is therefore an important part of the health check.

Benefits of screening

With the examination and tests completed, the family doctor should have a precise awareness of the person's physical, social and psychological well-being.

IDENTIFYING NEEDS
At this stage, health and social needs can be identified and a management plan agreed with the person involved. Available local social and support services

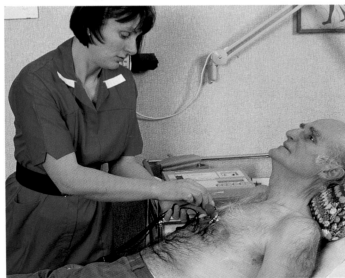

can be approached and if further investigation or hospital referral is required, this can be arranged.

Many people are found to be fit at annual checks; a third have a chronic disorder, often already known to the doctor, and a third require input from health and social care teams. If this is supplied promptly, hospitalization may be avoided and curative therapy can be instituted.

Annual health checks have uncovered a variety of needs, such as in vision and hearing, and simple chiropody problems that were crippling for the sufferer can now be dealt with early to maintain mobility.

ACCESS TO SUPPORT
All those who reach the age of 75 should accept the offer of an annual health check from their GP and ensure that the service offered is adequate and meets their expectations. Regular assessment can bring early preventative medical intervention.

For some people, participation may well prove to be life-saving; for others, it will bring access to needed professional support and for many it will merely confirm their own perception of well-being.

During electrocardiography, which is usually part of the check-up, electrodes are placed over the chest. These pick up signals from the heart, which are recorded by the ECG machine.

Index

A

abnormal heart rhythms 46–9
ACE inhibitors 63, 65, 75, 81
acute arthritis 26–7
age-related visual disorders 122–5
age spots 21
ageism 14
air travel, hazards of 168, 169
alcohol 160–1
  and atherosclerosis 54
  and cardiomyopathy 65
  and gout 154
  and heart disease 74
Alzheimer's disease (AD) 84–5, 86–8
andropause 12–13
aneurysms 79
angina 50–3
angiotensin-converting enzyme
  (ACE) inhibitors 63, 65, 75, 81
antibiotics
  for chronic bronchitis 149
  for endocarditis 67
  for pneumonia 151, 153
anticoagulants
  for angina 53
  for cardiomyopathy 65
  for deep vein thrombosis (DVT) 83
antidepressants
  Alzheimer's disease and 89
  for depression 101
arrhythmia 46–9
arthritis
  acute arthritis 26–7
  osteoarthritis (OA) 32–5, 131, 137
  rheumatoid arthritis (RA) 28–31, 137
  and sexual activity 165
aspirin
  following a stroke 104
  for heart disease 75
ateriosclerosis see atherosclerosis
atherosclerosis 54–5
  vascular dementia and 90–1

B

baldness 20
Baltimore Longitudinal Study 15
beta-blockers
  for angina 53
  for cardiomyopathy 65
  for heart disease 75
  for hypertension 81
bisphosphonates
  for osteoporosis 39
  for Paget's disease 41
bladder
bladder cancer 114–15
  the effects of ageing on 19

urinary incontinence 138–41
blood pressure, high see hypertension
bone scans 112
bones see also joints
  acute arthritis 26–7
  bone density and ageing 21
  mobility problems and 134–7
  osteoarthritis (OA) 32–5, 131, 137
  osteoporosis 28, 36–9, 137, 147
  Paget's disease 40–1
  rheumatoid arthritis (RA) 28–31, 137
bowels, healthy 160
bradyarrythmias 46, 49
brain disorders see mental health;
  nervous system
brain function, changes in 17, 18, 84–5
breast cancer 116–17
breathlessness, arrhythmias and 47
bronchitis 148–9
bunions 133

C

CAD (coronary artery disease) 72
calcitonin, for Paget's disease 41
calcium, and osteoporosis 39
callosities 131
cancer
  bladder cancer 114–15
  breast cancer 116–17
  exercise and 158
  kidney tumours 118–19
  lung cancer 110–13
  prostate cancer 106–9
cardiac arrest 51, 56–9
cardiomyopathy 64–5
cardiovascular disease, preventing 72
carers 85
cataracts 18, 120–1, 124–5
cells, ageing of 16, 18
chemotherapy
  for bladder cancer 115
  for lung cancer 113
  for prostate cancer 109
chiropody see foot disorders
cholesterol, high
  atherosclerosis and 54
  preventing cardiovascular disease 73
chronic bronchitis 148–9
cognitive behavioural therapy 101
Colles' fractures 37, 39
complementary therapies, for
  osteoarthritis (OA) 35
corns 131
coronary artery disease (CAD)
  72, 74–5
CT scans, for lung cancer 112
cystectomy, for bladder cancer 115

D

deep vein thrombosis (DVT) 82–3, 169
defibrillators 49, 65, 77
dementia 17, 84, 90–3
  see also Alzheimer's disease (AD)
depression 100–1
  dementia and 93
  and malnutrition 147
  sex and 165
DEXA scanning 38
diabetes 142–3
  atherosclerosis 54, 55
  cataracts 120
  exercise 158
  eyesight 124
  foot disorders 131, 132
  heart attacks 57
  heart disease 74
  sexual activity 165
diet 160
  angina and 53
  atherosclerosis and 54
  diabetes and 142, 143
  heart disease and 74
  malnutrition 144–7
  osteoarthritis and 35
  osteoporosis and 39
  prostate cancer and 106
disability, and sexual activity 165
diuretics
  for heart failure 63
  for hypertension 81
dizziness, arrhythmias and 47
Doppler ultrasonography 83
'dowager's hump' 21, 37
DVT (deep vein thrombosis) 82–3, 169

E

ears
  hearing, changes in 17, 18, 22
  hearing loss 128–9
  tinnitus 22, 129
education, in retirement 163
emphysema 148
endocarditis 66–7
environmental factors, ageing and 17
erectile assistance 166
exercise 156–9, 161
  angina and 53
  to assist with mobility 136
  atherosclerosis and 54
  cancer and 158
  chronic bronchitis and 149
  diabetes and 143, 158
  following joint replacements 44–5
  heart disease reduced by 74
  to help with depression 101

improving mental health 159
osteoarthritis (OA) and 35
osteoporosis and 37, 39
pelvic floor exercises 140, 141
eye problems
  age-related visual disorders 122–5
  cataracts 18, 120–1, 124–5
  changes in eyesight 17, 18
  glaucoma 124–5, 126–7
  macular degeneration 124–5
  rheumatoid arthritis and 28
  temporal arteritis and 94–5
  treating progressive blindness 124–5

F

falls, dangers of 135, 158
family history *see* genetics
feet
  foot disorders 130–3
  mobility problems 136
fertility, loss of 10, 19
floaters, in the eye 123
fungal infections, of the feet 132
further education 163

G

genetics 161
  age-related visual disorders 122
  ageing and 18
  Alzheimer's disease 87
  atherosclerosis 54
  breast cancer 116
  cataracts 120
  deep vein thrombosis (DVT) 83
  diabetes 142
  heart attacks 57
  Huntington's disease 98–9
  kidney tumours 118
  osteoarthritis (OA) 32
  Paget's disease 40
  prostate cancer 106
  rheumatoid arthritis (RA) 28
glaucoma 124–5, 126–7
gout 154–5
  and arthritis 26
  and foot disorders 131
grandparents 11, 163

H

hair
  changes in 16
  the effects of ageing on 20
health, maintaining 160–1
hearing
  changes in 17, 18, 22
  hearing loss 128–9
  tinnitus 22, 129
hearing aids 129
heart, the *see also* hypertension
  abnormal heart rhythms (arrhythmia) 46–9
  angina 50–3

atherosclerosis 54–5, 90–1
cardiomyopathy 64–5
coronary artery disease (CAD) 72, 74–5
deep vein thrombosis (DVT) 82–3, 169
the effects of ageing on 19
endocarditis 66–7
exercise and 159
heart attacks 51, 56–9
heart disease, reducing the risk 74–5
heart failure 60–3
myocarditis 68–9
pacemakers 49, 65, 76–7
pericarditis 70–1
prevention of cardiovascular disease 72–3
rheumatoid arthritis (RA) and 28
height, changes in 16, 21
heparin
  for angina 53
  for deep vein thrombosis (DVT) 83
high blood pressure *see* hypertension
hip fractures 39
hip replacements 42–5
hormonal therapy, prostate cancer 109
hormone replacement therapy (HRT) 10
  and breast cancer 116
  and deep vein thrombosis (DVT) 82
  and heart disease 74
  to protect against osteoporosis 39
  and sexual activity 167
Huntington's disease 98–9
hypermetropia 123
hypertension 78–81
  atherosclerosis and 54, 55
  eyesight and 124
  heart attacks and 57
  heart failure and 61
  preventing cardiovascular disease 73
  strokes and 104, 105

I

immobility, and deep vein thrombosis (DVT) 83
immune system, the effects of ageing on 19
impotence 166–7
incontinence 138–41
ingrowing toenails 132
inherited illness *see* genetics
insomnia 170–1
ischaemic heart disease 57, 61
isotope bone scans 41

J

joints
  gout 154–5
  joint replacements 42–5
  mobility problems 134–7
  non-inflammatory joint disorder 27

K

kidneys
  the effects of ageing on 19
  kidney tumours 118–19
knee replacements 43–5

L

laser eye surgery 125
Lewy body dementia 91
life expectancy 16, 24–5, 134, 159
lung problems
  chronic bronchitis 148–9
  the effects of ageing on 19
  emphysema 148
  lung cancer 110–13
  pneumonia 150–3
  pulmonary embolism 82
  rheumatoid arthritis (RA) and 28

M

macular degeneration 124–5
magnetic resonance imaging (MRI) scans 55
  for lung cancer 112
  for prostate cancer 107
male mid-life transitions 12–13
malnutrition 144–7
mammograms 117
manic depressive illness 100
mastectomy 117
melatonin 25
memory tests 173
menopause 10–11
mental ability, changes in 17
mental health *see also* nervous system
  Alzheimer's disease 84–5, 86–8
  brain function, ageing and 84–5
  dementia 17, 84, 90–3
  depression 93, 100–1, 165
  exercise and 159
  'mid-life crisis' 12–13
  mobility problems 134–7, 147
MRI scans *see* magnetic resonance imaging (MRI) scans
muscles, mobility problems and 134–7
myocardial infarction (MI) 51, 56–9
myocarditis 68–9
myopia 123

N

nephroblastomas 118, 119
nervous system
  changes in 17
  Huntington's disease 98–9
  Parkinson's disease 96–7
  stroke 102–5
  temporal arteritis 94–5
'Nobel Prize' syndrome 9
non-inflammatory joint disorder 27

non-steroidal anti-inflammatories
  (NSAIDs)
    for gout 155
    for osteoarthritis (OA) 35
    for pericarditis 71
    for rheumatoid arthritis (RA) 31
nursing homes 85

O

old age, entering 14–15
oophorectomy 117
osteitis deformans *see* Paget's disease
osteoarthritis (OA) 32–5, 137
  foot disorders 131
osteomalacia 26
osteoporosis 36–9, 137
  and malnutrition 147
  and rheumatoid arthritis (RA) 28
overflow incontinence 138, 139
oxygen therapy 149

P

pacemakers 49, 65, 76–7
Paget's disease 26, 40–1
palpitations 47, 68
Parkinson's disease 96–7
pelvic floor exercises 140, 141
pericarditis 70–1
physical exercise *see* exercise
physiotherapy
  for chronic bronchitis 149
  following a stroke 104
  joint replacements and 42, 44–5
  for osteoarthritis 35
  for Parkinson's disease 97
pneumonia 150–3
polymyalgia rheumatica 27
presbyacusis 18, 22, 128–9
prostate cancer 106–9
prostate gland, the effects of
  ageing on 19
psoriasis, and foot disorders 131
psychotherapy, for depression 101
pulmonary embolism 82

R

radiotherapy
  for bladder cancer 115
  for lung cancer 113
  for prostate cancer 108
relationships 162
  entering middle age 9
  sexual activity 164–7
  at the time of the menopause 11
renal tumours 118–19

retirement, enjoying 162–3
rheumatoid arthritis (RA) 28–31, 137
rickets 26

S

SAD (seasonal affective disorder) 101
scans
  bone scans 112
  CT scans 112
  DEXA scanning 38
  Doppler ultrasonography 83
  isotope bone scans 41
  magnetic resonance imaging (MRI)
    scans 55, 107, 112
  ultrasound scans 27, 55, 112
screening 161, 172–3
  mammograms 117
  for prostate cancer 109
seasonal affective disorder (SAD) 101
senile dementia 17, 84, 90–3 *see also*
  Alzheimer's disease (AD)
senses, deterioration of 17
sex therapy 167
sexual activity 164–7
sick sinus syndrome 46
sight *see* eye problems
Sjogren's syndrome, rheumatoid
  arthritis (RA) and 28
skin
  changes in 16
  the effects of ageing on 20–1
  urinary incontinence and skincare
    141
sleep patterns 170–1
smell, deterioration of 17, 23
smoking 160
  and angina 53
  and atherosclerosis 54
  and bladder cancer 114, 115
  and foot disorders 131
  and heart attacks 57
  and kidney tumours 118
  and lung cancer 110
  and osteoporosis 39
  preventing cardiovascular disease 73
social life, in retirement 163
spinal fractures 37, 39
spondylosis 33
stature, changes in 16
steroids
  for osteoarthritis (OA) 35
  for rheumatoid arthritis (RA) 31
  for temporal arteritis 95
stress, depression and 101
stress incontinence 138, 139

strokes 102–5, 136
subacute bacterial endocarditis (SBE)
  66–7
supplements, dietary 145
swimming 157

T

tachyarrythmias 46, 49
tamoxifen 117
taste, reduction of 17, 23
temperature extremes, avoiding
  161, 168
temporal arteritis 94–5
testosterone
  decreases in 12
  and prostate cancer 109
  and sexual activity 167
thrombolytic therapy 83
TIAs (transient ischaemic attacks) 102
tinnitus 22, 129
toenails 130, 132
total incontinence 138, 139
touch, the sense of 23
transient ischaemic attacks (TIAs) 102
travel-related illness 168–9

U

ultrasound scans
  for acute arthritis 27
  for atherosclerosis 55
  Doppler ultrasonography 83
  for lung cancer 112
urge incontinence 138, 139
urinary incontinence 138–41

V

vascular dementia 90–3
vasodilators
  for heart failure 63
  for hypertension 81
viagra 166
vision *see* eye problems
vitamins 145

W

warfarin, for deep vein thrombosis
  (DVT) 83
weight
  atherosclerosis and 54
  changes in 16
  deep vein thrombosis (DVT) and 83
  exercise and 158
  heart disease and 74
Wilms' tumours 118
wrinkles 20–1